CLINICAL REASONING IN
OCCUPATIONAL
THERAPY

ANNE CRONIN, PhD, OTR/L, ATP, FAOTA, and
GARTH GRAEBE, MOT, OTR/L

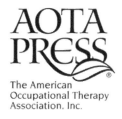

AOTA
PRESS
The American
Occupational Therapy
Association, Inc.

AOTA Vision 2025
Occupational therapy maximizes health, well-being, and quality of life for all people, populations, and communities through effective solutions that facilitate participation in everyday living.

Mission Statement
The American Occupational Therapy Association advances occupational therapy practice, education, and research through standard-setting and advocacy on behalf of its members, the profession, and the public.

AOTA Staff
Charles M. Partridge, *Interim Executive Director and Chief Financial Officer*
Christopher M. Bluhm, *Chief Operating Officer*

Chris Davis, *Associate Chief Officer for AOTA Press and Content Strategy*
Caroline Polk, *Digital Manager and* AJOT *Managing Editor*
Ashley Hofmann, *Development/Acquisitions Editor*
Barbara Dickson, *Production Editor*

Rebecca Rutberg, *Director, Marketing*
Amanda Goldman, *Marketing Manager*
Jennifer Folden, *Marketing Specialist*

American Occupational Therapy Association, Inc.
4720 Montgomery Lane
Bethesda, MD 20814
Phone: 301-652-AOTA (2682)
Fax: 301-652-7711
www.aota.org
To order: 1-877-404-AOTA or store.aota.org

Disclaimers
This publication is designed to provide accurate and authoritative information in regard to the subject matter covered. It is sold or distributed with the understanding that the publisher is not engaged in rendering legal, accounting, or other professional service. If legal advice or other expert assistance is required, the services of a competent professional person should be sought.
—*From the Declaration of Principles jointly adopted by the American Bar Association and a Committee of Publishers and Associations*

It is the objective of the American Occupational Therapy Association to be a forum for free expression and interchange of ideas. The opinions expressed by the contributors to this work are their own and not necessarily those of the American Occupational Therapy Association.

ISBN: 978-1-56900-388-6
Library of Congress Control Number: 2018935360

Cover design by Debra Naylor, Naylor Design, Inc., Washington, DC
Composition by Manila Typesetting Company, Makati City, Philippines
Printed by P. A. Hutchison, Lancaster, PA

Contents

About the Authors

Anne Cronin, PhD, OTR/L, ATP, FAOTA, is a graduate of the University of Missouri's Division of Occupational Therapy. Her first job as an occupational therapist was in a residential facility for adults with developmental disabilities (DDs). This was a wonderful springboard to developing the "out-of-the-box" clinical reasoning that she now tries to encourage in her occupational therapy students. Since then, Anne has worked in several settings and completed a doctoral degree in medical sociology.

Now a professor of occupational therapy at West Virginia University (WVU), Anne is involved in teaching occupational therapy and works extensively in interprofessional teaching and clinical settings. Anne is interested in research and scholarship supporting occupational therapy practice in the areas of DDS and assistive technology (AT). In addition to her passion for occupational therapy, Anne Cronin is an avid reader and artist.

Garth Graebe, MOT, OTR/L, holds a bachelor of science degree in economics. After working in business as an investment broker and branch office manager, he returned to school and earned his master's degree in occupational therapy at WVU. As an occupational therapist, he has worked with clients across the lifespan, with the majority of his clinical work in the areas of gerontology and mental health. Garth is currently an assistant professor and the clinical director of the faculty outpatient occupational therapy clinic, where he is responsible for the development of the clinic and delivery of occupational therapy services through the WVU therapy group practice.

Garth's interests lie in the areas of AT, mental health, and oncology. A skilled craftsman and volunteer in the community, Garth has been instrumental in supporting local charities and a WVU Division of Occupational Therapy initiative to design and build modified ride-on cars for local children with movement impairments.

Rondalyn Whitney, PhD, OTR/L, FAOTA, graduated from Samuel Merritt College, where she honed her skills in using a critical reasoning approach to both traditional and cutting-edge occupational therapy intervention. Most of her professional work has focused on the health and well-being of families living with DDS particularly autism, attention deficit disorders, and challenges of sensory integration and processing.

Rondalyn, a native West Virginian, focuses her research on the needs of rural Appalachian families. Her occupational roles include academic, researcher, writer, mother, wife, sister, daughter, friend, bread baker, and committed upcycler. Rondalyn is an enthusiastic advocate for the science of occupation—the importance of helping students and fellow practitioners learn to appreciate the importance application of evidence and the focus on meaningful outcomes.

When out of the office, Rondalyn can be found volunteering in after-school programs, teaching all-abled students how to build real-world solutions for health needs by creating adaptive equipment from toilet paper rolls, plastic milk cartons, and other castoffs otherwise headed for the landfill.

Figures, Tables, Exhibits, Case Examples, and Practice Wisdom

Case Examples

Practice Wisdom

Introduction

Anne Cronin, PhD, OTR/L, ATP, FAOTA, and Garth Graebe, MOT, OTR/L

One of the biggest challenges for novice practitioners is that people don't fit the prescribed clinical picture as it is taught in school. People mess things up, clouding the clinical picture with their personal histories, interests, comorbidities, and lifestyle choices. Occupational therapy practitioners' ability to provide safe, high-quality care can depend on their ability to flexibly reason, think, and judge, putting the client first.

Clinical reasoning is a practitioner's ability "to think in action" (Benner, Hooper-Kyriakidis, & Stannard, 2011, p. 3). *Thinking in action* means that practitioners have the ability to focus and filter clinical cues and medical data to recognize what is most and least important and identify the actual presenting problem. The systematic use of clinical reasoning strategies streamlines and supports the use of responsible and cost-effective interventions.

In teaching critical thinking and clinical reasoning to occupational therapy students for more than 20 years, patterns emerged. First, students often have difficulty identifying relevant clinical data in real-world situations. Most teaching texts that include case studies tailor those cases to the topics they are trying to teach. Although the cases help make a concept clearer, they do not present students with the baggage and extraneous data that occur during a real client intake interview. In this text, all cases are fully developed, including "extraneous" data for readers to sift.

Second, many clinical reasoning texts describe essential concepts such as *evidence-based practice* and *narrative reasoning,* but they do so through broad discussion. In this text, we look at clinical reasoning as a path to follow rather than an ideal. To that end we have organized this book sequentially, paving the path, one step at a time, to build readers' ability and confidence to think in action and reason, not only during the intake interview but also as a situation changes, and integrate broad concepts throughout the text.

Coming from different clinical and scholarly backgrounds, the authors spent many hours challenging each other's thinking and discussing ways to help students and novice practitioners understand the "big picture," the *person* in the context of occupation. In doing so, we felt that students would learn to convincingly communicate that occupational therapy is an essential science-driven service.

It is important to broaden the discussion of clinical reasoning beyond just a discussion of research validation (or lack of it) of particular interventions. Therefore, in this text we prioritize clients and their occupations to support the American Occupational Therapy Association's (AOTA's) Vision 2025: "Occupational therapy maximizes health, well-being, and quality of life for all people, populations, and communities through effective solutions that facilitate participation in everyday living" (AOTA, 2017).

This text is also deliberately aligned with the *Occupational Therapy Practice Framework: Domain and Process* (3rd ed., *OTPF–3;* AOTA, 2014) to help learners center reasoning on the "the therapeutic use of everyday life activities (occupations) with individuals or groups for the purpose of enhancing or enabling participation in roles, habits, and routines in home, school, workplace, community, and other settings" (AOTA, 2014, p. S1).

Responding to feedback from students and educators, we have tried to limit the use of discipline-specific jargon in favor of language that is widely used in both society and clinical settings. We find that students and novice practitioners become overly attached to professional jargon. For example, it is common to hear occupational therapists say that a person has "sensory issues" and expect that the phrase *sensory issues* is uniformly understood by all. On a more academic level, variation in the terminology of theories or frames of reference by authors make understanding these theories more confusing and harder to apply.

The text is organized into 3 parts. Part I, "Occupational Perspective for Clinical Processing," introduces clinical reasoning as a process and discusses its importance to occupational therapy practice. It includes basic definitions and explores how the *OTPF–3* supports clinical reasoning.

Part II, "Frames of Reference," presents some common frames of reference that are widely used in occupational therapy practice and that illustrate the roles of theory, science, and research in occupational therapy reasoning. The chapters in this section are intended to be read in sequence, deepening the discussion and of evidence-based practice and clinical reasoning. Each chapter includes a clinical case example, review of the literature, and practice examples related to the presented frame of reference.

Part III, "Intervention," discusses occupation-focused clinical reasoning. Occupation-focused models are presented as overarching guides to the occupational therapy process. This section has a particular emphasis on the intervention stages of the occupational therapy process and the professional considerations related to intervention implementation, communication, and outcome measurement.

Appendixes include the *AOTA Occupational Profile Template*, which is used throughout this text, and a summary of frames of references. Throughout the text, case examples facilitate practical learning. A uniform format for clinical cases was used so they could be used independently of the chapter in which they are introduced. At the end of each chapter, learning activities challenge readers to thoughtfully integrate what they are learning into their own ways of reasoning.

The goal of this text is to foster evidence-informed, client-centered, and cost-effective clinical reasoning in occupational therapy practice. We hope to inspire skilled communicators who will lead the profession in clinical practice, scholarship, and professional advocacy.

REFERENCES

American Occupational Therapy Association. (2014). Occupational therapy practice framework: Domain and process (3rd ed.). *American Journal of Occupational Therapy, 68*(Suppl.), S1–S48. https://doi.org/10.5014/ajot.2014.682006

American Occupational Therapy Association. (2017). *Vision 2025.* Retrieved from https://www.aota.org/AboutAOTA /vision-2025.aspx

Benner, P., Hooper-Kyriakidis, P., & Stannard, D. (2011). *Clinical wisdom and interventions in acute and critical care: A thinking-in-action approach.* (2nd ed.). New York: Springer.

PART I.

Occupational Perspective
for Clinical Reasoning

Overview of the Clinical Reasoning Process

Anne Cronin, PhD, OTR/L, ATP, FAOTA, and Garth Graebe, MOT, OTR/L

1

CHAPTER HIGHLIGHTS

- Describes how clinical reasoning helps both occupational therapy practitioners and the profession.
- Explains a working hypothesis in clinical reasoning.
- Applies problem-solving strategies in clinical reasoning, including using algorithms and heuristics as problem-solving tools.
- Promotes client-centered collaboration to guide clinical reasoning.
- Distinguishes between occupation-focused models and frames of reference in the clinical reasoning process.
- Describes the interplay between interprofessional collaborative practice and occupational therapy reasoning.

KEY TERMS AND CONCEPTS

Algorithm
Basic assumptions
Biomechanical frame of reference
Clinical hypothesis
Clinical reasoning
Collaborative reasoning
Diagnostic reasoning
Domain
Family-guided routines

Family-guided routines-based intervention
Focus
Frame of reference
Function–disability continuum
Heuristics
Insight
Interprofessional collaborative practice
Knobology

Medical diagnosis
Model
Occupation-focused models and frameworks
Occupational profile
Paradigm
Postulates of change
Problem solving
Theory
Trial and error

In all areas of practice, occupational therapy professionals are faced with complex questions regarding clinical reasoning, such as

- Who needs intervention and why?
- What are the expected outcomes of intervention?
- How should the outcomes be documented?
- What approaches to intervention are most effective in addressing the client's goals?
- What is the best way to ensure that desired outcomes are reached within the constraints of limited visits or limited opportunities for participation within the clinical setting?

Effective practitioners should be confident that they can respond to these questions, assimilate new information, make reasoned clinical decisions and give plausible reasons for these decisions, argue well, and advocate for both the profession and the client. This chapter introduces the clinical reasoning process and explains why it matters and is a focus of study in occupational therapy. The chapter discusses the terminology and process used in clinical reasoning.

INTRODUCTION TO CLINICAL REASONING

Clinical reasoning is not simply *diagnostic reasoning,* a term commonly used in medicine that involves the recognition of clinical patterns and the establishment of expected clinical trajectories based on disease or impairment (Elstein, 2009). Strong clinical reasoning skills are an attribute of expert practitioners. Unsworth (2001) described *experts* as people who possess a strong knowledge base that enables them to compare a current problem with their recollections of past cases. Experts are also better able to filter information so that they use less irrelevant information when making decisions.

The terms *clinical reasoning, clinical judgment, problem solving, decision making,* and *critical thinking* are often used interchangeably. In this text, the term *clinical reasoning* is defined as the process by which occupational therapy practitioners collect information, process this information, come to an understanding of a client's needs and values, and then plan and implement interventions in a reflective process consistent with the *Occupational Therapy Practice Framework: Domain and Practice* (OTPF–3; American Occupational Therapy Association [AOTA], 2014). This book is intended to teach novice practitioners the use of tools and strategies to organize and enhance clinical reasoning to help them advance toward the level of expert practitioner. The strategies presented can also help expert practitioners expand into new areas of practice.

Although much of the focus of this text is directed at the level of client-based care, practitioners also need to make decisions about many other factors in the course of their practice. Clinical reasoning is essential in all aspects of the occupational therapy role, not just in clinical care. This book also includes discussion of some of the common frames of reference used in the profession and decision-making challenges faced by practitioners.

Much of what is learned in professional education programs is diagnostic reasoning. This information is essential and provides the foundation for effective clinical reasoning. However, clinical reasoning goes beyond learning the basic protocols that guide care based on a medical diagnosis that is focused on a disease or medical condition. In the real world, occupational therapy clients have a collection of strengths and limitations that extend beyond the boundaries of diagnosis, resulting in patterns of strengths and limitations that may not be captured in a discussion of "the usual."

In addition, although the focus of this book is on reasoning that occurs in the context of the clinical encounter, clinical reasoning has a broad impact at all levels of professional practice. Case Example 1.1 is referred to throughout this chapter to highlight this impact.

In Case Example 1.1, Matthew was referred for limitations in hand function as a result of carpal tunnel syndrome (CTS), so the occupational therapist begins with a medical diagnosis. A *medical diagnosis* is "the formal identification by a medical provider (usually a medical doctor) of a condition, disease, or injury made by evaluating the symptoms and signs presented by a patient" (*American Heritage Science Dictionary*, 2015).

The practitioner considers Matthew's medical diagnosis, follows up with an assessment of hand function, and notes that Matthew has Grade II CTS, including weakness of the thenar muscles (but not atrophy), numbness and tingling, and a decrease in grip and pinch strength. In understanding the medical diagnosis (i.e., CTS) and the grade of severity attached to it (Grade II), the practitioner can use clinical reasoning to shortcut the assessment process and focus on the issues commonly associated with this diagnosis.

The use of shortcuts reduces the need for extensive questioning and can make the evaluation process more focused and efficient. This clinical reasoning approach, beginning with a medical diagnosis and subsequent evaluation that focuses on gathering information specific to the client, supports the development of a working clinical hypothesis for occupational therapy. A *clinical hypothesis* is a possible explanation for the limitations in occupational performance and participation made on the basis of limited presenting evidence and serves as a starting point to guide the evaluation process.

DIAGNOSTIC REASONING AND HEURISTICS

Diagnostic reasoning includes all of the information gathered by the occupational therapy practitioner regarding a specific diagnostic condition. In-depth diagnostic reasoning provides data to jump-start the clinical reasoning process. Diagnostic reasoning is only one tool that offers a shortcut to the expert practitioner. Other tools include theory, frames of reference, and data-driven decision making.

This use of shortcuts in reasoning is called *heuristics* by cognitive scientists. *Heuristics* are strategies that serve

CASE EXAMPLE 1.1. MATTHEW: WRIST CTS

Matthew, age 45 years, was referred to occupational therapy because of concerns regarding numbness and weakness in his right (dominant) hand secondary to CTS. This condition has led to limited hand skills that affect his performance in self-care and the supported employment program where he works.

Matthew was diagnosed with spastic quadriplegia as a child and is functioning at Level 3 on the Gross Motor Function Classification Scale (Palisano et al., 1997), meaning that he is able to sit on a regular chair but may require pelvic or trunk support to maximize hand function. He can move in and out of the chair using a stable surface to push on or pull up with his arms. Mathew walks with a rolling walker indoors and is usually transported in a wheelchair when traveling outdoors on uneven terrain. He works in the local newspaper office in a supported employment arrangement. He is involved in managing the mail, the copy machine, and the paper shredder and in restocking the office supply inventory in the storeroom. He uses his walker with a basket to transport materials in the office and has a sturdy chair with arms available for his use during other tasks.

Matthew's referral to occupational therapy is for hand therapy for CTS. Based on this diagnosis alone, the occupational therapy practitioner can generally expect success using a standard carpal tunnel treatment protocol. This referral begins the inductive reasoning process that will guide the occupational therapy evaluation process.

> **PRACTICE WISDOM 1.1.** Knobology
>
> "*Knobology* is a 'tongue-in-cheek' term for the study of application without theory . . . the term for students and clinicians who want to know only which knobs on a therapeutic modality to turn and are uninterested in why they are doing so. Not only would there be little advancement in medicine if all clinicians were knobologists, but patients would suffer from inadequate treatment. Don't be a knobologist!" *(Knight & Draper, 2012, italics added)*

as an aid to learning and problem solving by relying on familiarity with the condition or prior clinical experiences.

Clinical judgments based on heuristics are often accurate and appropriate. Intervention based on heuristics is likely to be effective in some clients, but consideration of individual factors such as the client's occupational history and experiences, patterns of daily living, interests, values, and needs that form a complete occupational profile (AOTA, 2014; see Appendix A, "Occupational Profile") are likely to greatly improve the efficacy of the intervention.

For example, in Case Example 1.1, the practitioner notes that Matthew has some additional complicating factors, most notably a preexisting condition of spastic quadriplegia. This chronic condition suggests that muscle tone and muscle activation patterns in the hand are likely to be atypical. It also causes the practitioner to extend the evaluation process beyond the usual because of Matthew's need to use his hands to assist mobility. In this case, restricting clinical reasoning to a heuristic approach to CTS would be faulty and lead to a poor clinical outcome. Such a restricted approach would be a form of *knobology,* or a lazy approach to clinical practice, as described in Practice Wisdom 1.1.

CLINICAL REASONING PROCESS

The clinical reasoning process has 5 steps (see Figure 1.1):
- *Step 1. Consider the client and the referral information:* This stage begins with first contact with the client. It requires consideration of the presenting strength and weaknesses of the individual within the context of information about condition and interventions from Step 1. Particular attention should be focused on any perceived incongruities, such as unexpected impairments or co-morbidities that were not included in the initial information.
- *Step 2. Develop clinical hypotheses to guide collection of cues and information:* In this stage, the practitioner uses occupational therapy clinical reasoning to identify potentially effective approaches to support client goals through occupational therapy intervention.
- *Step 3. Use targeted data collection and problem solving strategies to process information and evaluate the hypothesis:* Objective, measureable performance targets are identified and a data collection system is

established so the practitioner can trial the potentially effective approaches.
- *Step 4. Test and refine the clinical hypotheses:* Systematic review of client progress toward objective, measureable performance targets occurs. This allows for confirmation, alteration, or refutation of clinical hypotheses. This information moves the process back to Step 2 in which the strategies are refined or replaced based on the client data.
- *Step 5. Appraise the evidence:* This stage involves the assimilation of information from all sources to provide a foundation for decision making. Because reasoning is iterative, this can be both the start and the end of the process.

It is important to understand that the clinical reasoning process is a cycle; therefore, practitioners may find that a hypothesis is inaccurate or incomplete and will need to move back to Step 1 with the new information they have gathered.

Step 1. Client and Referral Information

The typical clinical reasoning process begins with a referral followed by a meeting between the occupational therapy practitioner and the client (see Step 1 in Figure 1.1). In Case Example 1.1, the first step of the process began with Matthew's referral for occupational therapy to treat the symptoms of CTS. The *occupational profile,* which includes compiled data on the client's needs, problems, and concerns about his or her performance in occupations (see Appendix A for a template), is developed on the basis of the information from all sources from Step 1 and the meeting with the client in Step 2 in which personal goals and concerns are explored.

Step 2. Clinical Hypotheses

To develop clinical hypotheses, Step 2 of the clinical reasoning process, the practitioner first develops a working hypothesis and uses it to lead the initial data gathering. In Case Example 1.1, as unique or distinctive aspects of Matthew and his impairments become clear, the practitioner must reflect on both standard protocols and alternative approaches to understand Matthew's participation impairments. This approach requires the use of problem-solving strategies to consider the information in context. These strategies require reflection and creativity and should be used to test clinical hypotheses (Step 3 of the process).

Step 3. Data Collection, Problem Solving, and Hypotheses Evaluation

In cognitive psychology, the term *problem solving* refers to the thought processes that people use to discover, analyze, and resolve difficulties. The thought processes used by occupational therapy practitioners in clinical settings depend on both the nature of the problem being addressed and the expertise of the clinician. As noted in

FIGURE 1.1.   **5-step clinical reasoning process.**

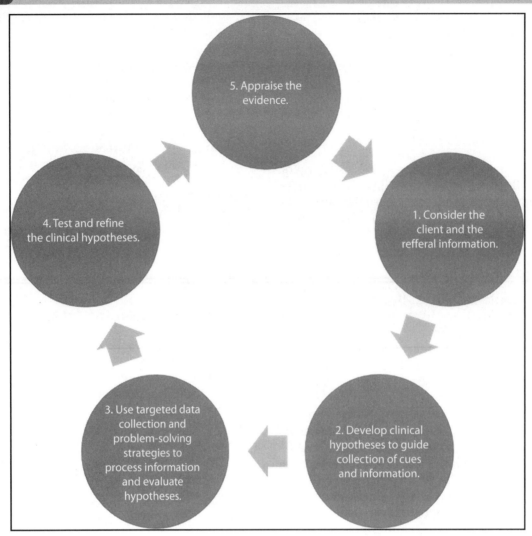

Cherry (2015), the literature describes 4 main types of problem-solving strategies:

1. Algorithm
2. Heuristic
3. Trial and error
4. Insight.

Exhibit 1.1 provides definitions for these strategies.

In Case Example 1.1, analysis and evaluation of the presenting data suggest that Matthew's spastic quadriplegia is likely to negatively affect his ability to improve with a standard CTS intervention protocol. Therefore, the practitioner must keep in mind the standard CTS diagnostic information and then hypothesize how it might be affected by spasticity. Because spasticity is a condition in which certain muscles are continuously contracted in a manner that interferes with normal movement, the practitioner must gather careful data on muscle tone, movement patterns, and range of motion (ROM) before establishing an intervention strategy.

The working hypothesis must be altered to respond to Matthew's individual needs. For example, Matthew may be unable to tolerate a standard wrist stabilization splint, he may have a greater than average problem with edema because the combination of spasticity and pain greatly limits his hand function, and he may be unable to perform a standard home exercise program as a result of his atypical movement patterns.

The working clinical hypothesis that is developed in Matthew's case is that spasticity is a significant factor and must be addressed while providing interventions for the acute CTS episode. Some intervention goals will be consistent for both spasticity and CTS (i.e., to maintain or improve ROM and mobility). Other intervention goals will need adaptations (i.e., the use of specific strengthening exercises and temporary splints). Yet other interventions, such as the use of cold packs, which may result in increased spasticity, may be excluded.

- **Algorithm:** An algorithm uses a formula or step-by-step procedure that will always produce a correct solution. Although an algorithm guarantees an accurate answer, it is not always the best approach to problem solving. It works best for well-defined problems that are consistent in their features. It is not practical or efficient for many clinical situations because the variability of individual goals, values, impairments, and contexts makes algorithms excessively long and complex.
- **Heuristic:** A heuristic is a general rule that may or may not work in certain situations. Unlike algorithms, heuristics do not always guarantee a correct solution. However, using a heuristic allows clinicians to simplify complex problems and reduce the total number of possible solutions to a more manageable and time-efficient set.
- **Trial and error:** Trial and error involves trying several solutions and ruling out the ones that do not work. This approach can be time-consuming by itself, so it is typically used in clinical problem solving after narrowing down possible options using either heuristics or algorithms. Trial and error is often used in cases in which the problem is ill-defined or multiple interacting diagnostic conditions or challenging contextual factors are present.
- **Insight:** Insight is distinct from the other problem-solving strategies because it is not a structured reasoning process but a mental process that often happens outside of awareness as a sudden novel idea to address the problem. Clinical problems that trigger insight often require that something new and nonobvious must be done to address the issues. Insight is grounded in clinician knowledge and experience and is more likely to be used by expert clinicians.

Note. Strategies from Cherry (2015).

Step 4. Test and Refine Hypotheses

A typical occupational therapy evaluation process usually balances one or more of these clinical hypotheses and influences what the practitioner emphasizes as he or she identifies the multiple demands, required skills, and potential meanings of the activities and occupations of the individual (AOTA, 2014). The clinical hypotheses are modified and refined (Step 4 in Figure 1.1) as the occupational profile is further developed and forms a context for clinical reasoning.

The *OTPF–3* (AOTA, 2014) states that the

evaluation process is focused on finding out what a client wants and needs to do; determining what a client can do and has done; and identifying supports and barriers to health, well-being, and participation. Evaluation occurs during the initial and all subsequent interactions with a client. The type and focus of the evaluation differ depending on the practice setting. (p. S13)

It is during the evaluation process that clinical hypotheses are developed, tested, and refined by the occupational therapy practitioner. These hypotheses form a context

for further clinical reasoning. Each clinical hypothesis evokes a template of possible clinical findings against which the client's performance can be compared.

Using the clinical hypothesis in Matthew's case that spasticity must be addressed while providing interventions for the acute CTS episode, the practitioner should consider that hand and wrist spasticity usually occurs in the flexor muscles. If this is true in Matthew's case, the standard CTS protocol can be adjusted to emphasize strengthening in the extensor muscle groups and to use physical agent modalities (PAMs) to help address the over-contraction of flexor muscle groups. This is a simple and straightforward modification to better meet the client's unique needs.

Step 5. Appraise the Evidence

Appraising the evidence is important, and extensive discussion of this aspect of the clinical reasoning process takes place later in this text. At this point it is important to understand that appraising the evidence includes more than a search for confirmatory evidence. It requires exploration of current science and its applications that are specific to contextual and client factors affecting the hypothesis.

CLINICAL REASONING TERMINOLOGY

The clinical reasoning terminology used in this text—theory, paradigm, frame of reference, and model—is consistent with that used in the *OTPF–3* (AOTA, 2014). Some of the terms may be familiar to readers from other contexts.

An essential term to consider when discussing clinical reasoning is *theory.* This word has many meanings and is used widely in daily life and in science. At its most basic level, it is a supposition intended to explain something. In the clinical reasoning context, the basic definition of the term is consistent with its popular use: "a plausible or scientifically acceptable general principle or body of principles offered to explain phenomena" (Merriam-Webster, 2017). In occupational therapy, leaders in the field have developed a wealth of theory that can provide excellent supports in the clinical reasoning process. Occupational therapy theories are often complex and far more involved than the basic definition we are using for this clinical reasoning context.

Sometimes occupational therapy practitioners are confused by all the specific theories and theorists specific to the practice of occupational therapy and lose perspective of why these theories were developed in the first place. For this reason in this text the term *theory* refers to the simple definition of a supposition intended to explain something.

Paradigm

The overall context for the discussion of clinical reasoning is the philosophy, values, ethics, and science that make up the professional worldview of occupational therapy. This big picture is called the *paradigm* of occupational therapy. A *paradigm* is the generally accepted perspective of a particular discipline at a given time. The occupational therapy paradigm is well explained and presented in the *OTPF–3* (AOTA, 2014) and serves as the foundation for this text.

Because a paradigm is a philosophical and theoretical foundation that contains basic assumptions and ways of thinking, it provides a very broad framework that can include many specific theories and theoretical concepts. It is the paradigm that informs the consideration of theory. Theory leading to a clinical hypothesis reflects the individual reasoning of the practitioner working within the paradigm, but with a narrowed focus guided by a specific theory that is consistent with the paradigm.

Earlier in the chapter algorithms and heuristics were introduced. While a paradigm provides a broad umbrella that encompasses many theories, many aspects of clinical practice require applied clinical skills, such as the taking of vital signs or the assisted transfer of a person with weakness. These applied clinical skills may be isolated from either paradigm or theory. Algorithms are useful, but are potentially a variety of knobology. They make something happen and may be necessary, but they are not essential to either paradigm or theory.

The use of heuristics, in the form of standard protocols, may or may not reflect the paradigm of occupational therapy. Heuristics are short-cuts to provide appropriate care in a focused and efficient manner. The problem is that without a foundation in theory or science, heuristics do not ensure a correct conclusion and rely heavily on expertise and experience. A heuristic allows practitioners to include the knowledge gathered by others in clinical reasoning. Although we often think of clinical reasoning as an individual endeavor, it is inherently an interactive process that involves other people, and information and data produced by others.

For the purposes of this text, we challenge readers to think of the *OTPF–3* (AOTA, 2014) and the theories, models, and frames of reference described in occupational therapy textbooks as tools that allow you to learn from others and enhance the development of effective heuristic reasoning tools. In addition, these tools will help throughout the occupational therapy process—in the discovery of the underlying problem, the decision of which issues to prioritize in intervention, how to understand a problem in the context of the client, the exploration of effective and valid intervention options, and the actions needed to achieve the practitioner's and the client's goals.

Frame of Reference

In occupational therapy, a *frame of reference* is a set of assumptions or concepts, often drawn from theory or science, that explains how assessment and intervention work in routine practice. A frame of reference is action focused, whereas a theory reflects an ideal that includes scientifically acceptable general principles to explain phenomena of interest. Throughout this text, the frame of reference is a tool used to approach a narrowly focused clinical problem and identify strategies for intervention.

Model

A *model* is an abstract way of schematizing a process to generalize a foundational theory (or theories) to solve problems that are similar to, but outside, the focus of that theory. In some literature, the terms *model* and *frame of reference* are used interchangeably. In this text, a frame of reference draws from one theoretical foundation and is prescriptive of clinical actions. A model may amalgamate more than one foundational theory to guide reasoning, but it is not prescriptive of clinical actions. Within a model of practice, more than one frame of reference may be used.

OCCUPATIONAL THERAPY FRAMES OF REFERENCE

Mosey (1996) provided occupational therapy with one of the first definitions of *frames of reference* as a support to occupational therapy clinical reasoning. Applied frames of reference as described by Mosey (1981) have 4 basic elements:

1. *Focus* is the clearly defined domain, scope, or focus of concern in occupational therapy. It is usually defined in the frame of reference.
2. *Basic assumptions* are the guiding beliefs that lead the clinical reasoning process. They are the ideas and concepts that explain possible explanations for the patterns of performance and participation observed. They are often not clearly defined and must be critically explored to effectively apply the frame of reference.
3. The *function–disability continuum* is the expectation of what is normal or a best outcome versus what is a poor or limited outcome within the scope of a theory. This continuum is often described in terms of function (i.e., aspects of performance that are indicative of functional activity supporting occupation) and dysfunction (i.e., behaviors that are interfering or inhibiting functional performance, thus limiting occupational engagement), especially when the focus of the frame of reference is based in occupation.
4. *Postulates of change* are the explanations offered within the frame of reference about what is needed to cause change. These explanations are often described in terms of occupational engagement and participation, especially when the focus of the frame of reference is based in occupation.

Occupational therapy frames of reference allow occupational therapy practitioners to be collaborative in their clinical reasoning and to be reflective in their clinical practice and offer heuristic tools that add rigor and evidence to clinical reasoning. For each frame of reference introduced throughout this text, Mosey's (1981) 4 basic frame-of-reference elements will be outlined. A collection of the frames of reference that are discussed in this text can be found in Appendix B, "Summary of Frames of Reference."

Exhibit 1.2 lists the most common frames of reference used in occupational therapy practice. Many are presented in the context of case examples later in this text, but the focus is not to teach all possible frames of reference but to understand how to critically consider and apply frames of reference as a heuristic to support clinical reasoning.

Frames of reference can be drawn from any source. For example, what is known in the occupational therapy literature as the *biomechanical frame of reference,* which refers to an amalgam of basic science and exercise information that focuses on the capacity for functional motion, is drawn from basic science foundations in physics, anatomy, physiology, and kinesiology. This frame of reference is a good starting point because it is both concrete and foundational to occupational therapy practice. The biomechanical frame of reference has no single author or source and is not theoretical or occupation focused, but it does include the four basic elements of a frame of reference (Mosey, 1981; Exhibit 1.3).

The biomechanical frame of reference is highly science driven, and interventions based on this frame of reference are some of the best accepted and most widely respected in health care. It is an occupational therapy frame of reference because it is central to the field's understanding

---

EXHIBIT 1.3. **Basic Elements of the Biomechanical Frame of Reference**

- **Focus:** This frame of reference is widely applied in the treatment of musculoskeletal impairments.
- **Basic assumptions:** It is based on scientific knowledge about body function and structure and on the assumption that the voluntary movement that supports human function is built on the interactions of joint ROM, muscle strength, anatomical integrity, and the physiological functions that support endurance.
- **Function–disability continuum:** The typical or average state of bodily function supports engagement in desired movements. Any limitation of movement, strength, endurance, or physiologic stability that limits the use of a limb or produces incapacity to perform desired movements is an impairment.
- **Postulates of change:** Exercise or other specific interventions to support improved performance of the musculoskeletal system will result in improved ROM, strength, or endurance. Although specific functional skills and daily occupations are not a part of this frame of reference, it is believed that with improved musculoskeletal function, a person with musculoskeletal impairments will return to desired occupations.

Note. ROM = range of motion.

---

of human function, but it is not focused on occupation. Although it is described in the occupational therapy literature, this frame of reference is general and widely used by many health professionals. Therefore, if interventions based on the biomechanical frame of reference are used in a health care setting and do not have an occupational therapy perspective, they are indistinguishable from the interventions of other professions (e.g., physical therapy, nursing).

This situation may engender competition among professionals about to whom such interventions belong in order to secure their place in the health care arena. For example, an occupational therapy practitioner may become competitive rather than collaborate with other team members to ensure his or her place on the team if these interventions are not solidly based in occupational therapy. Another result is that the client is less likely to get the best possible care because of a lack of interprofessional collaboration. Moreover, if there is not a distinct value in involving a specific profession in a health care intervention, it is unlikely that the intervention will be ordered. If occupational therapy interventions are indistinguishable from another profession's (e.g., physical therapy) interventions, both the client and the professions are poorly served.

The *OTPF–3* (AOTA, 2014) describes the occupational therapy *domain* as "the profession's purview and the areas in which its members have an established body of knowledge and expertise" (p. S3). Therefore, although occupational therapy practitioners often use knowledge from many sources and apply knowledge used in other fields and by other professions to occupational therapy

---

EXHIBIT 1.2. **Common Occupational Therapy Frames of Reference**

- Behavioral or applied behavioral analysis
- Biomechanical
- Cognitive Orientation to daily Occupational Performance
- Cognitive rehabilitation
- Cognitive–behavioral
- Cognitive disabilities
- Coping model
- Developmental systems
- Developmental or neurodevelopmental
- Dynamic interactional
- Motor control and motor learning
- Neurodevelopmental treatment
- Neurofunctional approach
- Psychodynamic
- Rehabilitation
- Role acquisition
- Sensorimotor or psychomotor
- Sensory integration
- Sensory processing.

interventions, when they use information from the scientific literature, they must carefully consider it within the scope of the occupational therapy domain of practice. They must also consider how it might be used as a heuristic shortcut to support human occupation. Failure to do so results in clinical practice that is not occupationally grounded and that may not be valued as distinct from interventions provided by other professions. Therefore, this text focuses on the clinical reasoning process as a tool to better clarify and emphasize occupational therapy as a distinct and essential service across practice settings and disability considerations.

Occupation-Focused Frames of Reference and Models

Increasingly, the occupational therapy literature singles out conceptual models and frameworks that focus on occupation as an essential tool to guide clinical reasoning. These *occupation-focused models and frameworks* are characterized by attention to the client's body functions and structures while also considering skills, roles, habits, routines, and the contexts of the client's lifestyle. Occupation-focused approaches concentrate on achieving participation or engagement instead of medical impairments. The focus is on the client and the potential performance-enhancing effects of occupational engagement as a tool to support health, development, recovery of function, and satisfaction with participation in daily life activities. Occupation-focused approaches are valuable because they prioritize human occupation and help clarify the distinct emphasis on occupational engagement and participation that may not be as evident when using frames of reference that originate outside of occupational therapy.

Occupation-focused models and frameworks have emerged from the fields of occupational science and occupational therapy and are consistent with the paradigm of the profession from which they were developed. As tools that are distinct to occupational therapy, these occupation-focused approaches are generally superior to the more specific frames of reference listed in Exhibit 1.2, which, like the biomechanical frame of reference, may not be inherently occupation focused. Some examples of occupation-focused models and frameworks are the Model of Human Occupation and the Person–Environment–Occupation–Performance Model.

Although any frame of reference can support occupation, not all explicitly focus on occupation. The frames of reference that do not originate from within the fields of occupational therapy or occupational science must be considered in terms of human occupation to be consistent with the *OTPF–3* (AOTA, 2014). It is the clinical reasoning process that is essential in making occupational

therapy practice occupation focused, not necessarily the model or frame of reference. Occupational therapy practitioners use the clinical reasoning process to assess and adapt new knowledge and information from diverse backgrounds into occupation-focused strategies for intervention.

Frames of reference and occupation-focused frameworks and models are typically used in combination. Occupation-focused approaches help the clinician focus on factors beyond a client's specific medical or performance impairments. However, these approaches seldom offer the clear guidance on interventions for specific medical or performance impairments. For this reason, an occupation-focused approach to clinical reasoning that is applied to the common (non-occupation-focused) clinical frames of reference make up the bulk of this text.

The frames of reference and occupation-focused clinical reasoning strategies discussed in the cases presented in the following chapters were chosen on the basis of their relevance to the case presentation and their prevalence in the professional literature. The development of theory and the application of theory in clinical practice are dynamic and ongoing processes. This text is not intended as a complete source for all possible frames of reference or occupation-focused models. Rather, it is intended as a tool to teach occupation-focused clinical reasoning within an evidence-based framework, with a focus on the tools and resources most available to occupational therapy practitioners in their everyday practice.

COLLABORATIVE REASONING USED IN OCCUPATIONAL THERAPY

Collaborative reasoning is the assimilation of perspectives of key individuals in the clinical reasoning process. The client is the essential "key individual" in collaborative reasoning, and other key individuals may include the client's family, members of the health care or educational team, and employers (Kassirer, Wong, & Kopelman, 2010).

In Exhibit 1.4, specifics of Case Example 1.1 are reviewed and expanded to include Matthew's basic occupational profile. A careful review of this case reveals that the impact of CTS on Matthew's daily occupations is pervasive, and his needs extend far beyond the scope of the biomechanical frame of reference. The occupational therapy practitioner will use clinical reasoning, including an explicitly collaborative process between the practitioner and Matthew that addresses hand intervention and supports Matthew in the performance of his valued occupations in a safe and efficient way. The intervention program should include not only attention to the immediate medical problem but an analysis of performance patterns to help prevent further CTS problems as Matthew engages in daily tasks.

EXHIBIT 1.4.	Matthew's Occupational Profile		
Client	**Reason the client is seeking service and concerns related to engagement in occupations**	*Referral:* Referred to occupational hand therapy for CTS. *Impact on occupation:* This condition has led to limited hand skills that affect Matthew's performance in self-care and at the supported employment program where he works. At this time, he does not go to work and needs increased supervision and assistance in all other occupations.	
	Occupations in which the client is successful	Matthew managed basic ADLs prior to injury. Matthew helps with chores around the house. Matthew has been engaged in paid work in an office.	
	Personal interests and values	Matthew enjoys watching sports and playing with children and participates in occasional evening recreational programs at the community center.	
	Occupational history (i.e., life experiences)	Matthew was diagnosed with spastic quadriplegia as a child and is functioning at Level 3 on the GMFCS (Palisano et al., 1997), meaning that he is able to sit on a regular chair but may require pelvic or trunk support to maximize hand function. He is able to move in and out of the chair using a stable surface to push on or pull up with his arms. Mathew walks with a rolling walker indoors and is usually transported in a wheelchair when traveling outdoors on uneven terrain. He works in the local newspaper office in a supported employment arrangement. He is involved in managing the mail, the copy machine, and the paper shredder and in restocking the office supply inventory in the storeroom. He uses his walker with a basket to transport materials in the office and has a sturdy chair with arms available for his use during other tasks.	
	Performance patterns (routines, roles, habits, & rituals)	*Occupational roles:* Matthew's valued life roles include his role as a worker, a brother, an uncle, and a Pittsburgh Pirates fan.	
Environment		***Supports to occupational engagement***	***Barriers to occupational engagement***
	Physical (e.g., buildings, furniture, pets)	Home and work are accessible to Matthew with his walker.	Impairment limits Matthew's hand use.
	Social (e.g., spouse, friends, caregivers)	Matthew lives with his brother's family (including a wife and 2 small children).	
Context	**Cultural (e.g., customs, beliefs)**	No cultural issues were identified during this assessment.	
	Personal (e.g., age, gender, SES, education)	Age 45 years.	
	Temporal (e.g., stage of life, time, year)	Middle adulthood.	
	Virtual (e.g., chat, email, remote monitoring)	Matthew is able to use his mobile phone for communication and basic texting.	
Client goals	**Client's priorities and desired targeted outcomes**	Matthews goals are to regain hand function, regain independence in basic ADLs, and return to work.	

(Continued)

EXHIBIT 1.4.	**Matthew's Occupational Profile** *(Cont.)*

ANALYSIS OF PARTICIPATION

Basic ADLs

Eating/oral–motor	Matthew typically eats independently during mealtimes but now needs assistance in cutting food and with utensil use because of weakness and wrist pain.
Grooming	Matthew has needed only standby assistance in hair care and shaving using an electric razor. Because of his spasticity, he has limited shoulder and arm movement for performing these tasks. The assistance needed is to check for task completeness and to help with aspects of the tasks beyond his reach. He continues to need standby assistance with hair care but is unable to sustain a grasp on the electric razor at this time and has become dependent in this task.
Bathing/transfer	Matthew is independent in bathing and transfers. He showers using a shower chair, a handheld shower head, and grab bars. He continues to perform this task independently, although there are increased safety concerns because he is less able to use his right arm to assist in transfers.
Dressing upper body	Matthew is unable to manage any aspect of upper-body dressing at this time. He will extend limbs to assist.
Dressing lower body	Matthew has limited mobility in sitting but was able to perform lower-body dressing with elastic waist pants and the use of his walker for support in standing. At this time, he is unable to maintain a grasp on his clothing and is unable to don pants or socks. He has slip-on shoes that he can manage without the use of his hands.
Toileting	Matthew is able to sit on the toilet with the aid of side rails. Since developing CTS, he sometimes needs assistance with personal hygiene and handwashing.
Problem solving/memory	Matthew has a moderate cognitive impairment but understands the steps of the tasks that need to be done and the materials necessary for those tasks. He understands the safety issues and has been effective in the supported employment setting in performing a variety of structured tasks.
Comments:	Matthew needs minimal assist in all mobility activities including the use of a walker. He continues to be able to use the walker with his right wrist pain, but the pain limits his willingness to participate and has led to increased concerns about his judgment and safety.

IADLs

Community mobility	Matthew has a rolling walker, which he uses for short distances. He enjoys walking, but this activity has been limited because of right wrist pain. He is able to manage the walker using his left hand predominantly, but it is more difficult for him and makes his speed much slower. Since his wrist injury, Matthew has relied more on the use of a wheelchair pushed by others to get around.
Health management/prevention	Matthew understands his diet and medication routine, although these areas are physically managed by others. Matthew has enjoyed mall walking as exercise and will ask his family members to take him walking. He has discontinued this activity since his wrist pain developed. Matthew has some cognitive problems that limit his ability to plan and schedule tasks. He will need supervision to manage any home exercise program.
Home management	Matthew assists others in cooking, laundry, and household chores. With assistive technology, he is able to open and close the front door, use the phone, manage electronics in his home and workspace (e.g., lights, thermostat, TV, radio), and call for help. There has been no functional change in this area since the development of CTS.
Financial management	Matthew is dependent for paying bills and budgeting. There has been no functional change in this area since the development of CTS.
Leisure	Matthew watches TV, goes to activities at a recreation center, and spends time with family. Activities at the center have been limited only as a result of his increased use of the wheelchair.
Safety	Matthew seems to have adequate safety awareness and will vocalize when he is frightened or concerned.
Comments:	Matthew is not involved in child care or caring for others.

(Continued)

EXHIBIT 1.4.   Matthew's Occupational Profile *(Cont.)*

Motor and Praxis Skills	
Sitting (static/dynamic)	Matthew is able to maintain static sitting when placed in a supported seating system. He has limited weight shift ability during sitting and poor dynamic sitting because of the decreased use of his right arm. He requires external supports.
Standing (static/dynamic)	Matthew is unable to assume standing because of decreased use of his right arm. Once he is assisted into standing, he is able to independently maintain the position. He can bear partial (<30%) weight on his right arm when using the walker.
Joint stability and skeletal mobility	Matthew has mild to moderate flexion contractures in both lower extremities. He has had bilateral heel cord releases and is able to get solid foot placement for transfers. He has a mild scoliosis and limited lateral trunk mobility. His upper-limb ROM (passive) is within functional limits.
Place can on shelf	Matthew is unable to complete the task. He is unable to grasp and hold the can in his right hand. He can lift and carry the can to and from his lap for transportation. He relies on others to manage objects on shelves.
Retrieve item from floor	Matthew is unable to retrieve items from the floor, secondary to decreased trunk control.
Screw lid on jar	Matthew was unable to screw a lid on a jar even before the CTS because of tightness in his wrist and elbow flexors. He has poor sustained grasp and limited active wrist movement with no functional radial deviation.
Comb back of head	Matthew ducks his head forward and can smooth his hair with his right upper extremity.
Write name	Matthew can scrawl his signature with his right hand. He does not write often in his daily routine.
Lift grocery bag	Matthew is unable to lift a grocery bag.
Process Skills	
Energy for task	Matthew's energy varies with the amount of physical exertion required.
Coordination	Matthew's coordination is poor. He is able to move limbs independently with greater control on the right. He has limited ability to engage in bilateral tasks and limited ability to engage in tasks at midline. He is unable to cross the midline of the body and unable to sustain sequenced rhythmic motions. He is able to do work tasks with set-up and accommodations.
Manipulation	Matthew consistently prefers his right hand for skilled activity. Since the development of CTS, his grip strength is poor, and he is unable to sustain the grip.
Knowledge/organization of tasks	Matthew is able to function within familiar environments and organize familiar tasks. He has a moderate cognitive impairment and has difficulty understanding, organizing, initiating, and sequencing new tasks.
Adaptation/praxis	Matthew appears to understand the demands of a task and seems able to understand the steps of the task sequence with familiar tasks.
Communication and social skills	Matthew is nonverbal but is able to express basic wants and needs with an augmentative communication device and pointing. His receptive language is WNL, and he is pleasant and appropriate with peers and medical staff.
Cognitive and emotional regulation skills	Matthew is alert and oriented. He demonstrates effective emotional regulation skills.
Level of arousal/attention	Matthew can attend to familiar multitask daily routines. He is attentive in 1:1 settings.
Orientation	Matthew is alert and oriented to person, place, time, and event.
Energy and drive	Matthew is motivated to be more independent at home and to return to work.
Higher level cognition	Matthew has limited executive function skills because of his preexisting cognitive impairment. Supervision and support for these skills are available in his home and workplace.

(Continued)

EXHIBIT 1.4.	Matthew's Occupational Profile *(Cont.)*
Sensory–Perceptual Skills	
Sensory	Matthew has intact basic sensory function.
Self-perception	Matthew is aware of his body in space but tends to lean to the left because of postural control problems.
Pain	Matthew has pain in his right wrist with use and that wakes him up at night.
Skin integrity	Matthew's skin is intact.
Comments:	Matthew has pain, numbness, and tingling in his right wrist and hand, consistent with a diagnosis of CTS.

Note. Occupational profile template from American Occupational Therapy Association (2017). Analysis of participation format adapted from Skubik-Peplaski, Paris, Boyle, & Culpert (2009). ADLs = activities of daily living; CTS = carpal tunnel syndrome; GMFCS = Gross Motor Function Classification Scale; IADLs = instrumental activities of daily living; ROM = range of motion; SES = socioeconomic status; WNL = within normal limits.

Matthew's goals are to be pain free and to return to work and daily life. He would like to contribute more at home to his own care and household chores. Matthew's brother wants a worksite analysis to determine what Matthew is doing that caused the problem and to develop accommodations to the task to help prevent future problems. Using a collaborative approach, the practitioner will encompass Matthew's goals into the intervention plan and in the outcome measures to ensure that Matthew's priorities are respected.

INTERPROFESSIONAL COLLABORATIVE PRACTICE

Effective occupational therapy practitioners in today's health care climate must not only have skills in evaluation and intervention but also be effective communicators in interprofessional practice, understand objective data collection and documentation, and be effective in advocating for the client and for the profession. *Interprofessional collaborative practice* involves interaction and communication between varied professionals and the clients receiving health care (World Health Organization [WHO], 2010). Core ideals associated with interprofessional collaborative practice include client and family centeredness, community-oriented care, and relationship-focused service delivery (WHO, 2010). This approach is a standard of best practice in the profession of occupational therapy, and more generally across both health care and educational settings.

Occupational therapy practitioners must have the clinical reasoning skills to work effectively in interprofessional contexts. These skills include having the ability to clearly articulate the unique nature of occupation and the value of occupation to support performance, participation, health, and well-being that is consistent with evidence-based practice standards. In this text, discussion of several common frames of reference and occupation-focused models will build skills in targeting science-driven strategies to guide interventions and outcomes that will be distinctive in an interprofessional setting.

To support client goals and provide care that is safe, timely, and efficient, effective and equitable teamwork and interprofessional communication is especially important. The pressures to reduce costs while improving the quality of client care are leading many health care organizations to explore novel solutions (e.g., telehealth services) and to change established practice models to include point-of-service documentation.

Many new strategies that are being introduced use information and communication technologies that provide prompts and guides to ensure that all aspects of care are consistently documented. These new approaches offer some challenging choices. For example, with drop-down boxes to select pre-identified intervention goals, the rich process of client-centered collaborative care can be eroded. Through professional communication of the clinical reasoning process, this trend toward simplification can be addressed to best represent the client.

One of the challenges of interprofessional collaborative practice is having adequate opportunity for professional to interact regularly to build partnerships and to share knowledge that will advance clinical reasoning. The widespread use of information and communication technologies offers collaborative opportunities unconstrained by geography. Consultation and collaboration can now occur virtually and can be available to practitioners working in relative isolation.

Although technology offers many new tools and opportunities to support clients through collaboration, challenges to occupational therapy practice, particularly to intervention practices, are sometimes driven by external factors. For example, the rapid expansion of the use of PAMs in health care settings has been in part fueled by trends in reimbursement and in best practice impairment-specific intervention protocols. This trend has challenged practitioners to gain new skills and amend their interventions to accommodate new strategies.

In addition, trends are often data driven, responding to scientific evidence. For example, the trend toward interprofessionally collaborative, family-guided routines-based intervention has been supported by studies that found that "parents' perceptions of efficacy and satisfaction increased when interventions are embedded in family routines and settings" (Kingsley & Mailloux, 2013, p. 433).

Family-guided routines-based intervention is an interprofessional team–guided strategy that embeds intervention consistently by all family members and service providers throughout the day rather than in individual, isolated therapy sessions. *Family-guided routines* are functional and predictable activities that match the interests and individual schedules of the child and family. In this approach, the family guides the selection of routines and contexts for intervention. This process is initiated in the evaluation process with the completion of a routines-based interview. Case Example 1.2 shows the process of interprofessionally collaborative routines-based intervention.

The routines-based assessment process looks beyond child function to include aspects of family function. In Case Example 1.2, it is clear that the demands of caring for Kia have negatively affected the occupational performance of other family members. Ms. Doe has her sleep interrupted and has little time to meet the demands of her role as homemaker. In addition, some tension exists between Mr. and Ms. Doe because of his concerns for Kia's health, for his wife's health, and for the family finances.

In interprofessional collaborative practice, Kia's early intervention team would meet with the family and review family priorities. In this case, the top 3 priorities that the family identified were to improve Kia's eating so that she can get off the nasogastric tube and be able to eat table food, improve Kia's sleep patterns so that Ms. Doe can get more sleep, and improve Kia's ability to communicate. Note that the family did not identify motor function as one of the top goals. They want Kia to gain motor skills, but this area was not a current priority.

CASE EXAMPLE 1.2. KIA: EARLY INTERVENTION

Kia, age 17 months, offers an example of occupational therapy in early intervention practice in which the understanding of family roles and routines will be essential in providing effective intervention. Her occupational profile is shown in Exhibit 1.5.

EXHIBIT 1.5.	Kia's Occupational Profile		
Client	**Reason the client is seeking service and concerns related to engagement in occupations**	*Referral:* Kia was referred to the early intervention program by her pediatrician. Kia has many delayed developmental milestones and atypical movement patterns. *Impact on occupation:* Kia's mother reported that she has not had a complete night's sleep since Kia came home from the hospital because of Kia's need for night tube feeding. She also reported that Kia was not eating the same foods that her family eats during mealtime.	
	Occupations in which the client is successful	Kia has occupational roles appropriate to her age. The occupational roles affected the most are those of her parents.	
	Personal interests and values	Kia enjoys social interactions with her family, enjoys riding in the car, and likes watching children at the playground.	
	Occupational history (i.e., life experiences)	Kia was hospitalized for the first 4 months after birth because she had cardiac surgery. She has been diagnosed with failure to thrive associated with cardiac anomalies and a seizure disorder.	
	Performance patterns (routines, roles, habits, & rituals)	Kia has limited roles as an infant. Her routines are currently managed by the adults in her life.	
Environment		*Supports to occupational engagement*	*Barriers to occupational engagement*
	Physical (e.g., buildings, furniture, pets)	The family has supportive positioning equipment for Kia at home and for community mobility	
	Social (e.g., spouse, friends, caregivers)	Kia has a supportive family	

(Continued)

CASE EXAMPLE 1.2. KIA: EARLY INTERVENTION *(Cont.)*

EXHIBIT 1.5.	Kia's Occupational Profile *(Cont.)*		
Context	**Cultural** (e.g., customs, beliefs)	No issues related to culture or beliefs were identified during assessment.	
	Personal (e.g., age, gender, SES, education)	17-month-old female.	Kia's mother is age 18 years and has dropped out of high school.
	Temporal (e.g., stage of life, time, year)	Toddlerhood.	
	Virtual (e.g., chat, email, remote monitoring)	Not applicable to Kia's case.	
Client goals	**Client's priorities and desired targeted outcomes**	Kia's mother's greatest concern is for Kia to continue to gain weight so she can get off the tube feeding. She would like to be able to have the family eat the same foods at mealtime and not have to feed Kia different foods. She would also like Kia to sleep through the night and to gain skills in mobility and communication.	

ANALYSIS OF PARTICIPATION	
Basic ADLs	
Eating/oral–motor	Kia was able to drink about 1 oz of liquid from a spouted cup when it was held for her. She accepted a variety of pureed baby food by spoon, and she was able to move the food around in her mouth with her tongue. She had good lip closure. Kia was taking between 5–10 spoonfuls of food per meal when seated in an adapted high chair. When new textures or foods were introduced, Kia choked or gagged initially. It was not clear if her gagging and choking were the result of oral hypersensitivity caused by her nasogastric tube or the result of neurological problems. She held a spoon and waved it when it was placed in her hand; however, she was not controlling the spoon to scoop food or bring food to her mouth or to finger feed. Kia is fed every 3–4 hours during the day and is on a feeding tube at night.
Grooming	Kia cooperates during grooming tasks. She is age appropriate in this area.
Bathing/transfer	Kia played during bath time, reaching for and batting toys, touching pictures and making sounds, and watching and making sounds in response to what happened around her. She is dependent in all aspects of bathing.
Dressing upper and lower body	Kia is not able to assist with dressing because she has significant challenges in moving her arms and legs.
Toileting	Kia wears diapers. She is age appropriate in this area.
Problem solving/memory	Kia recognizes familiar people and routines, anticipating her parent's actions during ADL tasks.
Comments:	Kia wakes several times during the night, taking 10–15 minutes to get back to sleep.
IADLs	
No IADLs were considered in this case because of Kia's age.	
Motor and Praxis Skills	
Sitting (static/dynamic)	Kia is able to support her head well when sitting in an adapted seat, being held either in sitting or standing supported at her trunk, and laying on her tummy or side. She is able to balance momentarily when propped in the sitting position (hands on the floor or on her knees) but is not able to regain her balance or get herself into the sitting position. She lifts her head and uses her abdominals to help get to sitting. She is able to roll from her back to her stomach and moves short distances forward, sideways, and backward lying on her stomach (twisting her body to inch along).

(Continued)

CASE EXAMPLE 1.2. KIA: EARLY INTERVENTION (Cont.)

EXHIBIT 1.5. Kia's Occupational Profile (Cont.)

Standing (static/dynamic)	Kia stands with maximal support when positioned in an infant stander. When held in upright, she is able to bear some of her own weight. Kia is able to hold her head up when supported in a standing position.
Joint stability and skeletal mobility	Kia has normal joint stability and normal PROM.
Place can on shelf	—
Retrieve item from floor	—
Screw lid on jar	—
Comb back of head	—
Write name	—
Lift grocery bag	—
Coordination	Kia reaches with both hands and is able to move objects by swiping at them. She pats pictures and bangs toys. She moves with mid-range motions and has difficulty getting full active movement of her limbs. Kia has moderate spasticity in both lower limbs and mild spasticity in both upper limbs.
Manipulation	Kia was able to grasp toys and other objects that were placed in her hand but was not able to consistently open her hand to pick up an object by herself.
Comments:	Kia is able to roll by herself from her stomach to her back but with some difficulty. Kim was also able to roll from her back to her stomach. She moved short distances forward, sideways, and backward lying on her stomach, mostly by twisting her body to inch along, although she was trying to pull with her arms and to push with her legs. She was motivated to move to get her toys, although she was not able to move far.
Process Skills	
Energy for task	Kia is age appropriate in this area.
Knowledge/organization of task	Kia shows recognition of several toys and objects by looking at them when they are named.
Adaptation/praxis	Kia has not been assessed in this area. Her movement patterns are significantly limited because of spasticity.
Communication and social skills	Kia engages in imitative play by making throaty sounds following sounds made by others. She was not babbling or making consonant sounds. Ms. Doe reported that Kia sometimes used gestures and sounds to let people know when she wanted to be picked up, was full, or did not like a particular food. Kia enjoys being with adults and other children.
Cognitive and emotional regulation skills	Kia cries and fusses when she is not understood.
Level of arousal/attention	Age appropriate.
Orientation	Age appropriate.
Energy and drive	Age appropriate.
Higher level cognition	Age appropriate.
Comments:	—
Sensory–Perceptual Skills	
General sensory	Kia has intact basic sensory function.
Hearing and vision	Hearing and vision are intact.

(Continued)

CASE EXAMPLE 1.2. KIA: EARLY INTERVENTION *(Cont.)*

EXHIBIT 1.5.	**Kia's Occupational Profile** *(Cont.)*
Self-perception	Kia is age appropriate in this area.
Pain	Kia has intact pain sensation.
Skin integrity	Kia's skin is intact.
Comments:	—

Note. Occupational profile from American Occupational Therapy Association (2017). Analysis of participation format adapted from Skubik-Peplaski, Paris, Culpert, & Boyle (2009). — omitted due to Kia's age and developmental level (these omissions reflect the challenges of evaluation and intervention to support a dependent client without also evaluating the client's care providers) or nonapplicable; ADLs = activities of daily living; IADLs = instrumental activities of daily living; PROM = passive range of motion; SES = socioeconomic status.

Notes from Routines-Based Interview With Kia's Family

What are the daily routines and activities of your family (where and with whom Kia spends time)?

- During the week, Mr. Doe gets up at 6:30 a.m. to prepare for work. June (Kia's big sister) usually gets up at the same time, and Mr. Doe gets her breakfast. Kia and Ms. Doe are up by 7:30, the time Mr. Doe leaves for work. Ms. Doe then feeds Kia, and gets both girls dressed. Ms. Doe spends most of the time at home during the day with Kia and June. She is beginning to do some errands with the girls during the day now that Kia is healthy. She had been doing shopping at night when Mr. Doe could be at home with Kia.
- Kia eats small meals every 3–4 hours. She is tube fed twice a day, around 1:00 a.m. and around 1:00 p.m. She will be weaned from the lunch feeding within the next week or so. Ms. Doe prepares different foods for Kia than for the rest of the family.
- Kia likes to play on the living room floor with June. She does so several times a day.
- June plays with neighborhood children almost every day, and Kia likes to watch them play and seems to want to play with them.
- June usually naps around 2:00 p.m. everyday, and Kia naps around 3:00. Ms. Doe has about an hour each day to do chores at home when both girls are napping.
- Mr. Doe returns home at 5:30 p.m. Ms. Doe likes to have dinner ready for him when he arrives.
- After dinner, Mr. Doe plays with the girls while Ms. Doe cleans up the kitchen and then watches TV.
- June goes to bed at night around 8:00 p.m., and Kia goes to bed around 9:30. Mr. and Ms. Doe usually go to bed around 10:00.

Are there other routines or activities you would like to establish? They can be routines or activities that your family would like to do now or in the future.

- Ms. Doe would like the girls to be on the same sleep schedule so she has some time to herself and to do household chores.

- Ms. Doe would like Kia to be around children her own age, especially because she really enjoys watching June play with neighbor children.
- Ms. Doe would like to have more support from Mr. Doe and Kia's grandparents in caring for Kia and June. She is hoping that they will be more willing to help with Kia when she is able to eat table foods and not gag.

Who are the people and what are the toys, activities, routines, and places your child enjoys the most?

- Kia likes riding in the car. Kia likes to be read books by her grandparents. She also enjoys playing games with them (peek-a-boo, pat-a-cake).
- June likes to interact with Kia during playtime, showing her books and toys and attempting to engage her in play.
- Kia enjoys being with most adults, especially her grandparents. Ms. Doe's parents live close by and visit several times each week during the day. They almost always spend time with Kia and June after church on Sundays.

Which routines or activities are challenging for you or your child?

- Mealtime, nap time, and bedtime.

What are your family concerns related to your child's development (including anything your family identifies that would help to improve your ability to meet the needs of your child)?

- Kia gags and chokes when new foods or liquids are introduced, and Kia's mom has to spend a good amount of time working to help Kia overcome her dislikes of new foods and textures. Kia's mom is concerned about how long it will take to transition Kia to table food that the rest of the family eats.
- Kia and her sister are not on the same sleep schedule (going to bed, awaking in the morning, or napping during the day), so Kia's mom doesn't always finish

CASE EXAMPLE 1.2. KIA: EARLY INTERVENTION *(Cont.)*

all of her chores and is frequently tired because Kia does not yet sleep through the night.
- Several times a day, Kia cries and fusses because Kia's parents and sister do not always understand what she wants or needs.
- Mr. Doe and Kia's grandparents are "uncomfortable" feeding Kia and spending long periods of time caring for her. Mr. Doe is not home a lot because of his long hours of work.
- Kia attempts to initiate play with her sister but is unable to move very far around the living room on her own and is unable to tell her sister what she wants to play with.

What are your family resources, including family, friends, community groups, financial supports, that are helpful to you?
- Kia usually spends her day at home with her mom and sister.
- Kia's maternal grandparents spend time with Kia and her family almost every Sunday after the family returns from church. Her grandparents are helpful with Kia and June.
- Transporting Kia to the store, church, and so forth is easy.
- Kia spends about 30 minutes 2 times per day playing on the living room floor with her sister.

All team members (i.e., occupational therapy practitioner, physical therapist, dietitian, developmental specialist) are expected to build their interventions around supporting the family in moving toward these priority goals. In this case, the practitioner might help the family build mealtime and bedtime routines that are consistent and can be used to shape Kia's behaviors. Working with the dietitian, the practitioner could organize meals so that oral feeding precedes any tube feeding because Kia will eat more when she feels hunger. The practitioner could coach the family to use sensory supports to help Kia go back to sleep when she wakes. Working with the speech therapist, the practitioner could teach Mr. Doe interactive games that encourage communication and other developmental skills. This activity may help him feel more comfortable addressing Kia's special needs and will help reduce the strain on Ms. Doe. In addition, the practitioner could choose interactive games that support the development of hand skills—as a bonus rather than the priority.

In interprofessional collaborative practice, the clinical reasoning process is essential and must be extended to provide care that is respectful of the entire team and puts the client's priorities above those of the individual practitioners.

SUMMARY

As occupational therapy practitioners learn to analyze the many aspects of the clinical reasoning process, they should also become better able to articulate the unique value of occupational therapy in their professional documentation and other communications. Clinical reasoning and effective clinical communication can greatly improve practitioners' effectiveness in clinical settings. It can also improve their ability to develop working hypotheses both for individual clients and in challenging clinical situations, enhancing their effectiveness and guiding clinical research.

In this chapter, the cases of Matthew and Kia illustrated the development of a clinical hypothesis. In the

first case it was that Matthew's CTS interventions needed to be customized because of the spasticity he had in his arm before the development of CTS pain. In Kia's case it was that improvements in Kia's eating were essential to both Kia's development and to family function. Additional clinical hypotheses could be made related to other aspects of these cases.

Note that multiple possible clinical reasoning paths can be chosen for a particular hypothesis, and if client–practitioner collaboration is central to the clinical reasoning process, each of these paths can lead to a positive outcome. In addition, best practice and evidence-based practice, often emphasized by occupational therapy, are the end result of a thought process that reflects the unique needs and contexts of the individual client.

LEARNING ACTIVITIES

Consider the key aspects of clinical reasoning in Matthew's case. Review CTS and the common treatments for it. As Matthew's occupational therapy practitioner, you must first thoroughly understand the specific problem that he came to occupational therapy to address. Once you are well-schooled in interventions for CTS, you will engage in many forms of clinical reasoning. Answer the following questions to consider these forms of clinical reasoning more specifically:

1. As you prepare to assess and treat Matthew, you will need to start with a clinical hypothesis. List at least 1 hypothesis to begin your reasoning process.
2. Some clinical reasoning will be based on algorithms. Describe at least 1 algorithm-based clinical reasoning path that is appropriate to this case.
3. Some of your reasoning will be heuristic. Describe at least 1 heuristic-based clinical reasoning path that is appropriate to this case.
4. Trial and error is likely to be an important clinical reasoning strategy in Matthew's case. Why?

5. In Matthew's case, the occupational therapy practitioner used an explicitly collaborative process that includes the practitioner, the interprofessional team, and the client. How would you expect this process to influence the clinical reasoning process?

6. This chapter offered discussions of the biomechanical frame of reference. Describe how this frame of reference would be important in Matthew's case. Discuss how occupation-focused clinical reasoning could affect or alter your application of the biomechanical frame of reference to provide the most relevant intervention in Matthew's case.

7. Assuming that your first priority is to address Matthew's acute needs associated with CTS, what would be your next priority focus area to meet his goal of returning to work? Explain your choice.

8. The rehabilitation frame of reference would be a good adjunct to use with the biomechanical frame of reference with Matthew. Look up the rehabilitation frame of reference, and describe it in terms of focus, basic assumptions, function and dysfunction, and postulates of change.

9. As a learning tool, you should quiz yourself on definitions of the 4 basic elements of frames of reference because they will be used consistently throughout the remainder of this book.

REFERENCES

American Occupational Therapy Association. (2014). Occupational therapy practice framework: Domain and process (3rd ed.). *American Journal of Occupational Therapy, 68*(Suppl. 1), S1–S48. https://doi.org/10.5014/ajot.2014.682006

American Occupational Therapy Association. (2017). AOTA occupational profile template. *American Journal of Occupational Therapy, 71*(Suppl. 2), 7112420030. https://doi.org/10.5014/ajot.716S12

Cherry, K. (2015). *Problem-solving: Problem-solving strategies and obstacles.* Retrieved from http://psychology.about.com/od/cognitivepsychology/a/problem-solving.htm

Elstein, A. S. (2009). Thinking about diagnostic thinking: A 30-year perspective. *Advances in Health Sciences Education, 14,* 7–18. https://doi.org/10.1007/s10459-009-9184-0

Kassirer, J., Wong, J., & Kopelman, R. (2010). *Learning clinical reasoning* (2nd ed.). Philadelphia: Lippincott Williams & Wilkins.

Kingsley, K., & Mailloux, Z. (2013). Evidence for the effectiveness of different service delivery models in early intervention services. *American Journal of Occupational Therapy, 67,* 431–436. https://doi.org/10.5014/ajot.2013.006171

Knight, K., & Draper, D. (2012). *Therapeutic modalities: The art and science* (2nd ed.). Philadelphia: Lippincott Williams & Wilkins.

Medical diagnosis. (2015). In *American heritage science dictionary.* Retrieved from http://bit.ly/DoE129

Mosey, A. (1981). *Occupational therapy: Configuration of a profession.* New York: Raven Press.

Mosey, A. (1996). *Applied scientific inquiry in the health professions: An epistemological orientation* (2nd ed.). Bethesda, MD: American Occupational Therapy Association.

Palisano, R., Rosenbaum, P., Walter, S., Russell, D., Wood, E., & Galuppi, B. (1997). Development and reliability of a system to classify gross motor function in children with cerebral palsy. *Developmental Medicine and Child Neurology, 39,* 214–223.

Skubik-Peplaski, C., Paris, C., Boyle, D., & Culpert, A. (Eds.). (2009). *Applying the* Occupational Therapy Practice Framework: *Using the Cardinal Hill Occupational Participation Process in client-centered care* (2nd ed.). Bethesda, MD: AOTA Press.

Theory. (2017). In *Merriam-Webster online dictionary.* Retrieved from https://www.merriam-webster.com/dictionary/theory

Unsworth, C. A. (2001). The clinical reasoning of novice and expert occupational therapists. *Scandinavian Journal of Occupational Therapy, 8,* 163–173. https://doi.org/10.1080/110381201317166522

World Health Organization. (2010). *Framework for action on interprofessional education and collaborative practice.* Geneva: Author.

Clinical Reasoning and Occupational Therapy's Domain of Practice

2

Anne Cronin, PhD, OTR/L, ATP, FAOTA, and Garth Graebe, MOT, OTR/L

CHAPTER HIGHLIGHTS

- Describes the occupational therapy domain and applies it to the clinical reasoning process.
- Communicates the distinct role of occupation in the clinical reasoning process.
- Defines the key elements of the occupational therapy domain as presented in the *Occupational Therapy Practice Framework*.
- Applies the language of occupation-based reasoning.
- Explore the elements of the occupational therapy domain in a clinical reasoning context.
- Illustrates the use of the occupational therapy domain in clinical reasoning as a problem-solving tool.

KEY TERMS AND CONCEPTS

Attitudinal environment	Internet of Things	Reflection
Beliefs	Motor skills	Rituals
Body functions	Natural environment	Roles
Body structures	Occupation	Routines
Client factors	Performance patterns	Social environment
Cultural context	Performance skills	Social interaction skills
Domain	Personal context	Spirituality
Environment	Personal factors	Temporal context
Environmental factors	Physical environment	Values
Function	Process skills	Virtual context
Habits	Products and technology	

Occupational therapy is a global profession that champions the belief that occupation is central to health, participation, and life satisfaction. As the profession continues to grow and mature, the depth and scope of its clinical reasoning must balance the core values of the profession with the growing scientific advances that affect individual, family, community, and population health. The practice of occupational therapy should be reflective of the culture and needs of the community within which the occupational therapy practitioner works, and there are complex cultural influences in determining what is considered best occupational therapy in any given place and time.

Occupational therapy in the United States faces unique opportunities and challenges, and this text is designed to support clinical reasoning for practitioners working within the constraints of practice in the United States. To this end, this text has been built around the *Occupational Therapy Practice Framework: Domain and Process* (OTPF–3; American Occupational Therapy Association [AOTA], 2014) and illustrates clinical reasoning challenges and cases drawn from occupational therapy practice in the United States. The intent is not to exclude practitioners from the global arena or to propose that occupational therapy in the United States is superior to that in other places. The focus on the United States is simply to allow the authors to be very specific in the cases and challenges presented for students and practitioners in this country.

KEY ELEMENTS OF OCCUPATIONAL THERAPY'S DOMAIN

Since its beginnings, occupational therapy has been a profession focused on function. *Function* is defined by Merriam-Webster (2016) as "the action for which a person or thing is specially fitted or used or for which a thing exists." One of the goals of the *OTPF–3* (AOTA, 2014) is to provide a standard language and structure for occupational therapy across clinical, scientific, and policy arenas.

The *OTPF–3* is an independent document but is, in many ways, consistent with the *International Classification of Functioning, Disability and Health* (*ICF*; World Health Organization [WHO], 2001). The *ICF* is a classification system intended to standardize the way to describe "changes in body function and structure, what a person with a health condition can do in a standard environment (their level of capacity), as well as what they actually do in their usual environment (their level of performance)" (WHO, 2002, p. 2). Because familiarity with both the *ICF* and the *OTPF–3* is useful in clinical reasoning, this chapter elaborates on aspects from both systems.

The *domain* is "the profession's purview and the areas in which its members have an established body of knowledge and expertise" (AOTA, 2014, p. s3). Understanding the domain of occupational therapy is an essential first aspect of clinical reasoning. In a sense, the domain is the occupational therapy lens through which practitioners consider information in the clinical reasoning process. In the *OTPF–3* (AOTA, 2014), the domain of occupational therapy has five components (Exhibit 2.1):

1. Occupations
2. Client factors
3. Performance skills
4. Performance patterns
5. Context and environments.

Occupations

Occupations warrant some special attention. A common lament of occupational therapy practitioners is that most people in their communities do not know what practitioners do. Part of this problem is caused by the word *occupation* because it has many meanings and some meanings have a strong emotional context. For most Americans, the first thing that comes to mind when they hear the word *occupation* is work or employment. Not surprisingly then, one of the most common assumptions of laypeople is that occupational therapy practitioners are people who help people find jobs.

Here, *occupation* is defined as "a group of activities that has personal and sociocultural meaning, is named within a culture, and supports participation in society" (Cole & Creek, 2016, p. 13). Many additional eloquent definitions of occupation as the foundation for occupational therapy are in the *OTPF–3* (AOTA, 2014), which categorizes occupations as activities of daily living (ADLs), instrumental activities of daily living (IADLs), rest and sleep, education, work, play, leisure, and social participation. These occupations are key focus areas of the occupational therapy clinical reasoning process.

Client Factors

Client factors are defined in the *OTPF–3* as "specific capacities, characteristics, or beliefs that reside within the person and that influence performance in occupations" (AOTA, 2014, p. S7). In its discussion of client factors, the *OTPF–3* draws upon the *ICF* (WHO, 2001) classification system to describe body functions and body structures. *Body functions* are physiological in nature and organized by functional system, such as mental, cardiovascular, or movement-related functions (WHO, 2001). *Body structures* are anatomically categorized by body part, such as the nervous system or structures related to movement. Body structures and body functions are interrelated and often influence a person's ability to engage in desired occupations.

Another component of client factors is values, beliefs, and spirituality, in which the *OTPF–3* (AOTA, 2014) differs from the *ICF* (WHO, 2001) model (which describes these components as attitudes and lists them as an environmental factor). Values, beliefs, and spirituality are essential for understanding motivation. Case Example 2.1 returns to the case of Matthew, first presented in Chapter 1, and provides Matthew's client factors.

EXHIBIT 2.1.	Aspects of Occupational Therapy's Domain			
OCCUPATIONS	**CLIENT FACTORS**	**PERFORMANCE SKILLS**	**PERFORMANCE PATTERNS**	**CONTEXTS AND ENVIRONMENTS**
Activities of daily (ADLs)*	Values, beliefs, and spirituality	Motor skill	Habits	Cultural
Instrumental activities of daily living (IADLs)	Body functions	Process skills	Routines	Personal
Rest and sleep	Body structures	Social interaction skills	Rituals	Physical
Education			Roles	Social
Work				Temporal
Play				Virtual
Leisure				
Social participation				

*Also referred to as *basic activities of daily living (BADLs)* or *personal activities of daily living (PADLs)*.
Source. From "Occupational Therapy Practice Framework: Domain and Process (3rd ed.)," by the American Occupational Therapy Association, 2014, *American Journal of Occupational Therapy,* Vol. 68, Suppl. 1, p. S4. Copyright © 2014 by the American Occupational Therapy Association. Used with permission.

CASE EXAMPLE 2.1. MATTHEW: CLIENT FACTORS

Because **Matthew's** presenting referral is the result of the specific musculoskeletal problem of CTS, the occupational therapy practitioner must pay extensive attention to Matthew's body structure and function client factors. The client factors of values and beliefs are equally important because they allow the practitioner to understand what Matthew cares about and is motivated to work toward. Spirituality is not a factor that Matthew described as important on his occupational profile, so it will not be a focus for clinical reasoning. Exhibit 2.2 lists Matthew's client factors.

| **EXHIBIT 2.2.** | **Matthew's Client Factors** |

Body Functions

Neuromuscular and movement-related functions: functions of movement and mobility, including functions of joints, bones, reflexes, and muscles:

- Has spastic quadriplegia-type CP.
- Is able to sit on a regular chair but may require pelvic or trunk support to maximize hand function.
- Is able to move in and out of the chair using a stable surface to push on or pull up with his arms.
- Walks with a rolling walker indoors and is usually transported in a wheelchair when traveling outdoors on uneven terrain.
- Has CTS and tingling, numbness, weakness, or pain in the fingers or hand.

Body Structures

Structures related to movement:

- *Shoulder region:* Intact.
- *Upper arm:* Intact.
- *Forearm and hand:* Pressure on the median nerve caused by swelling or anything that makes the carpal tunnel smaller causes CTS.

Values

- Lives with his brother's family (including his brother's wife and 2 small children) and values the opinion of his brother and sister-in-law.
- Values his life roles as a worker, brother, son, and Pittsburgh Pirates fan.
- Cherishes his independence in the community and wants to contribute rather than be a burden in his home.
- Values the friends and social connections he has made through his work and through participation in recreational programs at the community center.

Beliefs

- If pain free, will be able to return to work and daily life.
- If pain free, will be able to contribute more at home to his own care and household chores.
- CTS developed as a repetitive strain injury related to his work.

Spirituality

Spirituality was not introduced by the client as either a support or a confounding consideration in achieving desired levels of occupational performance. Spirituality, in this instance, should be respected but does not require any unique considerations in this case.

Note. CP = cerebral palsy; CTS = carpal tunnel syndrome.

Values

Values are "principles, standards, or qualities considered worthwhile by the client who holds them" (AOTA, 2014, p. S7). Values often reflect sociocultural contexts and influence the person's priorities and actions in all aspects of daily life.

Beliefs

Beliefs are "cognitive content held as true" (AOTA, 2014, p. S7). Beliefs and values are often described together because they are often interrelated. A belief is a feeling of being sure that something is true. It may or may not be grounded in fact. A belief may reflect values. For example, an older woman may be proud of her home and value that it is well decorated to reflect her achievement and social status. The belief may follow that exterior modifications to the home to allow wheelchair access diminishes the perception that she is independent and able. In this scenario, the older woman may choose to be less independent to continue the appearance of independence. In addition, if clients are not intrinsically motivated to perform recommended therapy activities, their values and beliefs can be explored to help find a common ground between clients' medical needs and personal motivations.

Spirituality

According to the *Framework*, **spirituality** refers to a broad set of principles that transcends all religions and is the way people seek and express meaning and purpose (AOTA, 2014). It also encompasses people's sense of connectedness to something larger than themselves and gives life meaning. Like values and beliefs, spirituality affects occupations through its influence on motivation and personal volition (Humbert, 2016; Maley, Pagana, Velenger, & Humbert, 2016) and may affect a person's beliefs about the healing or rehabilitative process.

For example, a client may believe that he or she is experiencing pain as retribution for a bad deed or that prayer can replace exercise in the recovery process. These beliefs must be understood and respected to establish a true collaborative process. Finding common ground or compromising to reflect respect for personal beliefs, values, and spirituality is an essential part of the collaborative clinical reasoning process.

Performance Skills

Performance skills are "goal-directed actions that are observable as small units of engagement in daily life occupations. They are learned and developed over time and are situated in specific contexts and environments" (AOTA, 2014, p. S7). Performance skills may make up components of a more complex occupation. These skills are also interrelated, and change in one performance skill can affect other performance skills. *Performance*, in the context of occupational therapy, means choosing, organizing, and carrying out occupations in interaction with the environment (Cole & Creek, 2016). Performance skills are subdivided into motor skills, process skills, and social interaction skills (see Case Example 2.2 for a list of Matthew's performance skills).

Motor skills

Although basic motor development and musculoskeletal functions are considered to be client factors, performance skills are the client's demonstrated ability to use musculoskeletal functions. Motor skills are distinct from *motor behaviors* (i.e., any performance of movement that can be observed or documented) or *motor development* (i.e., acquisition of motor behavior that is heavily maturational in origin). **Motor skills** are performed movement abilities that have been developed through practice and learning. These skills include the ability to imitate, plan, and sequence movements in a desired pattern (AOTA, 2014).

Process skills

Process skills are cognitive and information-processing abilities that allow people to manage and modify actions. These abilities include pacing oneself in task performance, choosing performance strategies, and organizing a task into a logical sequence. Attention, memory, and perceptual skills are considered to be client factors that are foundational to the more complex process skills needed for the performance of daily occupations. For example, the ability to correctly start and stop an action requires intact attention and perceptual skills as well as the use of memory to define and delimit the task. Other complex process skills include planning for appropriate tools to complete a task and evaluating the effectiveness of performance as it is happening (AOTA, 2014).

CASE EXAMPLE 2.2. MATTHEW: PERFORMANCE SKILLS

An analysis of Matthew's performance skills (see Exhibit 2.3) gives the occupational therapy practitioner insight into his prior performance and the daily impact of his CTS. Because of this specific musculoskeletal problem, the practitioner must pay careful attention to how it affects Matthew's motor skills. Although another profession may focus exclusively on Matthew's motor skills, the *OTPF–3* (AOTA, 2014) guides the practitioner to look more broadly at Matthew's function. Therefore, the practitioner also evaluates Matthew's process and social interaction skills.

It is essential for the practitioner to understand Matthew's process and social interaction skills because he has an intellectual impairment that may significantly hinder his ability to follow a home-based exercise program, a commonly used intervention for CTS. Social interaction skills can be explored within the initial interview. Preferences in communication style, including the possible use of pictures or other communication supports, should be identified early in the clinical contact. Careful consideration of social interaction and process skills in the clinical reasoning process allow the practitioner to develop a home program that plays to Matthew's strengths and optimizes his recovery.

(Continued)

CASE EXAMPLE 2.2. MATTHEW: PERFORMANCE SKILLS *(Cont.)*

EXHIBIT 2.3. | Matthew's Performance Skills

Motor Skills
- Matthew's ability to change and maintain his body position as needed has been limited as a result of his inability to use his right arm in transfers and with his rolling walker.
- Although previously independent in transfers, Matthew now needs physical assistance in transferring himself.
- Before the development of CTS, Matthew had significant limitation in his ability to carry, move, or handle objects because of his poor bilateral coordination as well as impaired bilateral arm strength and AROM because of spasticity. This limitation is worsened by the CTS.
- Before the development of carpal tunnel syndrome, Matthew had significant limitation in his fine hand use. He has an imbalance of flexion and extension motor function in his hands, resulting in weak bilateral wrist and finger extension.
- Matthew is right-handed and had been able to isolate fingers and use a gross grasp pattern in daily tasks before the CTS. Currently, greater limitations in the use of his right hand have made it difficult for Matthew to isolate finger motions, pick up and grasp objects, and manipulate objects.
- Matthew is unable to assume standing because of the decreased use of his right arm. Once he is in standing, he is able to independently maintain the position. He can bear partial (<30%) weight on his right arm when using the walker.
- Matthew has been unable to use his walker well since the development of CTS and has spent a large portion of his day in a standard manual wheelchair that he is able to propel slowly using his feet.

Process Skills
- Matthew has a moderate cognitive impairment but understands the steps of work tasks that need to be done and the materials necessary for those tasks. He understands safety issues and has been effective in the supported employment setting in performing a variety of structured tasks.
- Matthew is able to function in familiar environments and organize familiar tasks.
- Matthew has difficulty understanding, organizing, initiating, and sequencing new tasks. To learn new tasks, Matthew needs specific instruction and the ability to practice new skills with an extended period of direct supervision.
- Once he learns a skill, Matthew is able to perform it in novel situations and contexts, but he has limited ability to modify task actions in response to unexpected problems.
- Matthew has adequate attention, memory, and perceptual skills for the performance of his desired occupations.
- Matthew understands the tasks and task sequences that make up his daily routine.
- Before the CTS, Matthew was able to independently carry out his daily routine using some adaptive devices and activity modifications.

Social Interaction Skills
- Matthew interacts effectively in 1:1 interactions, responding to his name, following 1-step directions, and appropriately drawing attention to himself when he needs help or clarification.
- Matthew is able to comprehend literal meanings of spoken messages.
- Matthew is nonverbal but is able to express basic wants and needs with a tablet-based AAC device and one-finger pointing.
- Since the development of CTS, pointing has become painful for Matthew and he has been communicating more with gestures and partner-assisted interpretation of his vocalizations.

Note. AAC = augmentative and alternative communication; AROM = active range of motion.

Social interaction skills

Social interaction skills are both verbal and nonverbal abilities that allow the person to communicate effectively with others, establish positive social relationships, and interact within the social and cultural expectations of the interaction context. The social interaction skill functions include a broad scope of specific skills that include following simple directions in a one-to-one interaction, participating productively in a conversation, and being able to convey simple instructions and to express needs and wants. Social interaction skills also can mirror emotional regulation skills. When people have challenges with emotional regulation, the greatest negative impact of poor self-regulation is manifested in poor social interaction skills. Effective social interaction skills result in a smooth sequence of social behaviors that are applied in a dynamic way across various social contexts.

Performance Patterns

Performance skills often serve as the building blocks for *performance patterns,* which are "the habits, routines, roles, and rituals used in the process of engaging in occupations or activities that can support or hinder occupational performance" (AOTA, 2014, p. S8). Performance patterns may include several performance skills in combination to complete needed or desired tasks. Performance patterns are complex and profoundly affected by social and cultural contexts. They are often highly valued and may be integral to a person's social and personal identity (see Case Example 2.3 for a discussion and list of Matthew's performance patterns).

Habits

Habits are a type of performance pattern that is learned through frequent repetition and becomes automatic. Habits do not require attention to perform and once learned may be difficult to change or alter. Habits become so automatic that often people with dementia, who lose memory, demonstrate them, such as the habit of using utensils while eating. Habits may be overlooked in a standard assessment because the client may not be aware of them. For example, Matthew may fidget when he is in stressful situations. He does not plan to fidget and he may not always be aware that he is fidgeting because this activity pattern has become a habit. It is common that

CASE EXAMPLE 2.3. MATTHEW: PERFORMANCE PATTERNS

The analysis of performance patterns is the point in this case where the distinct role of occupational therapy becomes most clear. Matthew's CTS has led to a broad scale of impaired performance patterns that is far different than the typical limitations associated with the syndrome (see Exhibit 2.4). Matthew is experiencing a profound disruption in his daily occupations from which it may be hard to recover. His loss of roles and social participation may lead to another debilitating problem, depression.

The occupational therapy practitioner should work with Matthew, his brother, and his employer to build compensations and supports that will allow him to function in his valued roles while recovering his hand function. Without support in this area, Matthew may not be able to easily transition back to his active lifestyle and work roles.

EXHIBIT 2.4.   Matthew's Performance Patterns

Habits
- Matthew relies on the use of his right arm in pushing to stand from a sitting position, guiding his rolling walker, and touching his AAC device to make choices. Because of his hand use limitations, he has also developed impaired performance patterns in the areas of mobility, communication, and social interaction.
- Matthew usually uses his right arm for utensil use in eating. He is having difficulty adjusting to alternative approaches to eating.

Routines
- Matthew had developed a morning self-care routine that allowed him to independently prepare for his daily activities. This routine involved right-hand use at every step, from turning off the alarm clock to closing the door as he leaves the house. Because of his difficulty problem solving in novel situations, Matthew has become dependent in basic ADLs secondary to CTS.
- Matthew has lost the structure that performance of routines and work provided to his days. He now has difficulty planning and initiating tasks and task sequences.

Roles
- Matthew's valued life roles include his family roles of brother, uncle, and household member who contribute to the completion of needed chores in the home.
- Matthew is an employee. He works in the local newspaper office in a supported employment arrangement, although he has not been able to work since the development of CTS.
- Matthew describes himself as a Pittsburgh Pirates fan. He continues to enjoy watching televised games with his family.
- Matthew's mobility and communication limitations as a result of CTS have caused him to stop attending the evening recreational programs at the community center, limiting his social participation and social roles.

Rituals
- Rituals are not likely to be affected in Matthew's case. He is still able to participate in family activities and celebrations, although his independence is limited.

Note. AAC = augmentative and alternative communication; ADLs = activities of daily living; CTS = carpal tunnel syndrome.

people become fully aware of their habits only when the habits are disrupted, for example, by injury, or when trying to change a behavior, such as smoking.

Routines

Routines are established sequences of occupations or activities that provide a structure for daily life (AOTA, 2014). Routines are coordinated actions that serve to plan, manage, and complete the requirements of day-to-day procedures or duties, such as budgeting time and making plans for separate activities throughout the day (WHO, 2001). Like habits, routines are familiar and preferred patterns of activities, but they are not unconscious and can be altered more easily than habits.

Roles

Roles are "social and cultural norms and expectations of occupational performance that are associated with the individual's social and personal identity" (Cole & Creek, 2016, p. 13). Roles are socioculturally influenced, but note that they may be further conceptualized and defined by each person. For example, the social expectation of a person in the role of student is that the person attends to and performs assigned learning tasks. This person may choose to conform to this role or to alter it. For example, he or she may choose to perform extra learning tasks or to study independently.

Rituals

Rituals are "symbolic actions with spiritual, cultural, or social meaning" (AOTA, 2014, p. S8). Although religious rituals are common and well understood, occupational therapy practitioners should consider a broad range of rituals when working with clients. A ritual is simply a ceremony or action performed in a customary way. A client might have a morning ritual of drinking coffee while reading the newspaper. Rituals often involve the family and community. For example, birthday, wedding, and graduation celebrations are social rituals that are widely observed.

Contexts and Environments

The word *context* has been used extensively in theory to describe the interrelated conditions that influence a person and the performance of occupations. The *ICF*, recognizing that function and participation are not only influenced by features intrinsic to the person but by other factors, uses the term **environment**, not *context*, to refer to the "physical, social and attitudinal environment in which people live and conduct their lives" (WHO, 2001, p. 22). In the *OTPF–3*, however, the terms *context* and *environment* are used interchangeably, recognizing both the language of theory and that of the international community (AOTA, 2014).

The context and environment can include the **physical environment**, which includes the natural (e.g., geographic terrain, plants) and built (e.g., buildings, furniture) surroundings in which daily life occupations occur, and the **social environment** that includes social attitudes as well as the presence of, relationships with, and expectations of persons, groups, and populations with whom clients have contact (e.g., availability and expectations of significant individuals, such as spouse, friends, and caregivers). See Case Example 2.4 for an analysis of Matthew's contexts and environments.

Environmental factors

The *ICF* explains that **environmental factors** "are external to individuals and can have a positive or negative influence on the individual's participation as a member of society, on performance of activities of the individual or on the individual's body function or structure" (WHO, 2001, p. 22) and classifies 3 types of environmental factors:
1. Products and technology;
2. Natural environment and human-made changes to the environment; and
3. Support and relationships, attitudes, services, systems, and policies. (WHO, 2002)

This *ICF* classification system is elaborated on in the next sections (except for services, systems, and policies in Category 3), and the environmental factor of attitudes is linked to the *OTPF–3's* cultural context (AOTA, 2014). Services, systems, and policies affect opportunities and resources available to support performance in daily occupations and are discussed in greater detail in Chapter 9, "Occupational Therapy Intervention Process," and Chapter 10, "Strategic Thinking and Outcomes in Occupational Therapy."

Products and technology. The *ICF* category of **products and technology** refers to the physical items that people come in contact with while completing their daily activities (WHO, 2001). These items can include fundamental needs such as food and medications or complex items such as medical technologies. Products or systems of products can be natural or human made. In addition, they can include both animate and inanimate elements of the natural environment. A service animal is an example of an animate element of the natural environment that supports the performance of daily activities. Rehabilitation equipment of all types from sock aids to smart home technologies would be inanimate elements of the natural environment.

Any product or technology can be assistive; however, the *ICF* defines *assistive products* and technology as "any product, instrument, equipment or technology adapted or specially designed for improving the functioning of a disabled person" (WHO, 2017).

Natural environment and human-made changes to the environment. The **natural environment** includes physical features of outdoor settings such as land forms,

CASE EXAMPLE 2.4. MATTHEW: CONTEXTS AND ENVIRONMENTS

Matthew has very supportive contexts and environments (see Exhibit 2.5). They offer a clear path for him to return to his daily functions if the impairments and disruptions of daily routines noted previously can be addressed.

EXHIBIT 2.5.   **Matthew's Contexts and Environments**

Environmental Factors

- *Natural environment and human-made changes to the environment:* Matthew had been able to manage in a modified physical environment before his injury. He has had mobility and intellectual limitations that have already been accommodated to his functional impairments. These modifications continue to be in place.
- *Products and technology:* Before his injury, Matthew used a rolling walker with a basket, supportive armchairs at work and at home, a touchscreen tablet–based AAC system, and a manual wheelchair. He was able to propel the manual chair independently for short distances using his feet. For long distances or on uneven surfaces, he was usually pushed in the chair by another person.
- *Support and relationships:* Before his injury, Matthew received both physical and emotional support from his family, employer, coworkers, and social group at the community center. These relationships had been well defined based on Matthew's prior level of independent functioning. Matthew has become more dependent in all ADLs, IADLs, and workplace activities as a result of his injury. This dependency will cause a need for renegotiation of support roles across contexts and environments.
- *Attitudes, services, systems, and policies:* Matthew was in a supportive environment regarding these aspects of the external environment before his injury. Currently, these environmental factors are not problematic.

Personal Context

- Matthew is a 45-year-old man who is supported by his brother for housing and basic needs in the home environment. He has an intellectual impairment that has limited his educational achievement and employment options.
- For Matthew, internal personal factors, such as personality, coping style, and overall behavior pattern, were not described. Although these factors are important to consider, when personal problems do not emerge in the occupational profile, it may reflect adequate resources in this area, which is the case for Matthew.

Temporal Context

- Matthew is in middle adulthood.
- Matthew has led a very structured adult life that has been organized into periods defined by routine activity (e.g., self-care, work, leisure). The loss of roles as a result of his injury has caused Matthew's day to become disorganized, and he no longer has an organized temporal context to guide his activity patterns.
- It takes Matthew longer than most people to perform both ADLs and IADLs.

Virtual Context

- Matthew is linked to the virtual context through his tablet-based communication device.
- Matthew also uses some variety of telephone-based communication device or a hand-held device to help prompt him in his daily tasks.

Note. AAC = augmentative and alternative communication; ADLs = activities of daily living; IADLs = instrumental activities of daily living.

---

distances between resources, animals, and disasters. The *ICF* lists the following as categories of the natural environment: physical geography, population, flora and fauna, climate, natural events, human-caused events, light, time-related changes, sound, vibration, and air quality (WHO, 2001). In addition, the term *natural environment* is sometimes used to describe the environment in which occupations are typically performed, in contrast to the clinical environment. The clinical environment often has greater structure and supervision available than the natural environment. However, a client's performance in the clinical environment may not be the same as in the actual context in which the client needs to function.

Support and relationships and attitudes. The category of support and relationships falls into the social environment, which includes the "people or animals that provide practical physical or emotional support, nurturing, protection, assistance and relationships to other persons, in their home, place of work, school or at play or in other aspects of their daily activities" (WHO, 2007, p. 205). The *ICF* lists the following as elements of support and relationships: immediate family, extended family, friends, acquaintances, people in positions of authority, people in subordinate positions, personal care providers and personal assistants, strangers, domesticated animals, health professionals, and other professionals (WHO, 2001).

The *ICF* includes an environmental context described as *attitudes* (WHO, 2001). This attitudinal context is similar to the cultural context described in the *OTPF–3* (AOTA, 2014):

- The ***attitudinal environment*** includes the "attitudes that are the observable consequences of customs, practices, ideologies, values, norms, factual beliefs and religious beliefs" (WHO, 2001).
- The ***cultural context*** in the *OTPF–3* includes "customs, beliefs, activity patterns, behavioral standards, and expectations accepted by the society of which a client is a member" (AOTA, 2014, p. S9).

The parallels between these two descriptions are clear. In both instances, the influences consist of people external to the person of interest. Cultural context could relate to ethnic heritage but can also include the unique culture within a given family or social group. For example, in Case Example 2.5, the role of gamer is important to Jamal. There is a distinctive gamer culture, and understanding this culture would be important in helping Jamal meet his goals through the occupational therapy process.

Personal factors

Personal factors are part of the ***personal context,*** which includes demographic features of a person, such as age, gender, social background, past and current experience, and educational level, that are not part of a health condition. Internal ***personal factors*** include intrinsic psychological and personality patterns such as coping styles, overall behavior pattern, and other factors that influence how disability is experienced by a person (WHO, 2002). It is often factors from the personal context that support decision making that best supports a client's needs, goals, and values.

Temporal and virtual contexts are personal factors because they provide a sort of infrastructure for occupational performance. Many tasks are tied to a specific time of day (e.g., breakfast) or must be completed within a specific time frame (e.g., crossing the street with a traffic signal). With the broad availability of information and communication technologies, the virtual context includes the needs and expectations for virtual connectivity in everyday activities.

Temporal context. The temporal context is elaborated upon in the *OTPF–3* (AOTA, 2014) because of the high regard occupational therapy practitioners have for temporal influences on clients. The ***temporal context*** includes the developmental stage of life and history (i.e., personal context in the *ICF;* WHO, 2001) as well as the time of day or year and the duration or rhythm of an activity (external environmental factors in the *ICF*). The temporal context also includes less tangible factors such as how long an activity is expected to take. This information can be important because a client may be able to perform a specific task or activity but choose not to do it because he or she thinks that it takes too much time.

Virtual context. A ***virtual context*** is described in the *OTPF–3* (AOTA, 2014) because of the growing role of the Internet and web-based services in all aspects of human occupation. The increasing automation of daily tasks and the growing Internet of Things (IoT) has made this context important to occupational therapy practitioners. The ***Internet of Things*** is "a system of interrelated computing devices, mechanical and digital machines, objects, animals or people that are provided with unique identifiers and the ability to transfer data over a network without requiring human-to-human or human-to-computer interaction" (TechTarget, 2016).

The virtual context is less about devices than about the virtual connectivity associated with devices. With current smart home technologies, cars, refrigerators, thermostats, television controls, and door locks are potentially part of the IoT. All a device needs is a sensor and a network connection to join the IoT. This virtual context is growing rapidly and thus is not clearly defined. In the near future, clients may have access to wearable devices such as fitness bands that monitor and report selected medical vital statistics. They may also have robots in the home, and have autonomous community mobility through self-driving automobiles and power wheelchair systems.

USING THE OCCUPATIONAL THERAPY DOMAIN IN CLINICAL REASONING AS A PROBLEM-SOLVING TOOL

It is important for occupational therapy practitioners to review all aspects of the occupational therapy domain during clinical reasoning, even if particular aspects of the domain are not problematic for their client. This analysis provides practitioners with a balanced view of the client's strengths and weaknesses as they work toward the best solutions for the client. Case Example 2.5 offers another case through which to explore the occupational therapy domain.

Case Example 2.5 provides the key elements of the occupational therapy domain (i.e., occupations, client factors, performance skills, performance patterns, contexts and environments) for Jamal. Consideration of the domain of occupational therapy is central to helping Jamal succeed in working toward his goals. A narrow focus on the performance of ADL and IADL rehabilitation goals would not adequately prepare Jamal to move forward into his desired adult roles.

In most practice settings, occupational therapy assessment must be focused to address the specific reason for referral. For example, a client referred for occupational therapy after a flexor tendon injury would not expect an

CASE EXAMPLE 2.5. JAMAL: DOMAIN OF PRACTICE

Jamal, age 17 years, was a well-adjusted, successful student before his injury in an automobile accident. Jamal has become a paraplegic with a L1 spinal cord injury (SCI). He is home from the rehabilitation center and facing the transition back to school. Although Jamal's injury was physical, many internal and external contextual factors make developing an intervention plan for Jamal challenging.

As the occupational therapy practitioner created an occupational profile for Jamal, he noted that Jamal's valued occupations included the independent performance of all ADLs and IADLs. He was in high school and had been working part-time after school to save for college. Since his injury Jamal's ability to engage in most of these occupations has been impaired. His client factors include that he is teenager living with his mother. He was a good student and had planned on continuing his education at the local community college. Details of Jamal's client factors, performance skills, performance patterns and context and environments are presented in Exhibit 2.6.

Jamal's goals are to be more independent at home to relieve the pressure on his mother. He would like to finish high school through an online correspondence program rather than go back to school. Jamal is interested in learning to drive a car using hand controls. Jamal is also interested in going to college in a couple of years and hopes to study computer science.

Jamal's mother wants to see him go back to his old school and reconnect with his friends. She wants him to develop the skills to support going to college, including driving and doing household chores. Jamal's mother is deeply religious and would like to see him reconnect with the teen group at church.

EXHIBIT 2.6.	Jamal's Occupational Profile	
Client	**Reason the client is seeking service and concerns related to engagement in occupations**	Jamal was referred to school-based occupational therapy for home-bound care before his return to school. He has difficulties with maintaining and changing positions, manipulation with movement, using materials, hygiene, clothing management, and endurance following a complete L1 SCI and resultant paraplegia. *Impact on occupation:* He no longer engages in any IADLs on a routine basis. The only face-to-face social contact that Jamal now engages in is during church attendance with his mother.
	Occupations in which the client is successful	Jamal performs his ADLs independently or with minimal assist Jamal has been keeping up with his schoolwork at home but does not want to return to the school environment. The only occupation that he reports that he is satisfied with since his return home is online gaming. He has an established game character, a guild, and a network of friends who he socially interacts with online.
	Personal interests and values	Online multiplayer gaming.
	Occupational history (i.e., life experiences)	Last year, when coming back from a trip to the beach with friends, Jamal was involved in an automobile accident. In the accident, Jamal was thrown from his car to the pavement, landing on his back and resulting in paraplegia. Jamal has just been discharged from the rehabilitation hospital to home and is starting back to school in 1 month at the change of term.
	Performance patterns (routines, roles, habits, & rituals)	Jamal's valued life roles include his role as a son, brother, gamer, uncle, and student. Since he has been away from school, Jamal's day has little structure or routine.

(Continued)

CASE EXAMPLE 2.5. JAMAL: DOMAIN OF PRACTICE *(Cont.)*

EXHIBIT 2.6.	Jamal's Occupational Profile *(Cont.)*		
Environment		**Supports to occupational engagement**	**Barriers to occupational engagement**
	Physical (e.g., buildings, furniture, pets)	Jamal lives with his mother in a house that she has remodeled so that the old family dining room is now Jamal's bedroom and bathroom and he does not have to go upstairs.	
	Social (e.g., spouse, friends, caregivers)	Jamal is the youngest of 4 children. His oldest sister is married and has two children of her own. He also has a brother and a sister in college.	Jamal does not want to return to a regular high school classroom with physical supports. He should be returning to the same class he should be in and has had academic support to keep up during his rehabilitation.
Context	**Cultural** (e.g., customs, beliefs)	No issues with culture, customs, or beliefs were identified during assessment.	
	Personal (e.g., age, gender, SES, education)	Age 17 years. Male. Currently attending high school.	
	Temporal (e.g., stage of life, time, year)	Period of transitioning to adult life roles.	
	Virtual (e.g., chat, email, remote monitoring)	Jamal is highly skilled in this area.	
Client goals	**Client's priorities and desired targeted outcomes**	Jamal wants to regain needed mobility and self-care skills to be able to attend community college as a student.	
	ANALYSIS OF PARTICIPATION		
	Basic ADLs		
Eating/oral motor	Jamal is independent in this area.		
Grooming	Jamal is independent in this area.		
Bathing/transfer	Jamal is independent in this area. He showers using a shower bench, a handheld shower head, and grab bars.		
Dressing upper body	Jamal is independent in this area.		
Dressing lower body	Jamal has limited mobility in sitting but is able to perform lower-body dressing in supine on his bed. This task takes about 5 minutes, and Jamal becomes frustrated with it and often asks for help. Jamal is able to don his shoes and socks with the use of a reacher.		
Toileting	Jamal has a neurogenic bladder and uses a catheter. He was taught catheter care and management in the rehab hospital and is managing this task well. He also has a bowel management regimen that he is learning, but he still has occasional accidents.		

(Continued)

CASE EXAMPLE 2.5. JAMAL: DOMAIN OF PRACTICE *(Cont.)*

EXHIBIT 2.6.	Jamal's Occupational Profile *(Cont.)*
Problem solving/memory	Jamal has no difficulty in this area.
Comments:	Jamal has demonstrated the needed skills to manage on his own, but the performance of his ADLs is time-consuming, and he becomes frustrated with his slow performance.
	IADLs
Community mobility	Jamal has an ultra-lightweight manual wheelchair that he is able to propel well. He has moderate endurance for this task but is expected to improve with practice.
Health management/prevention	Jamal understands his diet and medication routines and is able to manage them on his own.
Home management	Jamal had many household chores before his accident. He has not been involved in home management since his return from the rehab hospital.
Financial management	Jamal has a bank account and manages his spending money. His mother managed home finances before his injury and continues to do so.
Leisure	Jamal is a serious World of Warcraft player and spends time online interacting with friends in his guild. He has established his game character over the past 2 years and has a broad social network within the game. Jamal was active in his church's teen group before his injury. He still attends church with his mother but no longer participates in the teen group.
Safety	Jamal has no difficulty in this area.
Comments:	Before his injury, Jamal had a group of 4 friends he went out with most weekends. These friends were involved in his accident. His injuries were the most severe of any, and he has limited his contact with them since his return from the hospital. Jamal is not involved in child care or caring for others.
	Motor and Praxis Skills
Sitting (static/dynamic)	Jamal is able to maintain both static and dynamic sitting when placed in a supported seating system.
Standing (static/dynamic)	Jamal is unable to assume standing.
Joint stability and skeletal mobility	Jamal has full AROM in all joints above the level of his lesion. He has full PROM below the level of the lesion.
Place can on shelf	Jamal is limited to a wheelchair for mobility. He is able to grasp, hold, carry, and place the can with either upper limb, but he must use a countertop rather than a shelf.
Retrieve item from floor	When seated in a wheelchair, Jamal can reach items on the floor using a reacher.
Screw lid on jar	Jamal has no difficulty with this task.
Comb back of head	Jamal has no difficulty with this task.
Write name	Jamal has no difficulty with this task.
Lift grocery bag	Jamal's ability to do this task depends on the placement of the bag and whether or not it has handles. He is able to lift 15 lbs. but must lift from a seated position.
Coordination	Jamal has no difficulty with upper-limb coordination.
Manipulation	Jamal is right-handed and has no difficulty with this task.
Comments:	None.
	Process Skills
Energy for task	Jamal tires more easily than a typical 17-year-old, but his performance is within a functional range.

(Continued)

CASE EXAMPLE 2.5. JAMAL: DOMAIN OF PRACTICE *(Cont.)*

EXHIBIT 2.6. Jamal's Occupational Profile *(Cont.)*	
Knowledge/organization of task	Jamal has no difficulty with this task.
Adaptation/praxis	Jamal has no difficulty with this task.
Communication and social skills	Jamal has no difficulty with this task.
Cognitive and emotional regulation skills	Jamal has no difficulty with this task.
Level of arousal/attention	Jamal has no difficulty with this task.
Orientation	Jamal is alert and oriented to person, place, time, and event.
Energy and drive	Jamal is motivated to be more independent at home but is not motivated to go back to the school environment.
Higher level cognition	Jamal has no difficulty with this task.
Comments:	None.
Sensory–Perceptual Skills	
Sensory	Jamal has intact basic sensory function above the level of his lesion.
Self-perception	Jamal does not want his schoolmates to see him in the wheelchair.
Pain	Jamal has no difficulty with this task.
Skin integrity	Jamal's skin is intact.
Comments:	None.

Note. Occupational profile template from American Occupational Therapy Association (2017). Format for analysis of participation adapted from Skubik-Peplaski, Paris, Boyle, & Culpert (2009). ADLs = activities of daily living; AROM = active range of motion; IADLs = instrumental activities of daily living; PROM = passive range of motion; SCI = spinal cord injury; SES = socioeconomic status.

analysis of family routines as a customary part of his or her care. However, the occupational therapy practitioner should keep the larger domain picture in mind to aid in clinical reasoning. In the process of clinical hypothesis development and hypothesis refinement described in the next chapter, all aspects of the domain are drawn into the reasoning process.

REFLECTIVE PRACTICE

Integral to contemporary occupational therapy practice are evaluating and improving care in a constantly changing health care environment. Evaluating care requires occupational therapy practitioners to develop the ability to reflect on their practice in a critical and focused way. *Reflection* is a method of using experiential knowledge to enable professional and personal development while reinforcing continuous learning (Nicol & Dosser, 2016). In the clinical practice context, reflection has 3 components:

1. *Reflection before action:* Involves practitioners thinking about what they aim to achieve and understanding the strategies best suited for success. Reflection before action draws on practitioners' foundational knowledge and knowledge gained through experience in the practice context.

2. *Reflection in action:* Relates to practitioners' actions and reactions in real time as they provide occupational therapy interventions as well as participate in interprofessional communications, program planning, and advocacy activities. This type of reflection supports practitioners as they modify what they are doing while they are doing it, responding to emergent challenges. Reflection in action is thinking on your feet.

3. *Reflection on action:* Refers to the process of review, that is, looking retrospectively at what happened and analyzing information gathered regarding knowledge, new learning, and professional development. This type of reflection can help identify areas that require improvement or a change in approach or attitude.

PRACTICE WISDOM 2.1.   Reflection
"By three methods we may learn wisdom: First, by reflection, which is noblest; second, by imitation, which is easiest; and third by experience, which is the bitterest." —*Confucius (n.d.)*

McKay (2009) described *reflection* as "an essential component for the competent and capable therapist practicing in the 21st century" (p. 56). McKay noted that the ever-changing practice contexts, which are affected by health and social care systems focused on cost-effectiveness, require practitioners to use reflection as a link between theory and practice. For example, practitioners may face pressures to shorten the client's length of stay in the hospital or meet the client's needs in only 6 visits. They must balance the immediate pressures with an understanding of the science supporting a focus on participation rather than a focus on performance skills.

Reflection is essential to learning and to becoming more than a knobologist. Through learning about the clinical reasoning process, practitioners should be able to streamline their path to wisdom in the practice of occupational therapy. Practice Wisdom 2.1 reflects the importance of reflection in learning.

The inclusion of clinical case examples throughout this text is intended to support reader reflection. McKay (2009) supported telling stories as a means of reinforcing reflective practice. As readers read the cases throughout this text, they should let their minds form pictures and complete the scenarios. This exercise will help them think beyond the immediate data to encompass the occupational therapy domain.

SUMMARY

This chapter examined the language of occupation-based reasoning that is provided in the *OTPF–3* (AOTA, 2014). Although the *OTPF–3* is the foundational document used to guide this text and to offer a uniform language to support clinical reasoning, the reader should note that this document is a thoughtful compilation of ideas and terms from many sources. Much of the language defined in this chapter is drawn from WHO (2001, 2002) and global scholarship in occupational therapy and occupational science.

Using a common language, whenever possible, helps occupational therapy practitioners communicate clearly as they collaborate with others. It also helps practitioners present the unique nature of their clinical reasoning and occupation-based services in a manner that is understood by others. Whenever possible, definitions used in this text come from a generalized source such as a dictionary rather than from occupational therapy literature. This approach was thoughtfully applied to aid in supporting the use of common language.

The choice of language directs attention to what is considered significant in any situation. For example, in the learning activity regarding Jamal and adjustment to a new disability, the language you chose and the way you organized and presented facts reflected your reasoning process. The language practitioners use in professional communication informs others of their focus and of possible ways they may respond to the issues they identify. The occupational therapy domain as presented in the *OTPF–3* (AOTA, 2014) was drawn broadly from the best scholarship in the field of occupational therapy. The *OTPF–3* is not a theory or a model. It is a compilation of scholarship that has resulted in a tool that can serve as a foundational paradigm for occupational therapy and that can help practitioners see the whole client rather than just the client's clinical presentation.

Having a common language and a paradigm of thought are essential first steps in clinical reasoning. Note that in the process of identifying intervention priorities for Jamal, you have integrated his case information and developed a clinical hypothesis about what was most essential and valued by Jamal. Not everyone will make the same initial hypothesis or come to the same starting point for testing that hypothesis through assessment and intervention. It is important to be aware that clinical reasoning is a process. Experience and knowledge can make the first hypothesis more accurate much of the time, but all clinicians need to test their hypotheses and adjust them as they collect new data.

LEARNING ACTIVITIES

More than any other chapter in this text, this chapter provides many definitions of key terms to help you use the *OTPF–3* as a clinical reasoning tool. As a learning tool, quiz yourself on the terms listed at the beginning of the chapter because they will be used consistently throughout the remainder of the book.

Consider Jamal's case and the disconnect between his expectations and those of his mother. Jamal is convinced that he can meet his college preparation needs through online classes. As Jamal's occupational therapy practitioner, you must address both his concerns and those of his mother. Note that clinical reasoning often begins before client contact, with the chart review. Follow these steps to structure the clinical reasoning process.

1. As you prepare to assess and treat Jamal, you will need to start with a clinical hypothesis. List at least 1 to begin your reasoning process.
2. As a school-based practitioner, your intervention plan should focus on Jamal's needs to function in a learning environment. Make a table listing at least 3 priority intervention areas, and describe how they might affect Jamal's ability to participate in or benefit from educational instruction.
3. Some of your reasoning will be using a heuristic (mental general rule strategy) regarding interventions appropriate for people with new SCIs. Research the facts, and then describe your heuristic for treating a 17-year-old male postrehab with an L1 SCI, without considering the information about Jamal presented in Case Example 2.5.

4. Make a table of client factors for Jamal's case.

CLIENT FACTOR	JAMAL'S CHARACTERISTICS
Body Functions	
Body Structures	
Values	
Beliefs	
Spirituality	

5. Using the heuristic approach you designed in Question 3, you may meet Jamal's physical needs but will not address his occupational needs. The key to reflecting the full scope of the occupational therapy domain of practice in collaborating with Jamal and his mother will involve a careful consideration of contextual and environmental factors. Make a table of Jamal's contextual and environmental factors.

CONTEXTUAL AND ENVIRONMENTAL FACTOR	JAMAL'S CHARACTERISTICS
Natural environment and human-made changes to the environment:	
Products and technology	
Support and relationships	
Attitudes, services, systems, and policies	
Personal Context	
Temporal Context	
Virtual Context	

6. Use your findings for Questions 1–5 to identify what you think are the 3 priority areas of focus for designing an intervention plan for Jamal.

This learning activity used a typical rehabilitation condition with involved contextual and environmental factors. The domain of occupational therapy presented in the *OTPF-3* (AOTA, 2014) can be used to ensure that in a case like that of Jamal, you look beyond simplistic heuristic answers and build interventions that respect client concerns, values, fears, and dreams for the future.

REFERENCES

American Occupational Therapy Association. (2014). Occupational therapy practice framework: Domain and process (3rd ed.). *American Journal of Occupational Therapy, 68*(Suppl. 1), S1–S48. https://doi.org/10.5014/ajot.2014.682006

American Occupational Therapy Association. (2017). AOTA occupational profile template. *American Journal of Occupational Therapy, 71*(Suppl. 2), 7112420030. https://doi.org/10.5014/ajot.716S12

Cole, M., & Creek, J. (2016). *Global perspectives in professional reasoning.* Thorofare, NJ: Slack.

Confucius. (n.d.). *BrainyQuote.com.* Retrieved from https://www.brainyquote.com/quotes/quotes/c/confucius131984.html

Function. (2016). In *Merriam-Webster online dictionary.* Retrieved from http://www.merriam-webster.com/dictionary/function

Humbert, T. K. (Ed.). (2016). *Spirituality and occupational therapy: A model for practice and research.* Bethesda, MD: AOTA Press.

Maley, C. M., Pagana, N. K., Velenger, C. A., & Humbert, T. K. (2016). Dealing with major life events and transitions: A systematic literature review on and occupational analysis of spirituality. *American Journal of Occupational Therapy, 70*(4), 1–6. https://doi.org/10.5014/ajot.2016.015537

McKay, E. A. (2009). Reflective practice: Doing, being and becoming a reflective practitioner. In E. A. Duncan (Ed.), *Skills for practice in occupational therapy* (pp. 55–72). Edinburgh: Churchill Livingstone.

Nicol, J. S., & Dosser, I. (2016). Understanding reflective practice. *Nursing Standard, 30,* 34–40. https://doi.org/10.7748/ns.30.36.34.s44

Skubik-Peplaski, C., Paris., C., Boyle, D., & Culpert, A. (Eds.). (2009). *Applying the* Occupational Therapy Practice Framework: *Using the Cardinal Hill Occupational Participation Process in client-centered care.* Bethesda, MD: AOTA Press.

TechTarget. (2016). *Internet of things (IoT).* Retrieved from http://internetofthingsagenda.techtarget.com/definition/Internet-of-Things-IoT

World Health Organization. (2001). *International classification of functioning, disability and health.* Geneva: Author.

World Health Organization. (2002). *Towards a common language for functioning, disability and health, International classification of functioning, disability and health.* Geneva: Author.

World Health Organization. (2007). *International classification of functioning, disability and health: Children and youth.* Geneva: Author.

World Health Organization. (2017). *Assistive devices and technologies.* Retrieved from http://www.who.int/disabilities/technology/en/

Hypothesis Generation and Refinement

Anne Cronin, PhD, OTR/L, ATP, FAOTA, and Garth Graebe, MOT, OTR/L

3

CHAPTER HIGHLIGHTS

- Defines *diagnostic hypothesis generation*.
- Describes the use of frames of reference as heuristic shortcuts in clinical reasoning.
- Illustrates use of frames of reference to guide clinical reasoning.
- Identifies strategies to guide hypothesis refinement while considering the occupational therapy domain.
- Examines clinical decision making under conditions of uncertainty and in the presence of anomalous data.
- Describes the role of clinical pathways and functional outcome measures in clinical reasoning.

KEY TERMS AND CONCEPTS

Activity analysis	Compensation approach	Functional outcome measure
Analysis of occupational performance	*Current Procedural Terminology*	Heuristic shortcuts
	Development approach	Maintenance approach
Anomalous data	Diagnostic hypothesis generation	Medical diagnosis
Causal reasoning	Education approach	Peer review
Clinical pathways	Evidence-based practice	Reflection before action
Cognitive rehabilitation frame of reference	Expert	Remediation approach
	Frames of reference	

This chapter discusses hypothesis generation and refinement through Steps 2–5 of the clinical reasoning process:

- *Step 2.* Develop clinical hypotheses to guide collection of cues and information.
- *Step 3.* Use targeted data collection and problem-solving strategies to process information and evaluate the hypothesis.
- *Step 4.* Test and refine the clinical hypotheses.
- *Step 5.* Appraise the evidence.

Readers will gain an understanding of the terminology and process used in hypothesis generation to support clinical reasoning. The chapter focuses on a problem-solving strategy called *diagnostic hypothesis generation* as a clinical reasoning tool. Diagnostic hypothesis generation is a process described by Kassirer, Wong, and Kopelman (2010) as a systematic approach to problem solving that occurs during encounters with patients or clients and may involve all 4 types of problem-solving strategies described in Chapter 1, "Overview of the Clinical Reasoning Process":
1. Algorithm,
2. Heuristic,
3. Trial and error, and
4. Insight.

These problem-solving strategies help to organize this disparate information so that it can be critically considered through an evidence-based practice lens.

OVERVIEW OF DIAGNOSTIC HYPOTHESIS GENERATION

Diagnostic hypothesis generation is a science-driven process of brainstorming that leads to the development of a working clinical hypothesis that is grounded in both clinical cues and scientific data. In Case Example 1.1 in Chapter 1, the use of a medical diagnosis as a tool to begin diagnostic hypothesis generation was illustrated. A **medical diagnosis** is the label provided by the medical doctor to describe the cause of an individual's illness or impairment. Although other health professionals, including occupational therapists, "diagnose" within their domain of practice, the medical diagnosis is a protected label that is generated by licensed physicians derived from the summative process of physical examination, patient interview, laboratory tests, review of the patient's medical records, knowledge of the cause of observed signs and symptoms, and differential elimination of similar possible causes (Medical Diagnosis, 2003).

In the Learning Activities in Chapter 1, readers were guided to consider a clinical hypothesis that was influenced by the medical diagnosis. In Chapter 2, "Clinical Reasoning and Occupational Therapy's Domain of Practice," the case of Jamal was introduced (see Case Example 2.5). Although Jamal had a medical diagnosis, the key to effective intervention and collaboration was likely to come from either insight or trial and error as a problem-solving strategy.

In most cases, when clients begin occupational therapy intervention, they have a medical diagnosis that is included in the referral information. Referral information in clinical settings is often very specific about the medical issues and impairment that have led to the referral. This initial information is useful in beginning the clinical reasoning process, but without additional assessment and reasoning, it will not, by itself, lead to the best occupational therapy assessment and intervention.

For example, Jamal was a healthy young man who had successfully completed rehabilitation after a L1 spinal cord injury. He was referred for occupational therapy to help support him to transition back to school and resume his daily occupations. Jamal's avoidance of social settings and resistance to returning to school could not be explained by his medical diagnosis, so other aspects of clinical reasoning had to come into play.

In the United States and many other countries, the medical diagnosis is of great importance because it influences both the type and frequency of occupational therapy intervention that are funded by health insurance or other health programs. The medical diagnosis is an important context for clinical reasoning, but occupational therapy–specific diagnostic hypothesis generation is an equally important part of the occupational therapy process. Although common use of the word *diagnosis* implies a medical decision, it is important to understand that any diagnosis is a working hypothesis based on clinical reasoning, which clarifies the best treatment path.

Kassirer et al. (2010) described *diagnostic hypothesis generation* as a tool to "frame or constrain a patient's problem and provide a context (or problem space) for further diagnostic reasoning or exploration" (p. 9). As occupational therapy practitioners gain information about clients, they use exploratory problem-solving techniques to compare the client data against common patterns within their own knowledge and experience base. This allows the generation of a mental template of possible clinical findings against which their client's findings can be compared. From this comparision, hypothesis generation begins. Occupational therapy practitioners use the emergent hypotheses to guide the assessment process and begin a process of hypothesis testing that is unique to the client.

This diagnostic hypothesis generation process is an occupational therapy tool that guides the collection and assessment of new data and allows the working hypothesis to be retained, rejected, or refined throughout assessment and service delivery.

INFLUENCE OF CLINICAL EXPERIENCE AND EXPERTISE

Diagnostic hypothesis generation is influenced by clinical experience and by expertise. As occupational therapy practitioners gain experience in and knowledge about a practice area, they become more efficient at clinical reasoning. For example, in their basic education, all practitioners are taught about human development and how it affects performance. However, practitioners who have worked in an early childhood setting for several years have deepened their knowledge of development (and developmental milestones), and, subsequently, it becomes an automatic element of clinical reasoning. In this case, these practitioners might be considered expert practitioners.

An *expert* is "an individual having, involving, or displaying special skill or knowledge derived from training or experience" (Merriam-Webster, 2016). This expert early childhood practitioner has the ability to accurately judge developmental level and atypical aspects of development simply by watching a child play and interact with the parent, without asking the parent questions and without the use of a standardized test. This automaticity in clinical reasoning is not expected of new practitioners; however, they are expected to work toward developing expert clinical reasoning skills through additional study and practice. Another good path toward developing these skills is working with an experienced practitioner as a mentor.

Expert clinical reasoning is specialized. For example, the early childhood expert may not have expert skills in a hand therapy or geriatric setting. An expert occupational therapy practitioner in a hand therapy setting would be likely to follow a different reasoning path when working with Matthew (see Case Example 1.1 in Chapter 1) than an expert practitioner in a vocational rehabilitation setting. In addition, the practitioners who worked with Jamal (see Case Example 2.5 in Chapter 2) in the rehabilitation hospital probably did not encounter the challenges that the school-based practitioner now faces.

In all of the examples given, practitioners skilled in the clinical reasoning process may reach the same final intervention plan, although their paths to getting there may be completely different. This concept is important for the new practitioner to understand. There is often more than a single path to best practice in occupational therapy. In addition, the initial part of the diagnostic hypothesis-generation process often can widely differ depending on the practitioner's background, education, and expertise. Similarly, when using specific frames of reference there are often multiple options that can be appropriate for any given client or situation. Although excellent end results can be achieved by practitioners who start the diagnostic hypothesis generation process from different points, clinical reasoning skills will not be effective if the practitioner does not have adequate knowledge about the client's occupations, disease characteristics, or functional limitations.

GENERATING THE INITIAL DIAGNOSTIC HYPOTHESIS

In all aspects of life, people constantly generate hypotheses about how and why things happen the way that they do. A hypothesis can be simple, such as, "There is nowhere to park this morning because of the road construction." A person might make this hypothesis by observing the road crew and their machines that are located in the area where he or she usually parks. In this hypothesis, the person is responding to the cues he or she has gathered from the environment. A hypothesis occurs at both the beginning of the clinical reasoning process and at the start of research.

This same process is followed in the clinical setting. The occupational therapy practitioner who received the referral for Matthew (Case Example 1.1 in Chapter 1) noted that Matthew came to his appointment in a wheelchair, which led the practitioner to question what role carpal tunnel syndrome (CTS) played in Matthew's ability to get around. This cue alone led the practitioner to hypothesize that Matthew may be experiencing some unique functional challenges; therefore, the practitioner added some questions about Matthew's mobility to the initial interview and to the evaluation (see "Community Mobility" in Exhibit 1.4 in Chapter 1). The use of the wheelchair as a cue to alter the standard protocol reflects the expansion of a clinical algorithm for addressing CTS that clarifies the presenting problem.

The initial hypothesis is an educated guess, and most initial hypotheses need further refinement to reach the best explanation, and therefore the best solution, for a problem. As suggested by Albert Einstein (see Practice Wisdom 3.1), error and reassessment are always a part of

PRACTICE WISDOM 3.1. Further Refinement

If we knew what it was we were doing, it would not be called research, would it? —*Albert Einstein (n.d.)*

the clinical reasoning and research processes. In clinical reasoning, the evaluation process is used to help formulate one or more initial clinical hypotheses. Practitioners then test and refine these hypotheses until they are satisfied that they have reached the right answer for the client or clinical situation.

DEVELOPING CLINICAL HYPOTHESES: USING HEURISTIC SHORTCUTS

Kassirer et al. (2010) described *diagnostic hypothesis generation* as a cognitive process that assimilates data about a client into meaningful chunks, or units, of information that seem logically related. Hypotheses in a clinical encounter are generated rapidly, and some may be in conflict with each other; therefore, the clinician must explore the plausibility of each hypothesis in light of its consistency with existing data. An essential tool in the hypothesis-generating process is **heuristic shortcuts** (i.e., strategies that rely on familiarity with the condition or prior clinical experiences) to help streamline the questioning process.

For example, during an initial interview, an occupational therapy practitioner hears that a young child resists bathing and toothbrushing, is a picky eater, and only will wear long-sleeved shirts, and her immediate thought is, *this sounds like a sensory processing problem*. The mental jump to the label "sensory processing problem" is a heuristic shortcut. It is an informed idea that guides the interview in process so additional data through specialized assessment should be gathered to support or refute this idea.

As another example, consider a practitioner's understanding of common functional limitations associated with a specific medical diagnosis. This provides a heuristic shortcut that can streamline the assessment process. If the findings are consistent with the heuristic, then it is valid to procede with a standard assessment strategy on the basis of medical diagnosis. Some heuristic shortcuts can be learned through studying common features of a particular diagnosis. Most heuristic shortcuts are acquired through actual clinical experience and scientific reasoning. It is the effective generation and testing of heuristic shortcuts that distinguishes the expert practitioner from the novice.

Heuristic shortcuts (and other steps) for diagnostic hypothesis generation are explored using Case Example 3.1. Diagnostic hypothesis generation begins with the referral information, and in the case example, the practitioner is school based and working within an educational practice model. Because Brody was referred to occupational therapy in an early childhood setting, the practitioner does not have an in-depth medical diagnosis with which to begin the hypothesis generation process. However, the practitioner gathers information about Brody

CASE EXAMPLE 3.1. BRODY: EARLY CHILDHOOD CLINICAL REASONING

Brody, age 3 years, is transitioning from home-based early intervention to a preschool program for children with special needs. Brody's parents want him in this program so he can continue to receive therapies and to help him develop the skills he needs to go to school when he turns age 5 years. They are most interested in supporting the development of independent mobility and self-feeding skills. Exhibit 3.1 shows Brody's client factors, performance skills, performance patterns, and his context and environments as essential components of his occupational profile.

Using heuristic shortcuts, the occupational therapy practitioner begins to formulate a plan for Brody. Because of the preschool classroom setting in which Brody is being seen, his impairments involving school

function must be the primary focus. These impairments include difficulties in communication; social participation; gross motor play; and the use of fine motor skills to manipulate toys, and classroom materials and to benefit from the educational program. In addition, in a school setting, goal setting is a collaborative team process that includes family goals and considerations of all teachers and therapists who interact with Brody at school.

As the practitioner thinks more about a plan for Brody, many ideas spring to mind. In fact, there is far too much information to consider all of it right away. However, the use of heuristic shortcuts points the practitioner to Brody's age and the developmental demands in his daily life contexts as initial factors to consider. Because age is a factor in all areas of occupational therapy clinical practice, the practitioner

EXHIBIT 3.1.	**Brody's Occupational Profile**	
Client	**Reason the client is seeking service and concerns related to engagement in occupations**	Brody is transitioning out of home-based early intervention into a special needs preschool program and needs an IEP. *Impact on occupation:* Brody is limited in his ability to develop skills outside of the home environment. He can communicate clearly only with people who know him well. Brody's lack of motor control leads to limitations in play and school contexts.
	Occupations in which the client is successful	Riding tricycle, exploring.
	Personal interests and values	Social and sensory play. He likes rough-housing and riding his tricycle. The family has a strict "no screen time" for children who are below age 5.
	Occupational history (i.e., life experiences)	Brody was born prematurely with a Grade 2 periventricular/intraventricular hemorrhage. He currently presents with spastic diplegia with moderate spasticity in both lower extremities and fluctuating muscle tone (normal to mildly increased) in his upper body and arms. His motor skills are profoundly limited, with strong postural reflex patterns. When on the floor, Brody is independent in position change, but when he is in the stroller, he needs assistance. He has normal intelligence and spastic diplegic CP. He has been seen by occupational therapy, physical therapy, and speech therapy since birth.
	Performance patterns (routines, roles, habits, & rituals)	*Occupational roles:* Son, brother, student, explorer. Body's routines are currently managed by the adults in his life.
Environment		**Supports to occupational engagement** / **Barriers to occupational engagement**
	Physical (e.g., buildings, furniture, pets)	Brody's family has supportive positioning and mobility devices to help him. / His physical limitations limit his mobility, self-care, and play opportunities.
	Social (e.g., spouse, friends, caregivers)	Brody is the youngest in a large family (5 kids), and there are many activities to entertain him. / Brody does not like to be left out or left alone. He manages transitions well as long as they do not involve separating him from the fun.

(Continued)

CASE EXAMPLE 3.1. BRODY: EARLY CHILDHOOD CLINICAL REASONING (Cont.)

EXHIBIT 3.1. Brody's Occupational Profile (Cont.)

Context	Cultural (e.g., customs, beliefs)	His parents have a strict rule of no television or video games for all of the kids except for Saturday mornings.	The family supports competitive athletics, and because Brody cannot participate, he is often left on the sidelines.
	Personal (e.g., age, gender, SES, education)	3-year-old boy.	
	Temporal (e.g., stage of life, time, year)	Toddlerhood.	
	Virtual (e.g., chat, email, remote monitoring)	Not applicable to Brody at this time.	
Client goals	Client's priorities and desired targeted outcomes	Brody's parents are most interested in supporting the development of independent mobility and self-feeding skills.	

ANALYSIS OF PARTICIPATION

Basic ADLs

Eating/oral–motor	Brody is beginning to finger feed, but he does not have a fine grip pattern and often crushes food in his hand.
Grooming	Brody cooperates with hand washing, face washing, hair care, and toothbrushing. He does not perform these activities himself.
Bathing/transfer	Brody cooperates with transfer. His parents sit him in a plastic laundry basket in the bathtub for bathing to help manage his postural control. Brody enjoys bath time and will splash and place his arms underwater when asked to rinse. He is dependent on others in performing this task.
Dressing upper body	Brody cooperates with dressing by pushing his arm through a sleeve. He is dependent on others in performing this task.
Dressing lower body	Brody will independently remove shoes and socks. He cooperates with diapering and lower-body dressing but is dependent on others in performing this task.
Toileting	Brody is able to sit on the toilet with back support and side rails. He is able to indicate a need to toilet but is dependent on others to get him on the toilet, clean him, and remove him from the toilet. He wears diapers at night and most of the time during the day.
Problem solving/memory	Brody has typical problem-solving and memory skills for his age.
Comments:	Toilet training has not been a focus for the family.

IADLs

Community mobility	Brody has a tricycle and a posterior walker for independent mobility. He has a jogging stroller for trips in the community but is unable to get in and out of his stroller without assistance. Brody travels in a regular car seat. He requires adult assistance and supervision in all aspects of community mobility.
Health management/prevention	Brody is age-appropriate in being dependent on adults in this area.
Home management	Brody is age-appropriate in being dependent on adults in this area.
Financial management	Brody is age-appropriate in being dependent on adults in this area.
Leisure	Brody is an active child who enjoys floor play with his family. He enjoys movement toys that he can ride. Brody likes listening to stories and "helping" in the kitchen.

(Continued)

CASE EXAMPLE 3.1. BRODY: EARLY CHILDHOOD CLINICAL REASONING *(Cont.)*

EXHIBIT 3.1.	**Brody's Occupational Profile** *(Cont.)*
Safety	Brody is age-appropriate in being dependent on adults in this area.
Comments:	None.
Motor and Praxis Skills	
Sitting (static/dynamic)	Brody presents with moderate spasticity in both lower extremities and generalized trunk weakness. He is unable to sit without support. When positioned on a solid seat with armrests, he is able to maintain the position for up to 5 minutes. His strong postural reflex patterns interfere with his control in sitting.
Standing (static/dynamic)	Brody is able to stand in a standing frame but does not like to do so because he likes to be active on the floor. He is unable to stand independently.
Joint stability and skeletal mobility	Brody has normal ROM in all joints. He has tightness and limited AROM in his hip, knee, and ankle flexors. He has poor active midrange control in his upper limbs.
Place can on shelf	This test was adapted to have him place a 1-inch cube on a table. He was able to perform the task with his left hand using a circuitous arm movement and a resisted release pattern.
Retrieve item from floor	When seated on the floor, Brody is able to push and swat nearby toys. When seated in a supportive chair, he is able to use a gross palmar grasp to grab and hold items.
Screw lid on jar	Brody is unable to do this.
Comb back of head	Brody is unable to do this.
Write name	Brody is unable to do this.
Lift grocery bag	Brody is unable to do this.
Coordination	Brody uses his arms in a unilateral pattern and is unable to perform bimanual tasks such as buttoning and cutting. He uses his legs reciprocally in the walker, but this action is slow and effortful.
Manipulation	Brody can hold an object in the palm of his hand and has a generalized but functional reach pattern but is not consistently able to release or place objects.
Comments:	Brody scores at a 6-month level on the developmental assessment's physical development subtest. When held upright, he will bear some weight on his legs, and when pulled to sitting, he is able to keep his head in line with his body. He is able to sit with low back support, and on the floor, he is mobile by rolling.
Process Skills	
Energy for task	Brody is age-appropriate in this area.
Knowledge/organization of task	Brody has average intelligence and is able to perform cognitive tasks in the classroom without a problem.
Communication and social skills	Brody communicates with gestures, facial expressions, and some vocalizations. His communication is clear to people he knows well, but he is poorly understood by new people. Brody is able to understand and follow discussions.
Cognitive and emotional regulation skills	Brody is more impulsive than expected for his age and becomes frustrated easily.
Level of arousal/attention	Brody attends well for his age.
Orientation	Brody is age-appropriate in this area.

(Continued)

CASE EXAMPLE 3.1. BRODY: EARLY CHILDHOOD CLINICAL REASONING *(Cont.)*

EXHIBIT 3.1. Brody's Occupational Profile *(Cont.)*	
Energy and drive	Brody is age-appropriate in this area.
Higher level cognition	Brody is age-appropriate in this area.
Comments:	When items requiring physical coordination were removed, Brody scored at the 24-month level for socioemotional skills on the developmental assessment. He understands the concept of sharing, family rules, and routines. He enjoys simple make believe and laughs at incongruous events.
Sensory–Perceptual Skills	
General sensory	Brody has intact basic sensory function.
Hearing and vision	Brody has normal vision and hearing. Brody has difficulty visually tracking a moving object (e.g., a ball being thrown to him).
Self-perception	Brody is age-appropriate in this area.
Pain	Brody is age-appropriate in this area.
Skin integrity	Brody's skin is intact.
Comments:	None

Note. Occupational profile template from American Occupational Therapy Association (2017a). Format for analysis of participation adapted from Skubik-Peplaski, Paris, Boyle, & Culpert (2009). ADLs = activities of daily living; AROM = active range of motion; CP = cerebral palsy; IADLs = instrumental activities of daily living; IEP = individualized education plan; SES = socioeconomic status.

considers Brody's age an important element of the occupational therapy plan. In reasoning through a problem, people tend to use chunks of logically related information, such as age related performance expectations. In this case, because the school function demands are age-related, it is logical for the practitioner to make them a focus of the assessment process.

The practitioner's original emphasis on age and developmental demands in daily life contexts leads the focus to Brody's specific patterns of performance and how these patterns affect his participation at school and home. As age-related developmental demands are contextually influenced, factors such as culture, socioeconomic status, and parent education affect what performance is expected of Brody in his school and home environments.

One of the first diagnostic hypothesis that can be made on the basis of Brody's performance patterns is that many of his difficulties are in motor control. What leads the practitioner in this direction is knowing the typical motor abilities of 3-year-old children and understanding motor impairments that result from spasticity. It may be that in Brody's home environment, modifications have been made so that the impact of his motor impairments are minimized, while at school he is in an environment that has not been customized to his needs. Effective diagnostic hypothesis generation must look across environmental contexts.

from an interview with and assessment of him along with discussions with his parents and teachers and then reviews all of the information.

DEVELOP CLINICAL HYPOTHESES TO GUIDE INFORMATION COLLECTION

After occupational therapy practitioners formulate a working hypothesis (Step 2), they usually must refine it as they further evaluate clients and develop intervention plans. Refining the initial diagnostic hypothesis can include determining an approach to occupational therapy, determining whether the working hypothesis is correct, collecting data, and modifying the hypothesis.

Determining an Approach to Occupational Therapy

Exhibit 3.2 reviews 5 broad approaches to occupational therapy services:
1. Remediation
2. Maintenance
3. Compensation
4. Development
5. Education.

EXHIBIT 3.2.	Broad Approaches to Occupational Therapy Services
APPROACH	**CLINICAL STRATEGY**
Remediation (rehabilitation)	Training in specific tasks based on analysis of valued tasks that have been lost or altered.
Maintenance (prevention of decline)	Task analysis, practice, and compensatory strategies are used to optimize function.
Compensation	Use of alternative strategies or devices when the potential for improvement in tasks is limited or when a highly valued task is above the current level of performance.
Development (habilitation)	Training in specific tasks within a developmental sequence.
Education (promotion of positive health behaviors)	Instruction in relation to safety, independent living, or life quality for the client and family.

Note. Adapted from Robnett & Kaminski (2014).

These approaches are useful for occupational therapy practitioners to consider when developing an evaluation plan. Case Example 3.1 is used in this section to explain the process practitioners use to choose an approach.

Brody's occupational therapy practitioner has determined that his motor impairments are caused by his neurological condition of spastic diplegia, not by a problem with his ability to learn or by a problem with the family's ability to teach the needed skills. In addition, the practitioner thinks about what is known about Brody, that is, he has not lost skills. This understanding leads the practitioner to dismiss the remediation approach, at least for now. The *remediation approach* involves training the client in specific tasks based on analysis of valued tasks that have been lost or altered, usually as a result of acquired injury or disease.

Because Brody is very young and his potential for improvement seems good, the practitioner also dismisses the maintenance approach. The *maintenance approach* assumes that skills are unlikely to increase and that task analysis, practice, and compensatory strategies can be used to optimize function.

The *compensation approach* involves the use of alternative strategies or devices to allow a person to perform a highly valued task that he or she cannot currently perform independently. For example, because Brody's neurological impairment has limited his ability to learn movements typically, he uses a posterior walker to help him walk, which is a highly valued task. Note that compensations, such as the walker, can be a temporary bridge to task performance while a client develops a needed skill or it can be a long-term solution if the client will not be able to acquire a needed skill on his or her own.

The working hypothesis used by Brody's practitioner is that the motor limitations Brody demonstrates in his daily occupations are caused by neurologic impairments. Science suggests that although he is likely to gain motor skill, he will do so more slowly than the typical child, and he may need to develop specialized strategies to accommodate his unique neuromotor difficulties (Morgan et al., 2016).

Therefore, Brody's practitioner determines that he may benefit from external supports (i.e., compensations) in performing desired occupations to help him gain function while his motor skills are slowly developing. In addition, his occupational profile indicates that compensations have been effective with Brody in the past and therefore should continue to be used going forward. Using this information leads the practitioner to implement the compensation approach.

The *development approach,* which focuses on training in specific tasks within a developmental sequence, seems an obvious choice to use with a very young child such as Brody. The practitioner would like to support age-appropriate skill acquisition so that Brody can participate in school and recreational activities with his same-age peers. The development approach requires the practitioner to gather in-depth data about typical motor skills used by 3-year-old children and compare those skills to Brody's current skills. Using the development approach allows the practitioner to further refine the hypothesis.

The *education approach* focuses on instruction to support the safety, health, and life quality for the client and family. The education approach would be useful for Brody's practitioner to use to teach support strategies to his family and teachers but is not likely to be an effective approach for direct intervention with Brody because he does not have consistent muscle control. His performance problems are not related to not knowing what to do or how to do it. Instead, he understands what needs done but has difficulty acting on this knowledge.

After considering the 5 occupational therapy approaches, Brody's practitioner determines that the compensation and development approaches seem to be immediately useful to guide clinical reasoning. Choosing the approaches to be used for Brody puts his practitioner at Step 2 in the clinical reasoning process. The reasoned hypotheses are that

- Brody's motor impairments reflect atypical patterns of motor development that stem from neurological damage and are unlikely to completely resolve, and
- Brody is in the process of maturing and developing skills, and his overall motor skills can be expected to improve.

These hypotheses offer a path from which to begin targeted data collection (Step 3). Remember that the clinical reasoning process is a cycle; therefore, practitioners may find that a hypothesis is inaccurate or incomplete and will need to move back to Step 1 with the new information they have gathered.

Determining Whether the Working Hypothesis Is Correct

Occupational therapy practitioners need to plan a focused strategy to determine whether their working hypothesis is correct to guide a client's intervention. Three possible strategies are

1. Refer to assessments they know about and determine what might be useful,
2. Refer to a resource book describing pertinent tests (e.g., Asher, 2014), or
3. Use a frame of reference.

The first 2 strategies are likely to lead practitioners to test assessments that are based on typically developing children. Therefore, available assessments may not be effective in testing a working hypothesis about children with disabilities. For example, for Brody, these tests would confirm that he has significant delays, which would not be new or helpful information because it is already known. Both of these strategies reflect variations of a trial-and-error problem-solving approach, which can be time consuming and inefficient. Strategy 2, however, could provide information about the scope of assessments in a particular area (e.g., for Brody, for motor assessments), which could lead practitioners to some useful tools to support data collection. Therefore, this strategy offers some promise.

The third strategy, which is the recommended approach, is to use frames of reference to shortcut the clinical reasoning process. *Frames of reference* are a set of assumptions or concepts, often drawn from theory, which can guide the occupational therapy process. Frames of reference are a valuable heuristic tool. For example, by choosing a frame of reference that offers guidance on improving upper-limb function, Brody's practitioner can make assessment decisions and test the working hypothesis. Table 3.1 lists commonly cited frames of reference used by occupational therapy practitioners to treat people with developmental motor impairments.

Brody's occupational therapy practitioner reviews the frames of reference. The practitioner then reflects on the previous hypothesis generation activity for Brody, which included consideration of his age and the belief that his motor impairments reflect atypical patterns of motor development that stem from neurological damage that are unlikely to completely resolve.

In addition, Brody is in the process of maturing and developing skills, and his overall motor skills can be

TABLE 3.1. Frames of Reference for Developmental Motor Impairments	
FRAME OF REFERENCE	**DESCRIPTION**
Biomechanical (Fabrizio & Rafols, 2014)	Focuses on ROM, strength, and endurance at the body function and structure levels. It is not specific to any particular age or developmental level.
CO–OP Approach (Dawson, McEwen, & Polatajko, 2017; Polatajko & Mandich, 2004)	An approach to skills development that includes client-chosen goals, dynamic performance analysis, cognitive strategy use, guided discovery, enabling principles, parent and significant other involvement, and structured intervention. It was developed from work with children but has been applied successfully to interventions with adults.
Developmental systems (Aldridge & Goldman, 2007)	Sometimes called the *skill acquisition frame of reference,* it was built on the work of psychologist Arnold Gesell and asserts that all children go through similar stages and sequences when learning skills. More recently, Gesell's work has been expanded and integrated with modern science to consider biological development, heredity, and evolution (Mandich, 2016). This frame of reference emphasizes the shared contributions of genes, environment, and epigenetic factors on developmental processes.
Motor learning (Sabari, Capasso, & Feld-Glazman, 2014)	Focuses on optimizing motor function through the use of science-driven data on movement and movement pattern acquisition. It was developed from work with adolescents and adults and has a strong science foundation.
NDT (Levit, 2014)	Built on the work of the Bobaths, a physician and a physical therapist working with children with CP. NDT offers insight into the development of atypical movement through comparison with patterns of typical motor performance (Milton & Logothetis, 2013).

Note. CO–OP = Cognitive Orientation to daily Occupational Performance; CP = cerebral palsy; NDT = neurodevelopmental therapy; ROM = range of motion.

expected to improve. Then, using clinical reasoning, the practitioner starts by removing the frames of reference that do not include developmental considerations. This strategy is simply to begin hypothesis testing; the occupational therapy practitioner may reconsider the biomechanical and motor learning frames of reference later in this process. Therefore, the following frames of reference are considered for Brody: the neurodevelopmental (NDT) approach, developmental systems approach, and Cognitive Orientation to daily Occupational Performance (CO–OP).

The NDT frame of reference is developmental and addresses atypical development. It is widely used in occupational therapy, especially in the treatment of people with atypical motor patterns. Because this frame of reference was developed specifically to consider the needs of children with CP, it seems especially relevant for Brody. The developmental systems frame of reference is widely used in early childhood educational settings and includes theories of learning and human development.

Compared with the NDT approach, the developmental systems approach explains delays in development but does not offer much insight into atypical developmental patterns, which are important in Brody's case. The CO–OP has specific applications to children. However, it has been used only to support motor skill acquisition, not to remediate atypical movement patterns.

After examining these 3 choices, Brody's practitioner chooses to focus on the NDT approach for initial hypotheses testing because it seems to be the best fit for Brody and to address goals important to the family. With this in mind, the NDT approach is used to guide assessment and intervention planning. The basic elements of the NDT approach are outlined in Table 3.2 (see Chapter 1 for a discussion of the 4 basic elements of a frame of reference).

Collecting Data

Reflection before action involves thinking about the data that you will need to gather during assessment to provide the foundation for building hypotheses to achieve functional outcomes. The hypotheses generated from the initial data reviewed by the occupational therapy practitioner provide questions that guide evaluation and additional data collection. Data should be collected on a goal that can be objectively measured, involves a daily life task, is valued by the client, and is consistent with the occupational therapy domain described in Chapter 2, "Clinical Reasoning and Occupational Therapy's Domain of Practice."

This type of assessment is called a *functional outcome measure.* This targeted data collection is the start of Step 3 in the clinical reasoning process. Although data collected will vary according to the client and his or her goals, occupational therapy practitioners should

TABLE 3.2.	Basic Elements of NDT Frame of Reference
ELEMENT	**DESCRIPTION**
Focus	The NDT approach, developed from work with children with CP, offers insight into the development of atypical movement through comparison with typical motor performance patterns.
Basic assumptions	The NDT approach assumes that • The brain is plastic and can be retrained to connect with a nonresponding or atypically responding muscle; • Through experience with normal movement patterns and input from vestibular, tactile, and somatosensory systems, the client can produce increasingly normal movement patterns; • Problems resulting from tone, balance, movement, and posture are also responsible for atypical movement synergies; and • Highly trained NDT therapists can assist in clients' functional movement by influencing the CNS through guided motor output and handling.
Function–disability continuum	The central concern of this frame of reference are clients with a neurological pathophysiology who present with the inability to control movement, decreased postural control, problems in tone and balance, and abnormal movement patterns. Because of the lack of control over their own movements, these clients have decreased participation in activities and life (i.e., dysfunction). Function is effective control of desired movements.
Postulates of change	Because of neuroplasticity, normal movement is possible in people with atypical movement patterns through the facilitation of normal movement patterns. Atypical movements cannot be overridden but are inhibited as much as possible during interventions. Treatment interventions are focused on repeating normal movement patterns to ensure motor performance, with therapist support to inhibit or limit abnormal movement influences. It is believed that the sensory experience of normal movement supports adaptive learning of movements in the future.

Note. CNS = central nervous system; CP = cerebral palsy; NDT = neurodevelopmental.

measure not only clients' general performance during therapy sessions but also their functional performance in valued occupations.

For example, for Brody, data collection using the NDT frame of reference involves careful qualitative analysis of upper-limb movements during therapy sessions. In addition, Brody's practitioner measures changes in the functional skill of self-feeding during routine meals and snacks because Brody's parents specifically identified self-feeding as a priority for them.

The data collected in this stage give objective information before moving to Step 4 of the clinical reasoning process, during which the clinical hypothesis is tested and further refined. If there is a clear gain in functional performance after the chosen intervention, it would be a reasonable assumption that the intervention is helping to resolve the problem. In this case, both the intervention and the data collection should continue.

If the data do not show clear improvement, the practitioner needs to reevaluate the hypothesis, the frame of reference, or both. It could be that the hypothesis is sound, but the choice of intervention is not correct for the situation. For example, the hypothesis for Brody appears to be correct. However, the intervention based on the NDT frame of reference did not result in improvement in Brody's performance, functional or otherwise.

Note that the NDT, although widely used, is an older frame of reference and does not have strong support in the scientific literature. It is human nature to stick to ideas and routines that have already been learned, as Brody's practitioner did, but sometimes new science challenges these ideas. Responsible occupational therapy practitioners have to be thoughtfully skeptical and motivated to keep up with current science. The NDT approach continues to be influential in clinical reasoning, but expert NDT practitioners now incorporate current motor control science into their clinical reasoning and intervention strategies. Therefore, although the NDT frame of reference seems a good fit for Brody, his practitioner should incorporate current evidence and not rely exclusively on this outdated approach.

Modifying the Hypothesis: Test and Refine

Diagnostic hypothesis generation is a dynamic process. As practitioners identify patterns in the data, they form hypotheses related to the patterns. Hypotheses must be tested systematically to ascertain their value (Step 4). Testing can occur through targeted assessment, but it also can be through a careful measure of client outcomes during the intervention process. For example, upon reflection about Brody's medical diagnosis (spastic diplegia with moderate spasticity in both lower extremities and fluctuating muscle tone [normal to mildly increased] in upper body and arms), Brody's practitioner completes targeted testing of muscle function and decides to

modify the original hypothesis because his arm function should be less impaired than it is, based on the original hypothesis.

The practitioner believes it is possible that Brody's upper-limb motor impairments may be aggravated by external contexts. As the youngest of 5 children, he usually has siblings around to do things for him and to bring him things he wants. This situation, in combination with his very limited independent mobility skills, may have led him to have fewer opportunities to develop upper-limb skills. Therefore, the practitioner develops a modified hypothesis that Brody's upper-limb motor limitations are caused by lack of access to movement and play opportunities and other external supports to facilitate the development of hand skills. Assessment data that are targeted to upper-limb function and hand use patterns will allow the practitioner to test this new working hypothesis.

Because Brody's practitioner has already dismissed the exclusive use of the NDT approach, another developmental approach is chosen for exploration, the developmental systems frame of reference. This approach is not incompatible with the NDT approach, but it focuses broadly on all aspects of development and their interrelationships. The practitioner repeats Steps 2–4 of the clinical reasoning process, refining both the clinical hypothesis and the intervention as she gains information. As before, the practitioner must be able to document progress on functional goals in the natural environment to meet client goals. If progress is not made in this area, then the hypothesis was incomplete or incorrect and additional problem solving is needed.

Note that that frames of reference are often used together as long as their assumptions are compatible. For example, the NDT frame of reference offered specific strategies to improve Brody's motor function. However, because Brody's practitioner did not see improved function in his desired performance area (i.e., self-feeding), she switched to the developmental systems frame of reference. This approach includes family characteristics and family stressors (Guralnick, 2001).

Therefore, using the developmental systems approach, Brody's practitioner worked with Brody's family to alter the home environment so that Brody was rewarded for independent upper-limb use, especially independent feeding. The practitioner continued to use the NDT approach to guide aspects of the intervention process, but the broader developmental systems approach carried Brody's skill development into functional performance domains.

EVIDENCE-BASED PRACTICE

Occupational therapy practitioners "integrating individual clinical expertise with the best available external clinical evidence from systematic research" (Law & McDermid, 2014, p. 3) is the ideal. *Evidence-based practice (EBP)* is the conscientious use of current best evidence to make decisions about client care and to expand the clinician's expertise through critical evaluation of the growing body of research available (Step 5).

In Brody's case, using EBP means critcally looking at intervention outcomes with the NDT approach and altering the central frame of reference guiding intervention decisions to one that results in positive, measureable functional outcomes. The use of the NDT approach alone could be supported if observable functional outcome goals were achieved with it. When progress is absent or very slow, other interventions or methods or options should come into play.

Occupational therapy practitioners have an ethical and professional obligation to make every effort to select interventions based on scientific principles that reflect the best knowledge in the field and that respect the client goals. To do so, practitioners must
- Read and understand scientific literature and
- Weigh scientific evidence against both historical treatments (e.g., the NDT approach) and anecdotal reports of others.

In practice, actual clinical cases rarely match the clinical controls used in scientific research, and there are many outside influences on the clinical reasoning process. Most clinical decisions contain an element of uncertainty, and practitioners may have one or more false starts as they assess the efficacy of selected interventions. (The section "Using Evidence: Evaluating Information Sources" later in this chapter provides more information on how to evaluate information.)

EBP is one of the essential tools for becoming an expert practitioner, but one of its challenges is that the body of evidence is continually growing and changing. Therefore, practitioners must include a current review of research evidence, personal experience, policy influences, contextual influences, and information from the client and family in the clinical reasoning process. EBP integrates this information and considers it within the unique circumstances presented by the client.

Although EBP is described as an ideal, it is only one component of the clinical reasoning process. No single source of evidence will give practitioners a single, clear path to resolve all problems for complete occupational participation. Research evidence, like all evidence gathered during the client assessment, needs to considered critically.

Clinical Pathways

In clinical settings, where clients often have similar medical conditions (e.g., stroke, spinal cord injuries), the rehabilitation team develops rules of procedure based on clients' diagnostic presentation. These rules have many labels—*clinical pathways, care pathways, critical pathways,* and *care maps*—but clinical pathways is used here. **Clinical pathways** are one of the main tools used to manage health care quality through the standardization of care processes by disease or disability using a decision tree. Clinical pathways reflect a review of the scientific evidence and best practices and the resulting decision tree reflects the available evidence.

Clinical pathways promote organized and efficient management of client care services, but they do not consider the client as an individual with unique needs and challenges and often do not consider aspects of uncertainty that can affect the client (e.g., depression, financial stress). Clinical pathways can be useful and supportive tools to guide the occupational therapy practitioner, but they do not replace the clinical reasoning process in occupational therapy practice.

Anomalous Data

When refining clinical hypotheses, occupational therapy practitioners must focus on the client and the his or her needs and note any client performance pattern that is anomalous. **Anomalous data** (or anomalous client performance) is information (or performance) that does not fit into the expected pattern.

Philosopher Thomas Kuhn (1962) explained the importance of anomalies in science, arguing that persistent anomalies play a key role in scientific revolutions. Since his seminal work on the history of science, many others have documented the importance of anomalous data in theory change among scientists.

Science educators Chinn and Brewer (1998) were interested in how to enhance science teaching through the exploration of anomalous data and identified 7 reactions to anomalous data in the students they studied. These reactions may also be seen in occupational therapy practitioners as they find confusing or conflicting information while searching for clinical evidence. Chinn and Brewer's reactions are
1. Ignore or exclude the data,
2. Reject the data,
3. Reinterpret the data,
4. Reconstruct the data,
5. Hold the data in abeyance (i.e., set it aside from immediate consideration),
6. Accept the data and make peripheral theory changes, and
7. Adopt the data and change theories (p. 627).

Table 3.3 displays the 7 postulated reactions to anomalous data and 3 types of responses to these reactions described in Chinn and Brewer's (1998) work.

It is natural for practitioners to gravitate toward information that is consistent with their current beliefs and values. It is also good for them to be skeptical of every "shiny new thing" that is introduced as a tool for clinical practice. This sketicism needs to be balanced with critical thinking and openness to innovation. The NDT frame of reference introduced in this chapter has been scientifically challenged, yet it is still used by

TABLE 3.3.	Responses to Anomalous Data		
REACTION	ARE DATA ACCEPTED AS VALID?	IS ANOTHER EXPLANATION ACCEPTED?	DO THE DATA CHANGE CURRENT THEORY?
Ignore or exclude	No	No	No
Reject	No	Yes	No
Reinterpret	Yes	Yes	No
Reconstruct	Yes	Yes	Partially
Hold in abeyance	Yes	Yes	Not at present
Accept	Yes	Yes	Partially
Adopt	Yes	No	Completely

occupational therapy practitioners. Few practitioners ignore or reject the new science of motor control, so what is seen clinically is both reinterpretation of the original constructs of the NDT frame of reference and peripheral changes to it to assimilate the new science of motor control.

One of the weaknesses of exclusive use of clinical pathways in occupational therapy practice is that lack of focus on individual client goals and the potential for inattention to anomalous data. As you gain skill in the hypothesis generation and hypothesis testing aspects of clinical reasoning, consideration of anomalous data will be important and help strengthen your abilities to become responsible evidence-based practitioners.

EVALUATION

The hypothesis generation process is supported through evaluation. Evaluation has been touched upon in earlier chapters with discussion of the occupational profile and the analysis of occupational performance. Occupational therapy evaluations result in the development of a plan of care, which reflects the practitioners' clinical reasoning and interpretation of the data.

The hypothesis generation process is heavily influenced by organizational and legislative directives. For example, practitioners must document evaluations in a manner that complies with pertinent regulations to ensure payment for services.

Although the guidance in documenting the occupational therapy process varies by setting and region, most practitioners in health care settings must use **Current Procedural Terminology (CPT)** in their documentation. *CPT* is a medical code set that is used by occupational therapy practitioners to report evaluation and intervention services to entities such as physicians, health insurance companies, and accreditation organizations (American Medical Association, 2017).

CPT guidance for reporting occupational therapy evaluation requires that each evaluation component for a code be documented (American Occupational Therapy Association [AOTA], 2017b). Using this information, the occupational therapy practitioner is then directed to report the level of occupational therapy evaluation (i.e., low, moderate, or high complexity or re-evaluation).

Having to determine the *CPT* evaluation level is a new requirement for occupational therapy practitioners, having gone into effect on January 1, 2017. Determining this level for each client requires practitioners to use clinical reasoning and expertise as well as client condition, complexity of clinical decision making, and clinical hypothesis generation based on the scope and nature of the client's performance deficits. In addition, the client's plan of treatment should reflect assessment of each of his or her identified performance deficits.

HYPOTHESIS REFINEMENT

This section explores the hypothesis refinement process in-depth, when heuristic shortcuts are inadequate. Consider the case of Surya in Case Example 3.2.

Hypothesis Generation

Hypothesis generation begins by reviewing Surya's referral information. Considering foundational information on traumatic brain injury (TBI), we know that distractibility, poor behavioral self-regulation, poor organization, and memory deficits are common sequelae of TBI experienced by people in the survivorship phase of recovery. Powell (2014) reports that the survivorship stage symptoms of mild TBI include "headache, dizziness, nausea, irritability, fatigue, and cognitive deficits such as impaired concentration, information processing speed, and memory" (p. 1064). Adults with mild TBI often return to normal functioning within 1–3 months (Powell, 2014).

Understanding of TBI survivorship offers a heuristic from which to generate these clinical hypotheses:
- Surya is early in the recovery process, and her need for support will be temporary.
- Surya may benefit from best practice strategies of occupational therapists intervening with persons with mild TBI, including establishing supportive routines, teaching the use of memory backups, and offering

CASE EXAMPLE 3.2. SURYA: TEEN WITH TBI

Surya, age 14 years, sustained a mild TBI 2 months ago following a cheerleading accident. She has been cleared for return to school but continues to have some residual deficits. Her teachers report extreme distractibility, poor behavioral self-regulation in the classroom, and difficulty with memory and organization of school work (see Exhibit 3.3).

EXHIBIT 3.3.	Surya's Occupational Profile		
Client	**Reason the client is seeking service and concerns related to engagement in occupations**	Referred to occupational therapy for assessment for a qualifying IEP meeting. Concerns reported by her teachers include extreme distractibility, poor behavioral self-regulation in the classroom, and difficulty with memory and organization of school work. *Impact on occupation:* Surya is in an 8th grade general education classroom. She is passive in the classroom and often tearful. She is frustrated because she has found that her ability to learn is changed (from her pre-injury abilities) and she is failing classes that were once easy for her. At home she is irritable and lashes out at her family in anger or hostility. Her grades at school have become steadily worse since returning to school.	
	Occupations in which the client is successful	Surya manages her basic ADLs and is beginning to regain some IADL skills	
	Personal interests and values	Surya wants to perform on the school cheerleading squad. Surya enjoys singing both in the school choir and with a community choral group as well as hanging out with friends. Surya loves animals and is interested in becoming a veterinarian.	
	Occupational history (i.e., life experiences)	Before her accident Surya helped around the family home, including supervising her younger brother, and was on the school cheerleading squad. She is responsible for taking care of the 2 family dogs. Surya is recently returned to school 2 months after a mild TBI. Although she was outgoing before her accident, currently she is quiet and shy. Although the physician reported that her recovery was complete and she was ready to return to school, the school is concerned and has asked for testing to consider special education supports for Surya.	
	Performance patterns (routines, roles, habits, & rituals)	Surya's valued roles include daughter, student, friend, sister, vocalist with a community choir, and pet owner.	
Environment		***Supports to occupational engagement***	***Barriers to occupational engagement***
	Physical (e.g., buildings, furniture, pets)	Surya has no difficulties with physical accessibility	
	Social (e.g., spouse, friends, caregivers)	Prior to her injury, Surya was a good student and had a small group of friends with whom she socialized at school and through social media.	

(Continued)

CASE EXAMPLE 3.2. SURYA: TEEN WITH TBI *(Cont.)*

EXHIBIT 3.3. Surya's Occupational Profile *(Cont.)*

Context	Cultural (e.g., customs, beliefs)	Surya's parent are both professionals who have immigrated to the United States from India.	Surya's parents expect academic excellence and have been distressed by her recent difficulties.
	Personal (e.g., age, gender, SES, education)	Age 14 years. Female. From an upper-income family.	
	Temporal (e.g., stage of life, time, year)	Adolescence.	
	Virtual (e.g., chat, email, remote monitoring)	Surya is able to access chat, email, and social media.	
Client goals	Client's priorities and desired targeted outcomes	Surya wants to get back to the lifestyle she experienced prior to her injury. She says that she doesn't want to be seen as a "freak" or to have her friends pity her. Her parents also want her to feel good about herself and to return to school. They expect her to perform well in her classwork. Surya's teachers want her to be more independent, and to learn to organize and sort things out on her own at school.	

Note. Occupational profile template from American Occupational Therapy Association (2017a). ADLs = activities of daily living; IADLs = instrumental activities of daily living; IEP = individualized education program; SES = socioeconomic status; TBI = traumatic brain injury.

school-specific stagies to help Surya plan, sequence, and persist with assigned classroom tasks.

These clinical hypotheses reflect foundational knowledge of TBI rehabilitation. The next step in clinical reasoning is to explore these initial hypotheses through targeted evaluation.

Evaluation

Evaluation "occurs during the initial and all subsequent interactions with a client" (AOTA, 2014, p. S13). The evaluation process consists of 2 components:

1. Occupational profile and
2. Analysis of occupational performance.

The ***analysis of occupational performance*** determines a client's ability to carry out desired daily occupations. This analysis identifies performance skills and patterns, activity demands, barriers, and contextual factors to guide selection of more specific performance assessment tools.

Through the occupational profile and analysis of occupational performance, we are looking for support that Surya's clinical presentation is consistent with the established clinical picture of mild TBI. For entry-level practitioners, the collection of an occupational profile as described in the *Occupational Therapy Practice Framework* (3rd ed.; *OTPF–3*; AOTA, 2014, 2017a) will provide the data needed to move the clinical reasoning process

forward. Here we will be decribing the process from the point of view of an entry-level practitioner.

The practitioner begins the evaluation process with a chart review which includes medical diagnostic information and current academic performance. Next, she interviews Surya about what she feels are her problems in school and her overall satisfaction with her performance and participation across activity settings. At this point the process of diagnostic hypothesis generation is well underway.

To test and refine the clinical hypothesis, the practitioner observes Surya's performance in the school setting. The primary assessment tool in this case will be observation of Surya performing tasks while the practitioner uses activity analysis to gain an understanding of her strengths and weaknesses. The *OTPF–3* describes ***activity analysis*** as examining

the demands of an activity or occupation to understand the specific body structures, body functions, performance skills, and performance patterns that are required and to determine the generic demands the activity or occupation makes on the client. (AOTA, 2014, p. S12)

Activity analysis is direct observation of the person performing a defined task. That task can be specifically chosen by the practitioner to challenge areas in which deficits are expected (on the basis of heuristic reasoning), or the task can be one that is valued by the client and reported to be problematic.

From the combined data gathered from the interview and activity analysis, the practitioner considers whether Surya's performance is consistent with expectations on the basis of the heuristic derived from the typical course of mild TBI. If the presentation is typical, the initial hypothesis seems to have been confirmed, and we could proceed with considering conceptual frameworks for organizing practice and then build support strategies that will help Surya for the next few month as her symptoms diminish and she regains her prior level of performance.

However, Surya's occupational profile reflects a greater scope of problems than typically expected based on our hypotheses from the foundational information on mild TBI. Her difficulties with behavioral self-regulation and impulse control are more marked than that commonly associated with mild TBI in adolescence. We must reflect on explanations for the full scope of presenting problems. Limiting ourselves to foundational knowledge, we could suggest that poor self-regulation and impulse control difficulties may be pre-existing problems that need not be included in this evaluation, but this approach will not help Surya benefit from intervention and is a clinical reasoning error. *When problems are not fully and consistently explained by the hypotheses, additional hypothesis refinement is needed.* New data are needed, and they require new interpretation, in light of existing information. This is the process of *hypothesis refinement.*

Hypothesis Evolution: Causal Reasoning

In Surya's evaluation, the occupational therapy practitioner finds all of the expected sequelae of mild TBI but at a greater level of impairment than expected; especially problematic are her poor judgment and impulse control, poor frustration tolerance, and performance anxiety. Surya's difficulties do not appear to be resolving but appear to be worsening. The initial hypotheses warrant support at school, but they would not support the ongoing need for special education supports and occupational therapy for Surya. Her difficulty and distress related to school are not fully addressed through the current hypotheses, and without further exploration into her performance, it is possible that Surya's difficulties will continue unaddressed until later when her progress in school is more profoundly affected.

An evolved hypothesis needs to be developed that addresses all of Surya's presenting strengths and weaknesses. Consider the second hypothesis: Surya may benefit from best practices strategies of occupational therapists intervening with persons with mild TBI, such as establishing supportive routines, teaching the use of memory backups; and offering school-specific stategies to help Surya plan, sequence, and persist with assigned classroom tasks. This hypothesis has some foundational use but does not fully address Surya's presenting level of performance deficits.

A good approach to refining a clinical hypothesis is the use of *causal reasoning,* which is an approach to problem solving that uses inductive reasoning using a process of elimination to evaluate potential hypotheses. Occupational therapy practitioners try to establish what is causing a certain limitation or performance pattern. If the correct cause is identified, then the presenting problem can be alleviated by isolating and treating the cause. In this approach, practitioners try to find the conditions under which a certain effect occurs and then isolate the causes that underpin and occur in every case. Causal reasoning shows that a certain cause or causes must be present for the effect to occur.

For example, Surya's difficulties with judgment, impulse control, poor frustration tolerance, and performance anxiety are very pronounced in the school environment but far less so in the home environment. Using causal reasoning, the occupational therapy practitioner should assess the context and environment within which Surya functions at school. It may be that school-specific factors are causing some of her impaired performance patterns.

Analysis of Occupational Performance

As previously described, analysis of occupational performance includes collecting and interpreting information to refine the clinical hypotheses and to specifically identify supports and barriers related to occupational performance. The end result of the analysis of occupational performance is to identify targeted outcomes for intervention. During the analysis of occupational performance, clinical data do not need to be accumulated in a fixed pattern, but it is typical to start with the client's history and follow up with information from an interview, physical examination, activity analysis, formal testing, and clinical observation. Using information from Surya's occupational profile, we can focus on her specific occupations and contexts that need to be addressed.

Data are gathered through several methods, including

- Observing Surya's performance during activities relevant to desired occupations, and
- Selecting and using specific assessments to measure performance skills and performance patterns, performance contexts, and activity demands that influence performance skills and performance patterns.

The choice of evaluation strategies is an essential part of the clinical reasoning process and and is influenced by frames of reference. The measurement and documentation of occupational performance skills involves a unique mix of tools, including tests, interviews, and observations for each case.

With information from multiple data-gathering methods, Exhibit 3.4 presents the compiled information the practitioner has gathered about Surya through assessment.

EXHIBIT 3.4.	Analysis of Surya's Occupational Performance

Basic ADLs	
Eating/oral–motor	Surya has no difficulty in this area.
Grooming	Although Surya has the ability to do basic tooth brushing, hair care, and personal hygiene, she has lost interest in her appearance and does not try and look her best.
Bathing/transfer	Surya has no difficulty in this area.
Dressing upper body	Surya has no difficulty in this area.
Dressing lower body	Surya has no difficulty in this area.
Toileting	Surya has no difficulty in this area.
Problem solving and memory	Surya understands the steps of the tasks that need to done when questioned but does not consistently initiate the tasks. She is distractible and loses her place in a multistep task or forgets what she was asked to do by the teacher. Surya has been unable to complete assignments at school when working independently.
Comments:	Surya has adequate large and small motor skills for all school tasks. She has some generalized weakness and in difficulties in coordination after her injury and has not regained her pre-injury motor skill level. Her current level of motor skill is adequate for the demands of her basic ADLs.
IADLs	
Community mobility	Surya can walk and run adequately for basic community mobility. Her movements are awkward, and she has difficulty with managing uneven or moving surfaces (e.g., escalator).
Health management and prevention	Surya has a home exercise program developed by the physical therapist at the rehabilitation center to help her regain strength and endurance. Surya understands this program but seldom initiates it. When prompted and supervised Surya will do the exercises but puts little effort in them. Surya has been excused from PE since returning to school.
Home management	Surya is pleasant and follows instructions to do chores and homework. Although generally compliant, she does not initiate or manage familiar routines without prompting. Surya assists appropriately in cooking, laundry, and household chores.
Financial management	Because of her age, this has not been identified as an area of concern.
Leisure	Previously Surya was a good student and active in after-school activities. She has not returned to her previous leisure activities of hanging out with her friends and singing in the choir. She currently spends most of her leisure time watching Netflix and surfing the web.
Safety	Surya has a good understanding of safety rules and procedures, but she is sometimes impulsive. She has forgotten to turn off appliances (e.g., iron, stove) since coming home from the hospital.
Comments:	Surya has returned to the care of the family pets and is doing well. She has not returned to pet-sitting or cheerleading.
Motor and Praxis Skills	
Sitting: static/dynamic	Surya can maintain static sitting on a regular chair or stool. She has good dynamic sitting.
Standing: static/dynamic	Surya can independently assume standing and maintain her balance in routine situations. Surya has demonstrated slowed equilibrium responses and mild dyspraxia when her balance is challenged.
Joint stability and skeletal mobility	Surya has full functional ROM and adequate joint stability at all joints.
Place can on shelf	Surya can complete this task starting from a sitting position, coming to stand, and placing the can.
Retrieve item from floor	Surya can complete this task from both sitting and standing positions.
Screw lid on jar	Surya can complete this task in both sitting and standing positions.
Comb back of head	Surya can do this, and uses her fingers to detect tangles. Surya can pull her hair into a neat ponytail.

(Continued)

EXHIBIT 3.4. **Analysis of Surya's Occupational Performance** *(Cont.)*

Writing	Surya can write her name with a pen and using a standard keyboard. She writes legibly, but her writing is very slow. When tested she was writing an average of 15 wpm. She is unable to write fast enough to take notes in class. Surya can operate the computer, using both the keyboard and the mouse. She types using the "hunt and peck" 2-pointer finger method and can type about 12 wpm.
Lift grocery bag	Surya is able to do this.
Coordination	Poor. Surya is able to move limbs independently and engage in simple tasks. She has difficulty with activities that require dynamic balance (e.g., running while kicking a ball). Her movements are slowed and she seems to need to closely attend to her actions. When she is distracted, she is very clumsy and poorly coordinated.
Manipulation	Surya consistently prefers her right hand for skilled activity. She has adequate grip strength for routine activities. She has difficulty with fine hand coordination in writing, keyboarding, and craft activities.
Comments:	Surya has normal postural tone. Her gross motor skill milestones are developmentally appropriate. She has a pattern of dyspraxia, which shows in slowed, uncertain movements. She can complete all tasks, but she does so with periods of motor incoordination, especially when she is multitasking.
	Process Skills
Energy for task	Surya is withdrawn and disinterested. She is physically able to do most tasks but often seems detached and does not exert herself more than she has to.
Knowledge/organization of task	Surya can function within familiar environments but needs assistance to organize even familiar multistep tasks. She often needs a 1:1 prompt to initiate tasks. She will work on tasks appropriately once started but stops again rather than asking for help or problem solving on her own.
Adaptation/praxis	Surya understands the demands of a task but seems unable to reliably sequence the steps or adjust her strategies when needed.
Comments:	None.
	Behavioral and Cognitive Skills
Communication and following social conventions	Surya's receptive and expressive language is WNL. She has difficulty with speed and organization in written communication.
Cognitive and emotional regulation skills	Surya is easily frustrated and responds with tears and angry outbursts when frustrated. She is impulsive in her work, often making errors and then giving up in frustration.
Level of arousal/attention	Surya is easily distracted, even in 1:1 settings.
Orientation	Surya is alert and oriented to person, place, time, and event.
Energy and drive	Surya is motivated to get back to "being herself" but is easily frustrated with poor task persistence.
Memory and understanding	Surya is able to understand and follow a series of 2 or more related instructions but does not anticipate problems and does not problem solve solutions when familiar strategies do not work. She has difficulty with short-term memory and has trouble keeping up with her school assignments and school materials.
Higher level cognition	Surya has difficulty with many EF skills, including keeping track of time, making plans, making sure work is finished on time, and looking for help or more information when it is needed.
	Sensory–Perceptual Skills
Sensory	Surya has intact basic sensory function, but she is near-sighted and wears contact lenses.
Self-perception	Surya has basic of awareness of body position in space and spatial relationships.
Pain	Surya does not report any pain.
Skin integrity	Surya's skin is intact.
Comments:	Surya has adequate visual–perceptual skills for the academic demands of school.

Note. Format adapted from Skubik-Peplaski, Paris, Boyle, & Culpert (2009). ADLs = activities of daily living; EF = executive functioning; IADLs = instrumental activities of daily living; PE = physical education; ROM = range of motion; WNL = within normal limits; wpm = words per minute.

Interpreting Assessment Data to Identify Performance Supports and Hindrances

Throughout the assessment process, practitioners must judge how to best support clients while meeting the needs of the context from which the referral emerged and in which clients need to perform. Surya's case occurs in a school setting for service provision, so the practitioner must focus on performance in the school environment and Surya's ability to access and learn. Failure to focus on performance in the school context is a point at which a clinical reasoning error could occur. Goals that would be supported in a medical environment may not be valid in an educational environment.

After reviewing the data from our evaluation, a systematic and science-driven way is warranted. Our foundational information on mild TBI is drawn from a highly respected source, but it describes TBI as it is experienced in adults, not in adolescents. The source also reflects a medical view of the impairments rather than an educational view of them. The following reflections exemplify using insight to refine the hypothesis:

- Surya's recovery might be influenced by her age.
- Is information on adult TBI valid in a young teen?

The assessment process must examine age-appropriate performance expectations. Failure to do this is another possible clinical reasoning error.

Let's now sort through the data to understand Surya's performance more completely so we can specify possible supports for and hindrances to her performance. By identifying Surya's strengths and weaknesses, we can organize the evaluation. Exhibits 3.5–3.7 take readers through this

process using the categories presented earlier in the analysis of occupational performance (Exhibit 3.4).

To interpret evaluation results in the analysis of occupational performance we need to look at both specific findings and patterns that are consistent across categories of those findings. Surya has the ability to independently perform all activities of daily living (ADLs) and instrumental activities of daily living (IADLs) tasks but does not consistently initiate these. She is easily distracted and does not always persist until a task is completed, and seems to have lost her motivation to perform grooming tasks. This analysis helps us understand Surya, but none of the weaknesses in ADLs or IADLs described here would specifically limit her school participation.

Surya has the basic motor and praxis skills to function in the school environment (Exhibit 3.5). Her slowed performance speed, especially in producing written work, will have challenges, but these can be addressed with assistive technology supports. Reviewing these first 2 aspects of her daily occupations, there are deficit areas, but they are mild deficits that can be accommodated until Surya's recovery progresses.

Prior to reviewing this final strengths and weaknesses table (Exhibit 3.6), the original plan, based on the foundational knowledge clinical hypothesis, seems appropriate. Surya has many strengths, and the limitations evident in this part of the review are easily addressed using assistive technology and classroom supports, but a more complex set of problems becomes evident in the behavioral and cognitive skills presented in Exhibit 3.7. Many of the problems (i.e., "weaknesses") suggest that Surya has social–emotional performance patterns that are not typical

EXHIBIT 3.5. Surya's Strengths and Weaknesses in ADLs and IADLs	
STRENGTHS	**WEAKNESSES**
Basic ADLs	
- Independent in eating/oral–motor. - Independent in grooming, bathing, dressing, and toileting. - Remembers how to do tasks and understands the steps of the tasks that need done when questioned.	- Has lost interest in her appearance and does not try and look her best. - Does not consistently initiate tasks. - Has impairments in short-term memory and will lose her place in a multistep task or forget what she was asked to do by the teacher.
IADLs	
- Can walk and run adequately for basic community mobility. - Has a home exercise program developed by the physical therapist at the rehabilitation center and understands this program. - Is pleasant and follows instructions to do chores and homework. - Has a history of consistent and varied leisure participation. - Has a good understanding of safety rules and procedures.	- Movements are awkward and she has difficulty with managing uneven or moving surfaces such as an escalator. - Seldom initiates the home exercise program. When prompted and supervised will do the exercises but puts little effort in them. - Does not initiate or manage familiar routines without prompting. - Has not returned to her previous leisure activities of hanging out with her friends and singing in the choir. - Currently spends most of her leisure time watching Netflix and surfing the Web. - Is sometimes impulsive. - Has forgotten to turn off appliances since she has been home.

Note. ADLs = activities of daily living; IADLs = instrumental activities of daily living.

EXHIBIT 3.6.	Surya's Strengths and Weaknesses in Motor and Praxis Skills
STRENGTHS	**WEAKNESSES**
▪ Has good dynamic sitting. ▪ Can independently assume standing and maintain her balance in routine situations. ▪ Has full functional ROM and general functional movement patterns are adequate to routine demands. ▪ Can legibly write her name both with a pen and using a standard keyboard. ▪ Can move limbs independently and engage in simple tasks. ▪ Is right-handed and has adequate grip strength for routine activities.	▪ Has demonstrated slowed equilibrium responses and mild dyspraxia when her balance is challenged. ▪ Handwriting and keyboarding are very slow. ▪ Is unable to write fast enough to take notes in class. ▪ Movements are slowed and she seems to need to closely attend to her actions. ▪ When distracted, is very clumsy and poorly coordinated. ▪ Is slow in performing tasks that require fine hand coordination.

Note. ROM = range of motion.

EXHIBIT 3.7.	Surya's Strengths and Weaknesses in Process, Behavioral, and Cognitive Skills
STRENGTHS	**WEAKNESSES**
▪ Will initiate tasks she is asked to do. ▪ Understands the demands of a task. ▪ Receptive and expressive language is WNL. ▪ Is alert and oriented. ▪ Is motivated to get back to "being herself." ▪ Can understand and follow a series of 2 or more related instructions. ▪ Has intact basic sensory function. ▪ Has basic intact awareness of body position, pain awareness, and visual–perceptual skills	▪ Is withdrawn and disinterested. ▪ Seldom initiates any behavior without a 1:1 prompt. ▪ Will work on tasks appropriately once started but stops again rather than asking for help or problem solving on her own. ▪ Is often unable to reliably sequence the steps or adjust her strategies when needed. ▪ Is impulsive in her work, often making errors and then giving up in frustration. ▪ Is easily frustrated and responds with tears and angry outbursts when frustrated. ▪ Does not anticipate problems and does not problem solve solutions when familiar strategies do not work. ▪ Has trouble keeping up with her school assignments and school materials. ▪ Has difficulty with many executive function skills, including keeping track of time, making plans, making sure work is finished on time, and looking for help or more information when needed.

Note. WNL = within normal limits.

of mild TBI but are greatly limiting her performance. These data lead the occupational therapy practitioner to consider the social–emotional performance patterns and refine the original hypothesis.

USING EVIDENCE: EVALUATING INFORMATION SOURCES

As occupational therapy practitioners refine the clinical hypothesis, their reasoning must be informed by the available evidence from a variety of sources. At this point, the practitioner should move beyond foundational knowledge and the basics learned during training to enter the profession. The conscientious use of current best evidence in making decisions about patient care and the expansion of a clinician's expertise through critical evaluation of the growing body of research that is available is called *evidence-based practice (EBP).*

Internet-Based Information

Easy access to information through the Internet has dramatically changed occupational therapy practice and has offered both supports and challenges to clinical reasoning. The occupational therapy practitioner can easily find information on the Internet, but there is too much to easily analyze and it is hard to know how accurate that information may be.

Rather than drown in information, a systematic approach can address concerns about the trustworthiness of information found through an Internet search. Some of these common concerns are summarized in Exhibit 3.8.

PRACTICE WISDOM 3.2.	Internet Information

"Getting information off the Internet is like taking a drink from a fire hydrant." —*Mitchell Kapor (n.d.)*

| **EXHIBIT 3.8.** | **Considering Internet-Based Information** |

There is no assurance of accuracy or quality when it comes to information found on the Internet.

Anyone can post anything.
- Individuals or businesses marketing to occupational therapy practitioners may publish unsupported claims as "facts" to promote their products.

Not all websites are created equal. They differ in quality, purpose, and bias.
- Websites that focus on a particular intervention are more likely to present that intervention in a positive light and to present competing interventions more negatively. This is true of websites targeting clients as well as those targeting practitioners.
- Websites that are supported by professional occupational therapy organizations (e.g., AOTA) are most likely to be committed to supporting practitioners and are likely to provide highly reliable information.
- Advertising is important. Some websites (including occupational therapy blogs) have sponsors who pay for specific content or advertisements to promote their products or ideas.
- Occupational therapy blogs and online communities of practice are growing. These newer information tools are often very easy to read and understand and more likely to tackle timely issues. The process of maintaining an active blog can be daunting, and increasingly popular blogs receive the financial support of advertisers to maintain that blog. This is not a problem, but readers should be aware that the information presented may not always be impartial.

Some websites are old, and their information is out of date.
- It is important to review the most current information available on the topic in which you are interested. Most responsible websites have a date posted somewhere that lets you know how old the information is. If you cannot find a date, you should not use the information.

Some online information is second hand.
- Information in online "encyclopedias" is often secondhand, compiled by an interested party, and may not reflect sound scholarship.
- Internet-based information sources and encyclopedias can be excellent for giving you an overview of an intervention, a medical condition, or a clinical challenge. It is important to take this overview a step further before using it in clinical reasoning. Practitioners should take the information from secondary sources and search it again through scholarly sources before accepting it as sound.

Note. AOTA = American Occupational Therapy Association.

Peer Review

For both online and more traditional sources of information, the gold standard used in considering the trustworthiness of information is whether the information has been subjected to a peer review process. *Peer review* is a process of evaluating information submitted for publication or presentation. When there is a peer-review process in place, the author (or presenter) of the information must submit it for review. In the case of a scientific journal, this means authors submit their articles to a journal editor who forwards it to experts in the field for review.

Because the reviewers specialize in the same scholarly area as the author, they are considered the author's *peers*. These reviews are usually "blind," meaning that the reviewers do not know the name of the paper's author so the review is impartial. These peer reviewers are charged with carefully evaluating the quality of the submitted manuscript. Because a peer-reviewed journal will not publish articles that fail to meet the standards established for a given discipline, peer-reviewed articles that are accepted for publication exemplify the best research practices in a field.

Peer-reviewed materials have some easily recognizable features. First, because peer review reflects a gold standard for information, professional associations are likely to rely on the peer review process to support their members. Because peer review has value, most publications or conferences using a peer review process will identify that in descriptions. If you use a search database (e.g., Google Scholar, CINAHL, Medline, PsycINFO), you can limit your search to scholarly or peer-reviewed publications.

There is a peer review process in place for many professional continuing education (CE) opportunities. People hoping to present at a conference with a peer review process must submit a proposal for consideration, and the merit of the presentation will be considered through peer review. Some peer review processes are more rigorous than others, with some scientific journals and some professional conferences warranting greater respect and prestige in their peer review process.

Looking for information that has been supported through peer review is an essential tool in building knowledge translation skills for clinical reasoning. Practitioners are expected to engage in ongoing CE to reinforce professional practice and maintain professional certification. As practitioners seek CE opportunities, they

EXHIBIT 3.9.	Clinical Hypothesis Evolution for Surya

- *Initial hypothesis:* Surya is early in the recovery process, and her need for support will be temporary.
- *Hypothesis evolution:* Surya is early in the recovery process. Due her age-related brain immaturity, her impairments may persist and grow over time.

should note whether the CE program has undergone a peer review process. CE aimed at teaching occupational therapy practitioners new techniques or introducing innovative products may serve the individuals marketing the technique or product more than practitioners who seek to build an evidence-based practice.

Exploring Evidence: Surya

Returning to the case of Surya, the practitioner needs to examine the published evidence on brain damage resulting from TBI in adolescents that considers the typical brain development in children and adolescents (Savage, 2012). It is best practice to focus on the most recent literature available because the state of science and knowledge change over time, making older data obsolete. This is true in Surya's case.

Older literature states that the increased plasticity of young brains makes them more adaptable and better able to fully recover from TBI than their adult counterparts. However, Babikian, Merkley, Savage, Giza, and Levin (2015) did a thorough review of the literature and found that

> while TBI is likely to affect the level of previously achieved functioning in children, it can also potentially impact the course and rate of future cognitive development moving forward. It is hypothesized that the pattern of poorer cognitive outcomes of childhood injury may be related to increased probability that there will be a disruption of acquisition and development of skills that were not achieved before the time of injury. Indeed, TBI may impede the future development of new skills, in addition to interfering with skills that were in process of being acquired at the time of injury. (p. 1851)

Babikian et al. offer an explanation that fits the data we have collected on Surya, but it can only guide our process toward creating occupational therapy goals in collaboration with the client that lead to desired outcomes. This new information leads us to reconsider the foundational clinical hypothesis we developed for Surya. Exhibit 3.9 presents our original and a refined clinical hypotheses incorporating the new evidence for this case.

ERRORS AND EXPERTISE

With our newly evolved hypothesis, we are now at another point at which clinical reasoning errors can occur.

PRACTICE WISDOM 3.3.	Errors Are Part of Clinical Reasoning

"In all science, error precedes the truth, and it is better it should go first than last."—*Horace Walpole (n.d.)*

Errors are an essential and natural part of the clinical reasoning process.

Failure to consider new (or anomalous) evidence, or to take the time to look beyond foundational evidence, can lead to developing goals that do not fully address the scope of a client's needs. Such errors can lead to the inefficient provision of services. Practitioners making this type of error would set goals and perhaps even document progress, but Surya is likely to have new or persistent problems emerge after she is discharged from therapy. This could lead to a delay or inability to get her back into the therapy process to address the emergent issues.

An *expert* was described earlier as someone with special skill or knowledge derived from training or experience. An expert occupational therapy practitioner in the field of TBI would already understand the unique impact of TBI on the developing brain and could omit the first round of hypothesis refinement and move forward from this point.

Errors are inevitable, but for novice practitioners it is essential to carefully use established functional outcome measures to identify errors as early as possible. Novice practitioners should also consider the work of Chinn and Brewer (1998) and identify where their own reactions to data fall among the 7 reactions to anamolous data that they describe (i.e., ignore, reject, exclude, hold in abeyance, reinterpret, accept and make peripheral theory changes, accept and change theories).

CREATING COLLABORATIVE GOALS

Earlier this chapter discussed the goals reported by all of the key informants in Surya's case. Surya wants to get back to the lifestyle she experienced prior to her injury. She said that she doesn't want to be seen as a "freak" or have her old friends pity her. This goal, combined with the gathered clinical data, suggests that she is self-conscious and views her current performance negatively.

Surya's parents also want her to feel good about herself and to return to school and perform well in her classwork. They have been supportive but are taking a longer view than their daughter. With good school performance, she will have more and better options as she faces her adult life. The teachers at the school want to support Surya but have limited time and resources in the general educational classroom. They are looking for expert evaluation to help determine how best to support Surya so that she can succeed at school.

The essential purpose of the Individuals With Disabilities Education Improvement Act of 2004 (IDEA; P. L. 108–446) is to ensure students with disabilities have access to a free and appropriate public education. IDEA requires assessing students who may need special educational support. Part of this assessment involves colloborative goal setting. This legislation provides guidance on having a meeting that includes all of the school and family stakeholders in a child's life. In this meeting, the combined widom of the group guides the specification of educational and functional goals for Surya that are measureable and essential within the school environment.

After this meeting the following priority concerns were identified for Surya:

- Surya has difficulting planning and prioritizing her actions.
- Surya has trouble breaking a task down into simple steps.
- Surya has difficulty detecting errors in work.
- Surya is hypercritical of herself and does not take constructive criticism well.

It was also noted that she was easily distracted, and when distracted would lose her place in the task at hand, aggravating the concerns identified by the team. The result of this meeting was a recommendation that Surya receive occupational therapy support in the school setting. The practitioner must now explore her clinical hypotheses and delineate potential intervention approaches on the basis of best practices and available evidence to support Surya. The result of this exploration should include identifying functional outcome measures that reflect the identified collaborative goals.

USING THE HYPOTHESIS FOR INTERVENTION PLANNING

Repeating the sequence introduced earlier in the chapter, consider the broad categories of occupational therapy services that might be offered to Surya: remediation, maintenance, compensation, development, or education. The school team's priority is to get Surya's school performance improved rapidly to help her regain confidence and the prior quality of her learning. All parties understand that she is still in the recovery process following her TBI and expect her to slowly regain skills. The overall consensus is to give her tools to get by, to help her consistently use those tools, and to support her as she recovers.

The development approach seems a good first choice for Surya because of her age and it respects the role of neuroplasticity in supporting her recovery, but it has a medical focus that may prioritize different skills than those needed in the school setting. Looking at the other choices, the remediation approach also seems to be a good option because her skills are so greatly limiting her participation, and this approach is sensitive to her

school-related performance needs. The maintenance approach does not fit this case, and there is no expectation of a decline in skills.

The compensation approach also has potential if it can allow Surya to immediately perform skills rather than waiting for neural recovery. The compensation approach is also sensitive to her school-related performance needs, but if given a compensation tool, it may be that Surya may not develop some underlying skill that she needs. Finally, the educational approach, which focuses on health promotion and developing positive health behaviors, could be good to consider in the future, but a focus on health behaviors is not a priority at this time.

Understanding these broad categories in clinical reasoning helps focus the intervention planning. These categories are not necessarily exclusive of one another, and it is appropriate at this point to keep the development, remediation, and compensation approaches in mind as we look for a frame of reference to guide us forward. Chapters 4–7 discuss how to review and consider frames of reference as part of the clinical reasoning process, but for now we omit this discussion and identify the *cognitive rehabilitation frame of reference* as the conceptual guide for this case (see Exhibit 3.10). This frame of reference was chosen because it supports both the remediation and compensation approaches, the 2 strongest approaches to support Surya. It does not have a developmental component, so developmental aspects will need

---

EXHIBIT 3.10. Elements of Cognitive Rehabilitation Frame of Reference in Occupational Therapy

- **Focus:** Emphasizes the neuroscientific understanding that every intentional act results from a dynamic balance among all brain structures, and the functional nervous system as a whole can be disturbed by a lesion in one area.
- **Basic assumptions:** Addresses cognition (i.e., acquisition, organization, use of knowledge), perception, visual–motor organization, thinking operations (i.e., executive functions), memory, attention, and concentration.
- **Function–disability continuum:** Function is reflected in effective cognitive function for the tasks of everyday life. Dysfunction occurs following injury or disease and results in poor performance due to poor cognitive function.
- **Postulates of change:** Improvements in function can be achieved through a combination of cognitive retraining and use of compensation for cognitive deficits.
- **Component-specific training:** Components (i.e., perception, visual–motor organization, thinking operation, memory) are trained using specific tools in a structured environment. As the person achieves success, the difficulty of tasks is increased, considering changes to the task and its context. The person is trained in both problem solving and compensatory strategies appropriate for the performance of targeted daily life tasks.

to be considered in addition to the cognitive rehabilitative frame of reference.

For a frame of reference, the cognitive rehabilitation model seems promising for Surya because it offers specific strategies that can immediately lead to improved function in the school environment. We acknowledge that as an adolescent, tasks and expectations must be adapted to focus on skills appropriate to her developmental expectations and the school context. Our evolved clinical hypothesis is that Surya is early in the recovery process and her impairments may persist and grow over time due her age-related brain immaturity.

Using the cogntive rehabilitation frame of reference we have plan for addressing the problem, and this is added to the hypothesis. The refined hypothesis is: *Surya is early in the TBI recovery process and due to her age-related brain immaturity, her impairments may persist and grow over time.* Surya's impairments are hypothesized to be largely due to difficulties with cognitive function that can be treated through use of cognitive retraining and compensatory strategies.

Use of the cognitive rehabilitation model not only provides focused treatment strategies but also guides us to evaluation strategies. Few tests of cognitive function are standardized for adolescents, but the School Function Assessment (SFA; Coster, Deeney, Haltiwanger, & Haley 1998) addresses specific issues of performance in the school setting and documents the types of task supports currently provided to the student. A limitation of this test is that it is aimed more at students with chronic disabilities and does not address some of the complex performance expected of adolescents in typical school environments.

In a developmental context, adolescent neurodevelopment is characterized by the maturation of the prefrontal cortex and the refinement of executive function and self-regulation skills. The term *executive function* refers to neurocognitive processes involved in goal-directed behavior, including working memory, attentional flexibility, and inhibitory control (Vilgis, Silk, & Vance, 2015). It is well documented that problems in executive function are common and persistent long term after pediatric TBI (Kurowski et al., 2013).

Because the SFA does not specifically test executive functions, additional testing should also be considered. The cognitive rehabilitation model offers insight into additional testing tools that may be beneficial. We have chosen the Multiple Errands Test–Revised (MET–R; Morrison, et al., 2013) as a tool that, with slight modification for the school environment, may be useful with Surya as an adjunct to the SFA. The MET–R was designed to be used with adults who experienced a mild stroke, not adolescents with mild TBI, but its focus is on executive function, and this is the constuct we need more information on to best understand Surya. It is a clinical judgment that we make: This tool might be useful if

given in this atypical manner. It is our expectation that the use of these 2 assessment tools will give a picture of Surya's strengths and weaknesses in the school setting that is both efficient and defensible.

With this information, specific functional, measurable, and educationally relevant goals and interventions can be developed that will help Surya gain self-awareness, challenge her level of thinking, and practice using compensatory strategies to help her perform needed tasks as she recovers function. It is through functional goal setting and data collection on those goals that the greatest test of the revised clinical hypothesis occurs. If progress in the targeted functional and measureable goals is documented, the hypothesis stands, but it may still be refined as more information is gathered. If progress is not documented, then a clinical reasoning error has been made and the process needs to be reinstated, including all of the additional data gathered in the first trial.

Error may be a part of the process. Error should be eliminated as much as possible but should also be faced directly when it occurs. Thorough original data gathering and strong evidence-based reasoning reduces the liklihood of error. Expertise allows a more streamlined process but does not eliminate the possibility of error. It is important to limit error to the greatest extent possible, but it is also important to recognize errors early and use them as a source of data to refine the clinical hypothesis.

SUMMARY

This chapter reviews hypothesis generation and refinement. After the initial hypothesis is generated, occupational therapy practitioners usually follow a process to refine it as they gain more information about the client. In effective clinical reasoning, data drive the process. For Brody, if motor learning or CO–OP had been chosen as the first frame of reference, his occupational therapy practitioner would still have gathered functional outcome data and refined his or her clinical hypothesis. The end result of the process, regardless of the starting point, should lead to an intervention that is acceptable to the client and result in measureable functional change in valued areas of occupation.

The expert practitioner is likely to have a more streamlined clinical hypothesis process, with better-informed decisions made early in the process, than the novice practitioner. Error is part of the process in hypothesis generation. Error offers valuable data but also adds time to the process. Becoming well versed in frames of reference can support and improve practitioners' clinical hypothesis generation and reduce the time it takes to develop an effective and meaningful intervention process for clients.

The clinical expert remains an expert only if he or she continually reviews the literature for new or expanded knowledge in the area of their expertise. A person who is a novice in a particular practice area or with the treatment of a particular condition can use evidence and conceptual models such as frames of reference and theories to help them reason at a more expert level.

Evidence is seldom available on exactly the client conditions for which you are looking. Practitioners must understand their clients as individuals and in searching the literature consider their particular needs. From this point forward in the text we will expect that evidence-based considerations will be a component of all clincal reasoning. We also begin to explore and consider some distinct frames of reference in the context of available evidence.

LEARNING ACTIVITIES

1. This chapter examined the case of Brody and focused on motor impairments, but other important impairments were not discussed. Review Brody's occupational profile in Exhibit 3.1, and list 2 areas in the occupational therapy domain in which compensation would be good for Brody.
2. A strong evidence-based frame of reference that might support Brody is the motor learning frame of reference. Research this frame of reference, and define its focus, basic assumptions, function–dysfunction continuum, and postulates of change.
3. More than one frame of reference can be used with a client if their assumptions are compatible. Chapter 1 presented the biomechanical frame of reference, which is an evidence-based approach that supports improved motor function. Is it compatible with both the NDT and the developmental systems frames of reference? Explain your reasoning.
4. School-based occupational therapy practitioners should focus intervention plans on students' needs to function in a learning environment. List at least 3 priority areas for Brody, and describe how they might affect Brody's ability to participate in or benefit from educational instruction.
5. The priorities listed in the previous question are likely to differ from the priorities Brody's parents listed. Because goal setting needs to be collaborative, write an argument to support your priorities as you present them to Brody's parents.
6. Brody has significant impairments in communication and social interaction that were not addressed in this chapter. Occupational therapy will collaborate with his school team and his family to support skill development in these areas. It is likely that his speech therapist will suggest the use of an augmentative communication device, and occupational therapy will be involved in helping integrate the use of the device in the school and home settings. Search *augmentative communication devices* on Youtube.com, and watch preschoolers operate

these devices. List 2 ways that you could incorporate the device you observed into activities that the family values.
7. Read the article by Stephens, Williamson, and Berryhill (2015). Consider the evidence on cognitive rehabilitation and discuss how it supports or alters your analysis of Surya's case.
8. Look up the cognitive disabilities frame of reference (Levy, 2018; Levy & Burns, 2005). This frame of reference was not used to address Surya's needs. Discuss why this frame of reference may or may not be an effective tool for Surya's case. Explain your answer by considering the focus, basic assumptions, function–dysfunction continuum, and postulates of change associated with the frame of reference to justify your answer.
9. Read the review article by Baker, Unsworth, and Lannin (2015). This article offers a different focus and type of consideration of functional limitations following TBI. What issues raised in this review would be important to consider for Surya, even if she is not planning to drive? Explain your answer.

REFERENCES

American Medical Association. (2017). *CPT® (Current Procedural Terminology): Use the Current Procedural Terminology (CPT®) code set to bill outpatient and office procedures.* Retrieved from https://www.ama-assn.org/practice-management/cpt-current-procedural-terminology

Aldridge, J., & Goldman, R. (2007). *Current issues and trends in education.* Boston: Allyn and Bacon.

American Occupational Therapy Association. (2014). Occupational therapy practice framework: Domain and process (3rd ed.). *American Journal of Occupational Therapy, 68*(Suppl. 1), S1–S48. https://doi.org/10.5014/ajot.2014.682006.

American Occupational Therapy Association. (2017a). AOTA occupational profile template. *American Journal of Occupational Therapy, 71*(Suppl. 2), 7002420030. https://doi.org/10.5014/ajot.2017.716S12

American Occupational Therapy Association. (2017b). *The new evaluation codes: What are performance deficits?* Retrieved from https://www.aota.org/~/media/Corporate/Files/Advocacy/Federal/coding/Performance-Deficits-new-CPT-evaluation-codes.pdf

Asher, I. E. (Ed.). (2014). *Asher's occupational therapy assessment tools: An annotated index* (4th ed.). Bethesda, MD: AOTA Press.

Babikian, T., Merkley, T., Savage, R., Giza, C., & Levin, H. (2015). Chronic aspects of pediatric traumatic brain injury: Review of the literature. *Journal of Neurotrauma, 32*, 1849–1860. https://doi.org/10.1089/neu.2015.3971

Baker, A., Unsworth, C. A., & Lannin, N. A. (2015). Determining fitness to drive: A systematic review of the methods and assessments used after mild traumatic brain injury. *British Journal of Occupational Therapy, 78*, 73–84. https://doi.org/10.1177/0308022614562405

Chinn, C. A., & Brewer, W. F. (1998). An empirical test of a taxonomy of responses to anomalous data in science. *Journal of Research in Science Teaching, 35,* 623–654. https://doi.org/10.1002/(SICI)1098-2736(199808)35:6<623::AID-TEA3>3.0.CO;2-O

Coster, W., Deeney, T., Haltiwanger, J., & Haley, S. (1998). *School Function Assessment (SFA).* San Antonio, TX: Pearson Education.

Dawson, D. R., McEwen, S. E., & Polatajko, H. J. (Eds.). (2017). *Cognitive Orientation to daily Occupational Performance in occupational therapy: Using the CO–OP Approach to enable participation across the lifespan.* Bethesda, MD: AOTA Press.

Einstein, A. (n.d.). *Brainyquote.com.* Retrieved from https://www.brainyquote.com/quotes/albert_einstein_148837

Fabrizio, A., & Rafols, J. (2014). Optimizing abilities and capacities: Range of motion, strength, and endurance. In M. Radomski & C. Latham (Eds.), *Occupational therapy for physical dysfunction* (7th ed., pp. 589–613). Philadelphia: Lippincott Williams & Wilkins.

Guralnick, M. (2001). A developmental systems model for early intervention. *Infants and Young Children: An Interdisciplinary Journal of Early Childhood Intervention, 14,* 1–18. https://doi.org/10.1097/00001163-200114020-00004

Individuals With Disabilities Education Improvement Act of 2004, 20 U.S.C. § 1400 (2004).

Kapor, M. (n.d.). *BrainyQuote.com.* Retrieved from: https://www.brainyquote.com/quotes/mitchell_kapor_163583

Kassirer, J., Wong, J., & Kopelman, R. (2010). *Learning clinical reasoning* (2nd ed.). Philadelphia: Lippincott Williams & Wilkins.

Kuhn, T. S. (1962). *The structure of scientific revolutions.* Chicago: University of Chicago Press.

Kurowski, B. G., Wade, S. L., Kirkwood, M. W., Brown, T. M., Stancin, T., Cassedy, A., & Taylor, H. G. (2013). Association of parent ratings of executive function with global- and setting-specific behavioral impairment after adolescent traumatic brain injury. *Archives of Physical Medicine and Rehabilitation, 94,* 543–550. https://doi.org/10.1016/j.apmr.2012.10.029

Law, M., & McDermid, J. (2014). *Evidence-based rehabilitation: A guide to practice* (3rd ed.). Thorofare, NJ: Slack.

Levit, K. (2014). Web A: Optimizing motor behavior using the Bobath Approach. In M. Radomski & C. Latham (Eds.), *Occupational therapy for physical dysfunction* (7th ed., pp. 643–665). Philadelphia: Lippincott Williams & Wilkins.

Levy, L. (2018). Neurocognition and function: Intervention in dementia and the Cognitive Disabilities Model. In N. Katz & J. Toglia (Eds.), *Cognition, occupation, and participation across the lifespan: Neuroscience, neurorehabilitation, and models of intervention in occupational therapy* (4th ed.). Bethesda, MD: AOTA Press.

Levy, L. & Burns, T. (2011). The Cognitive Disability Model reconsidered: Rehabilitation of adults with dementia. In N. Katz (Ed.), *Cognition and occupation across the life span: Models for intervention in occupational therapy* (3rd ed., pp. 407–441). Bethesda, MD: AOTA Press.

Mandich, M. (2016). Classic theories of human development. In A. Cronin & M. Mandich (Eds.), *Human development and performance throughout the lifespan* (2nd ed., pp. 38–59). Boston: Cengage Learning.

Medical diagnosis. (2003.) *Miller-Keane Encyclopedia and dictionary of medicine, nursing, and allied health* (7th ed.). Retrieved from http://medical-dictionary.thefreedictionary.com/medical+diagnosis

Merriam-Webster. (2016). *Expert.* Retrieved from http://www.merriam-webster.com/dictionary/expert

Milton, Y., & Logothetis, A. (2013). An occupational therapy practice initiative using the Bobath Concept: A collaborative partnership with higher education. *British Journal of Occupational Therapy, 76,* 452–455. https://doi.org/10.4276/030802213X13807217284224

Morgan, C., Darrah, J., Gordon, A. M., Harbourne, R., Spittle, A., Johnson, R., & Fetters, L. (2016). Effectiveness of motor interventions in infants with cerebral palsy: A systematic review. *Developmental Medicine and Child Neurology, 58,* 900–909. https://doi.org/10.1111/dmcn.13105

Morrison, M. T., Giles, G. M., Ryan, J. D., Baum, C. M., Dromerick, A. W., Polatajko, H. J., & Edwards, D. F. (2013). Multiple Errands Test–Revised (MET–R): A performance-based measure of executive function in people with mild cerebrovascular accident. *American Journal of Occupational Therapy, 67,* 460–468. https://doi.org/10.5014/ajot.2013.007880

Polatajko, H., & Mandich, A. (2004). *Enabling occupational in children: The Cognitive Orientation to daily Occupational Performance (CO–OP) approach.* Ottawa, ON: CAOT Publications.

Powell, J. (2014). Traumatic brain injury. In M. Radomski & C. Latham (Eds.), *Occupational therapy for physical dysfunction* (7th ed., pp. 1042–1075). Philadelphia: Lippincott Williams & Wilkins.

Robnett, R., & Kaminski, T. (2014). Client factors in occupational performance functioning. In K. Jacobs, N. McRae, & K. Sladyk (Eds.), *Occupational therapy essentials for clinical competence* (2nd ed.). Thorofare, NJ: Slack.

Sabari, J., Capasso, N., & Feld-Glazman, R. (2014). Optimizing motor planning and performance in clients with neurological disorders. In M. Radomski & C. Latham (Eds.), *Occupational therapy for physical dysfunction* (7th ed., pp. 614–676). Philadelphia: Lippincott Williams & Wilkins.

Savage, R. (2012). *The developing brain after TBI: Predicting long-term deficits and services for children, adolescents, and young adults.* Retrieved from http://www.international brain.org/articles/the-developing-brain-after-tbi/

Skubik-Peplaski, C., Paris, C., Boyle, D. & Culpert, A. (Eds.). (2009). *Applying the* Occupational Therapy Practice Framework: *Using the Cardinal Hill Occupational Participation Process in client-centered care* (2nd ed.). Bethesda, MD: AOTA Press.

Stephens, J. A., Williamson, K. C., & Berryhill, M. E. (2015). Cognitive rehabilitation after traumatic brain injury: A reference for occupational therapists. *OTJR: Occupation, Participation and Health, 35,* 5–22. https://doi.org/10.1177/1539449214561765

Vilgis, V., Silk, T. J., & Vance, A. (2015). Executive function and attention in children and adolescents with depressive disorders: A systematic review. *European Child and Adolescent Psychiatry, 24,* 365–384. https://doi.org/10.1007/s00787-015-0675-7

Walpole, H. (n.d.). *Brainyquote.com.* Retrieved from https://www.brainyquote.com/quotes/quotes/h/horacewalp161868.html

PART II.

Frames of Reference

Psychodynamic and Developmental Systems Frames of Reference

Anne Cronin, PhD, OTR/L, ATP, FAOTA, and Garth Graebe, MOT, OTR/L

4

CHAPTER HIGHLIGHTS

- Explores key elements of the psychodynamic frame of reference within occupational therapy's domain.
- Describes the function–dysfunction continuum within the psychodynamic frame of reference.
- Provides an evidence-based consideration of the state of the science supporting the psychodynamic frame of reference.
- Illustrates use of the psychodynamic and the developmental systems frames of reference in case examples.
- Reflects on evidence-based practice and the use of frames of reference.
- Defines key elements of the developmental systems frame of reference within occupational therapy's domain.
- Explores the elements of the developmental systems frame of reference in a clinical reasoning context.
- Describes the function–dysfunction continuum within the developmental systems frame of reference.

KEY TERMS AND CONCEPTS

Attachment theory	Ego psychology	Maturation
Creativity	Frames of reference	Nonlinear thinking
Development	Half-life of knowledge	Psychodynamic frame of reference
Developmental systems theory	Hasty generalization	Superego
Ego	Id	Theory

This chapter describes the psychodynamic and developmental systems frames of reference within the scope of the occupational therapy domain and process by introducing a formal review process that can be applied to other frames of reference commonly used in the profession. In Chapter 3, "Hypothesis Generation and Refinement," we introduced the use of frames of reference as heuristic tools in the clinical hypothesis generation process. ***Frames of reference*** are sets of assumptions or concepts, often drawn from theory, that can guide the occupational therapy process. They are built upon scientific and clinical knowledge from both within and outside the field of occupational therapy.

In this chapter the psychodynamic and the developmental systems frames of reference are presented together because they are complementary and widely used in occupational therapy practice. These frames of reference are so embedded in occupational therapy's domain that they are often not specifically identified in scientific papers or textbooks offering practice guidelines.

TERMINOLOGY

Earlier in this text ***theory*** was defined as a plausible or scientifically acceptable general principle or body of principles offered to explain phenomena ("Theory," 2016). In occupational therapy the term *theory* is used broadly to describe, explain, and predict behavior or relationships among concepts and events. This definition can be confusing because theory is often the foundation of both models and frames of reference and is not really distinct from either.

Throughout this text we preferentially use the terms *frame of reference* or *model* for the sake of clarity. The term *theory* is used to discuss ideas, especially those emerging from outside the profession of occupational therapy. For example, in this chapter the psychodynamic frame of reference (sometimes referred to as the *psychoanalytic frame of reference*) is introduced. This frame of reference has its origins in the theories of psychiatrists and psychologists Sigmund Freud, Carl Jung, Carl Rogers, and Abraham Maslow (Brown, Stoffel, & Muñoz, 2011).

Rather than focusing on the theories underlying the psychodynamic frame of reference, this chapter focuses on applying these theories for occupational therapy. The term *psychodynamic* is preferred because occupational therapy involves dynamic activity, and psychoanalysis primarily involves talk therapy and analysis (Fidler & Fidler, 1963). The psychodynamic frame of reference is a theoretical frame of reference with strong historical underpinnings, both in occupational therapy and in psychology, the field of its origin.

HISTORICAL PSYCHOANALYTIC THEORY

To apply the psychodynamic frame of reference appropriately, it is important to first understand the historical psychoanalytic theories that form its basis. Freud's (1923) original work on personality was based on a 3-part description of the mind's processes: (1) id, (2) ego, and (3) superego (Mandich, 2015).

Freud defined the *id* as primarily unconscious needs and desires. It is made up of primitive, often illogical biological drives and instincts that often conflict with the ego. The *ego* is the conscious mental process that is most observable to the outside world. It is learned through experience and is often considered the "self." The *super-ego* represents the part of the personality that strives for perfection, a moral compass that is based on the individual's belief system. Later psychoanalytic theorists believed that the ego was responsible for creating the personality and was separate and independent from the id (Brown et al., 2011). Figure 4.1 illustrates the evolution of Freud's theory to its application in present-day occupational therapy.

PSYCHODYNAMIC FRAME OF REFERENCE FOR OCCUPATIONAL THERAPY

Occupational therapy practitioners have long incorporated psychodynamic concepts to attempt to explain occupational behavior and guide therapeutic interventions (Wendland, 1956). The psychodynamic frame of reference is drawn from the theory that evolved from the work of Freud, Jung, Rogers, Maslow, and others. The *psychodynamic frame of reference* theorizes that behavior results from the conscious and unconscious, and structured activities enable exploration and expression through which the client can develop an understanding of themselves and others (Bruce & Borg, 2002). Fidler and Fidler (1963) theorized that people engage with others as well as objects to fulfill unconscious desires and objectives, firmly placing the psychodynamic frame of reference within the occupational therapy domain of practice.

This frame of reference has integrated contemporary science since 1963 and differs in many ways from the original theories underlying the frame of reference. The persistence of the use of this approach is explained by the clinical need to understand and explain human emotions (Cole & Tufano, 2008). The psychodynamic frame of reference proposes that behavior is influenced by the conscious and unconscious mind. For example, Cole (2012) suggests that irrational behavior (e.g., taking drugs, harming oneself) may be explained by exploring the unconscious in which past emotional conflicts and experiences drive current behaviors.

The psychodynamic frame of reference is often used in group-based activities and has a long history in occupational therapy practice, especially in mental health.

The occupational therapy psychodynamic frame of reference explains observed behavior as a manifestation of intrinsic mental processes that are difficult or impossible to objectively test and measure. This frame of reference is often used to help clients appropriately express emotions and facilitate creativity to support performance and participation. It is from this perspective that the basic assumptions of the frame of reference are derived (Exhibit 4.1).

As noted Exhibit 4.1, the Freudian idea of the *ego* is what most concerns occupational therapy practitioners, which has grown from the understanding of modern *ego psychology,* a contemporary approach that emerged from Freud's early work. Ego psychologists consider the

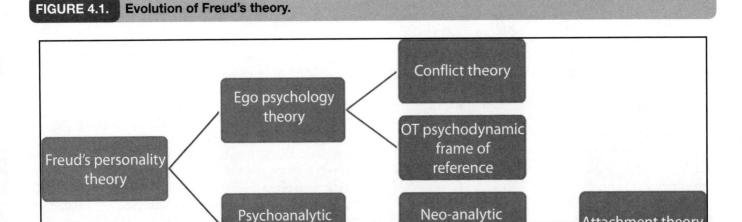

FIGURE 4.1. Evolution of Freud's theory.

Note. OT = occupational therapy.

EXHIBIT 4.1.	Psychodynamic Frame of Reference Elements as Used in Occupational Therapy

- **Focus:** In occupational therapy, this frame of reference focuses on emotional expression and motivation for engagement in occupation. Of the Freudian concepts, it is the ego with which occupational therapy practitioners have been most concerned.
- **Basic assumptions:** Individuals' occupational behavior reflects their interaction with both the external world and internal forces. Through a focus on activities to support aspects of ego functioning, improved performance can be elicited in the areas of social participation, relationship development and maintenance, self-awareness, and clarification of occupational goals and priorities.
- **Function–dysfunction continuum:** Function is portrayed by a strong sense of self that is free from conflicts and fixations, functioning well in the environmental contexts. *Dysfunction* is defined in terms of conflicts among the Id, ego, and superego. These conflicts can manifest as neurosis, psychosis, or character disorders that interfere with the ability to complete ADLs and to function as a participating member of society (Cole, 2012).
- **Postulates of change:** Through engagement in structured activities, occupational therapy practitioners strive to alter the function of the client through developing ego skills that enable clients to function optimally. Occupational therapy interventions guided by this frame of reference are based on activities that foster self-expression and motivation for engagement in occupations (Cole & Tufano, 2008). Interventions also focus on stress and coping skills to enable clients to express feelings in a safe environment and develop a positive self-efficacy (Brown et al., 2011).

ego as a defensive structure that is highly and inherently adaptive and can influence human development (Danzer, 2012). In this context, ego functioning relates to how well (or impaired) someone's thoughts, feelings, and actions work together to form a person's occupational behavior (Cole & Tufano, 2008).

The psychodynamic frame of reference with an ego-centric focus can be used to build on clients' strengths and helps them recognize their natural talents and abilities and cultural, creative, and spiritual practices (Danzer, 2012). By exploring internal resources, individuals can learn to cope with and work through external challenges. In 1973, Bellak, Hurvich, and Gediman identified 12 separate ego functions that form the foundation of ego psychology. These 12 functions are described in Table 4.1.

In the psychodynamic frame of reference it is assumed that by strengthening the ego's 12 functions the individual will develop a stronger sense of self and build on personal strengths to be better able to manage any remaining conflicts and fixations. The theory supporting the psychodynamic frame of reference proposes

that the ego, represented by the 12 ego functions listed in Table 4.1, can potentially affect intellectual function and the performance of daily occupations. By encouraging a sense of accomplishment through activities, occupational therapy practitioners can help clients achieve higher self-awareness and self-efficacy, which, in turn, helps to develop positive functions. As the ego functions develop, clients will, according to the psychodynamic frame of reference, be motivated to continue to engage in occupations that further develop their social participation, emotional expression, and relationship skills.

Creativity

Creativity, an adaptive trait in humans, is the ability to express through thoughts or actions originality or imagination to transcend everyday ideas, rules, or patterns. The psychodynamic frame of reference supports creative expression to help individuals learn to cope with and work through external challenges. Individuals who can respond to the unexpected with novel solutions are more likely to succeed and meet their daily needs. Physical, intellectual, and social impairments can cause people to focus inwardly and rely on the mundane, those things that are common and familiar. Strategies to support creative thinking and problem solving can support the remediation of these impairments.

Through creative endeavors, clients can explore new forms of self-expression, find tools for self-regulation, and practice problem solving. In many cases participation in creative activities helps to reduce anxiety and ease tension. Such outcomes can be powerful motivators for continued engagement in creative activities and provide an avenue for future ego skill development.

Llorens and Johnson, early leaders in occupational therapy, emphasize that practitioners must help to develop ego skills, provide a means to practice those skills, and support the mastery of those skills (Brown et al., 2011). They divided occupational therapy treatment groups into 3 stages:

1. *Evaluation:* Observation is used to enable the therapist to assess mood, relationships, motivation, performance, and skills among the group members.
2. *Convalescence:* Goals in this stage are to increase independence in functioning as both individuals and members of the group.
3. *Rehabilitation:* This stage emphasizes mastery of the task and the motivation to complete the task.

Attachment Theory

Attachment theory is a specialized subtheory within the psychodynamic frame of reference. Attachment theory was developed to explain infant behavior toward their attachment figure. Ainsworth (1973) and Bowlby (1969) were pioneers in researching this theory (Mandich, 2015). Attachment theory proposes that attachment

TABLE 4.1. 12 Ego Functions

EGO FUNCTION	LAY DESCRIPTION	FUNCTION	DYSFUNCTION
Reality testing	Accurate descriptions of the external and internal worlds.	Ability to self-examine one's thoughts and feelings and objectively compare them to what has actually occurred in the environment.	Hallucinations and delusions.
Judgment	Ability to plan a course of action and predict the outcome.	Accurately predicting the result of behaviors to help prevent negative consequences.	Poor judgment often leads to repeated patterns resulting in negative consequences.
Sense of self and the world	Insight or the awareness of what is influencing various behaviors.	Understanding the *why, how,* and *what* is what makes people feel the way they do in various situations.	Denial, no sense of who they are, or pretending to be someone they are not.
Autonomous functioning	Purposeful behavior and understanding of what can be controlled in the environment.	Goal-directed behaviors. Ability to control impulses and handle obstacles.	Individuals who feel they have no control over their life. They are victims of their circumstances.
Control of drive affect and impulse	The ability to modify impulsive reactions to situations.	Acts instead of reacts.	Often impulsive with poor inhibition abilities.
Object relations	An internal sense of self that manifests in the physical objects with which individuals surrounds themselves.	Understanding that objects do not define an individual.	Self-identity and self-worth defined by the clothes worn or brands chosen to own.
Thought processes	Ability to postpone instant gratification.	Waiting until environmental conditions are appropriate.	Acting on impulse regardless of environmental conditions.
Adaptive regression in the service of the ego	Regression to an immature stage of development to avoid anxiety or conflict.	When used in play and imagination, can be a force for creative expression as a coping mechanism.	Excessive eating, aggressive or compulsive behaviors.
Defensive functioning	Unconscious way to avoid conflicts.	Appropriate coping mechanisms. Anticipation, humor, and suppression are forms of adaptive defenses.	Denial, distortion of reality, acting out, or overemphasizing symptoms.
Stimulus barrier	Ability to manage environmental stimuli.	Ability to maintain attention and concentration in the presence of competing stimuli.	Being overwhelmed by the environment. A breakdown in the ability to function due to perceived overstimulation.
Synthetic integrative functions	Allows an individual to think, feel, and act in an acceptable manner.	Can get angry at someone they love. Although these feelings can conflict, they can be resolved over time.	Inability to resolve conflicting feelings. Panic attacks may be an expression of dysfunction.
Mastery competence	Ability to create solutions to environmental conflicts.	Self-confidence and self-efficacy.	Apathy, frustration, and loss of hope.

behaviors formed in infancy help shape the attachment relationships people have as adults.

Recent studies have criticized attachment theory because it does not reflect or account for differences in temperament that are genetic. Although it is acknowledged that attachment to others is central to individual well-being, attachment is not believed to emerge in infancy but grows over time to include extended family members and friends (Rholes & Simpson, 2004). Although the occupational therapy psychodynamic frame of reference presented here focuses on ego functions, it should be noted that persons with complex or disrupted social histories, such as refugees from war-torn areas, may have difficulty with attachment and with building relationships. Supporting emotional self-expression can help individuals with attachment difficulties gain the skills they need to connect socially.

State of Science and Evidence-Based Considerations

The psychodynamic frame of reference is drawn from theory. Theory and science inform each other, but a theory is an idea, not scientific evidence. The psychodynamic frame of reference grew from well-informed ideas, theory, and clinical observations. Unconscious thoughts and ideas, such as those considered in this frame of reference, can be scientifically studied only through a person's behaviors or verbal explanations.

The scientific method is not easily applied to the unconscious or the egocentric mental functions that are the foundation of this frame of reference. Indeed, Beck and Hurvich (1959) and Beck and Ward (1961) attempted to apply the scientific method to study the psychodynamics of depression. They failed to confirm their hypothesis that depression was the result of unconscious desires. Therefore, occupational therapy practitioners may be challenged to support this frame of reference as based in evidence.

For example, in seeking evidence in a literature search, using the search terms *psychodynamic* and *occupational therapy*, scholars will at first feel encouraged with nearly 175 records. Removing all duplicates and those not relevant to occupational therapy the search list is reduced to 42. This shortened list includes publications from 1956 through the present. As noted in Chapter 3, knowledge grows and changes, and it is important to look at the most recent evidence available. With this in mind, if we limit our list to only those papers published after 2005 and truly about occupational therapy practice, the list is shortened to 11 publications. This shows that there is continuing interest and exploration of this frame of reference, but the evidence is very limited. With another analysis of the search result list, we find that more than half (7) of the papers were published in the past 2 years, suggesting a resurgence in interest in this frame of reference.

As we consider the evidence supporting this frame of reference, let us choose a recent paper to analyze here. Sleight and Stein Duker (2016) wrote an opinion paper, *Toward a Broader Role for Occupational Therapy in Supportive Oncology Care.* It does not specifically mention the psychodynamic frame of reference but was included in our search because of its use of creative expression as an occupational therapy intervention tool. These authors define *supportive care* in oncology as "any treatment or service designed to help people cope with cancer and its psychological, physical, and emotional consequences" (p. 1). Activities that encourage emotional expression are considered to be supportive care within this definition.

This description is clearly consistent with the psychodynamic frame of reference. But is an opinion paper considered evidence?

Evidence-based practice standards focus on high-quality research studies but also incorporate evidence from clinical experience and expert opinion. None of the other recent papers in the search were specific research studies built around the psychodynamic frame of reference. This should lead us to consider that the evidence for this approach is weak. However, the paper by Sleight and Stein Duker (2016) focused on expressive emotional support without specific reference to the term *psychodynamic.*

If we expand our search by replacing the term *psychodynamic* with the term *expressive,* we see many more papers, some of which are true research papers. Of these we will review Cooper and Davis' (2016) paper, *Using Writing as Therapy: Finding Identity—An Evaluation of Its Effects Upon Clinical Outcomes and Service.* This is a well-organized study with 36 participants. Like the Sleight and Stein Duker (2016) article, the authors did not state that they were using a psychodynamic frame of reference, but the writing intervention strategy that they report is consistent with the frame of reference as we have presented it. This study has promising findings and could serve to support future interventions of this type.

There is little science supporting the psychodynamic frame of reference. In spite of this, this frame of reference has endured, with a presence in the occupational therapy literature for nearly as long as there has been occupational therapy literature. This frame of reference considers individual strength-based creative interventions that are aimed at emotional expression. There is no current research that specifically identifies itself as "psychodynamic," but there is current research in occupational therapy and other fields that supports the use of this frame of reference. Focusing on the essential aspects of creative expression and creative problem solving, there are some interventions described in the scientific literature that are consistent with the psychodynamic frame of reference.

Art-Based Activities as Psychodynamic Interventions Used in Occupational Therapy

Art has been shown to be beneficial in helping clients express themselves in a nonverbal manner (Thomas, Gray, McGinty, & Ebringer, 2011). Although occupational therapy practitioners are not art therapists, the use of arts and crafts as a tool is often used as a therapeutic activity for creative expression within the psychodynamic frame of reference. This frame of reference includes participation in daily occupations but does not include "talk" psychoanalysis, so occupational therapy practitioners do not interpret a client's art; rather, they rely on clients to interpret their own work.

When art is used in group settings, clients can, in addition to gaining insight from their own interpretation of their art, receive feedback from other group members. Expressive therapy through art activities have been shown to improve several mental illness symptoms in people of different ages (Slayton, D'Archer, & Kaplan, 2010). Use of art in occupational therapy can be either free form or guided.

For example, to encourage positive self-regard, an occupational therapy group in a psychiatric inpatient facility decided to make shamrocks as a project for St. Patrick's Day. Each group member was given a plain paper shamrock and instructed to write on the stem the words "I am lucky." They were asked to decorate the paper and write statements on each leaf describing what they feel makes them lucky. Participants were then asked to share their statements with the group. The therapist encouraged interaction among the group members and helped the participants come up with positive statements by asking open-ended questions. Group members expressed how the activity helped to remind them that there were many positive aspects of their lives that they took for granted.

Case Example 4.1 presents Benjamin, who was referred to occupational therapy in a mental health practice setting.

CASE EXAMPLE 4.1. BENJAMIN: USING THE PSYCHODYNAMIC FRAME OF REFERENCE IN OCCUPATIONAL THERAPY INTERVENTION

Benjamin, age 35 years, was divorced and diagnosed with schizoaffective disorder. He had great difficulty verbally expressing himself.

During Benjamin's occupational therapy evaluation (see Exhibit 4.2 for his occupational profile), he mentioned that his psychotherapist had suggested journaling as a means to access his unconscious mind. His coping skills were poor, and he often turned to illegal drugs. He stated that the only things that gave him any pleasure in life were his 2 young children. His goals from therapy were to gain independence in his daily life, get a job, and regain visitation rights with his children.

As he and his occupational therapist developed rapport, Benjamin shared some of his journal entries, which were very dark and foreboding. They reflected

EXHIBIT 4.2.	Benjamin's Occupational Profile	
Client	**Reason the client is seeking service and concerns related to engagement in occupations**	Referred to occupational therapy for impairments in basic organizational skills, self-regulation, and use of effective cognitive strategies to plan, sequence, and persist with daily obligations. *Impact on occupation:* Benjamin has drifted from an unskilled job to another, staying an average of 2 months in any single job. He becomes frustrated with problems at work and stops attending. When he is inevitably fired, he often turns to drugs and alcohol until he returns to the psychiatric hospital. He is currently homeless and lives either in shelters or on the street.
	Occupations in which the client is successful	Benjamin is independent in basic ADLs, although he does not always have the physical resources to complete these tasks.
	Personal interests and values	Benjamin is interested in his children and values his role as a father.
	Occupational history (i.e., life experiences)	Benjamin was diagnosed with schizoaffective disorder when he was age 23 years. At that time he was married and working as a department manager in a large grocery store where he had worked since high school. After his second child was born, he began to become increasingly depressed. He often turned to alcohol to help cope with the demands of a growing family and increased financial pressure. He was hospitalized several times for his alcohol abuse, leading to the loss of his job. His wife left him shortly after he lost his job. He has been drifting ever since.
	Performance patterns (routines, roles, habits, and rituals)	At this time, Benjamin's only valued life role is his role as a father. He does not value his role as an ex-husband, because he feels he has failed as a husband and provider. Although he had previously worked toward becoming a store manager for the grocery store chain, he has given up on this possible role.

(Continued)

CASE EXAMPLE 4.1. BENJAMIN: USING THE PSYCHODYNAMIC FRAME OF REFERENCE IN OCCUPATIONAL THERAPY INTERVENTION *(Cont.)*

EXHIBIT 4.2.	Benjamin's Occupational Profile *(Cont.)*		
Environment		*Supports to occupational engagement*	*Barriers to occupational engagement*
	Physical (e.g., buildings, furniture, pets)	Benjamin has no difficulties with physical accessibility.	Benjamin does not have a regular place of residence.
	Social (e.g., spouse, friends, caregivers)		Benjamin has very few friends, and those whom he identifies as friends are people with whom he drinks and does drugs.
Context	**Cultural** (e.g., customs, beliefs)	No cultural challenges were identified in the assessment process.	
	Personal (e.g., age, gender, SES, education)	35-year-old male. High school diploma. Currently living in poverty.	
	Temporal (e.g., stage of life, time, year)		Benjamin is in middle adulthood and is socially expected to have paid employment, have his own home, and support his children.
	Virtual (e.g., chat, email, remote monitoring)	Benjamin is able to use telephone and to type.	Does not have a regular access to virtual context.
Client goals	**Client's priorities and desired targeted outcomes**	Benjamin wants to be able to keep a job and get his own apartment. He would like to have a greater role in his children's lives.	
	ANALYSIS OF PARTICIPATION		
	Basic ADLs		
Eating/oral–motor	Benjamin has no difficulty in this area.		
Grooming	Benjamin has no difficulty in this area, but he often neglects to shave or comb his hair.		
Bathing/transfer	Benjamin has no difficulty in this area.		
Dressing upper body	Benjamin has no difficulty in this area.		
Dressing lower body	Benjamin has no difficulty in this area.		
Toileting	Benjamin has no difficulty in this area.		
Problem solving/memory	Benjamin does not like problems and has great difficulty making decisions, even simple ones. He often ignores problems or puts off things to avoid dealing with them. This has proven to be a dysfunctional pattern, leading him to conclude that no matter what he does, it will turn out badly.		
Comments:	Benjamin has given up on things he once found enjoyable. He lives in a revolving pattern of depression, homelessness, and drugs.		
	IADLs		
Community mobility	Benjamin has no difficulty in this area. He does not drive, nor does he own a vehicle, but he is able to walk or use public transportation as needed.		

(Continued)

CASE EXAMPLE 4.1. BENJAMIN: USING THE PSYCHODYNAMIC FRAME OF REFERENCE IN OCCUPATIONAL THERAPY INTERVENTION *(Cont.)*

EXHIBIT 4.2.	Benjamin's Occupational Profile *(Cont.)*
Health management/prevention	Lately, Benjamin has been more compliant with attending group therapy at the local mental health center and with taking his medications. He has a history of having periods of adequate health management followed by periods of noncompliance due to drug and alcohol abuse.
Home management	Benjamin does now have his own home.
Financial management	This is an area of concern due to Benjamin's disorganization and lack of steady employment.
Leisure	Benjamin is unable to identify any satisfying leisure activities.
Safety	Benjamin has no difficulty in this area.
Comments:	Benjamin often relies on others to manage his IADLs. The social workers at the hospital frequently help him get things back on track, but once he is discharged, his pattern of learned helplessness causes him to revert back to his dysfunctional ways.
	Motor and Praxis Skills
Sitting: static/dynamic	Benjamin has no difficulty in this area.
Standing: static/dynamic	Benjamin has no difficulty in this area.
Joint stability and skeletal mobility	Benjamin has no difficulty in this area.
Place can on shelf	Benjamin has no difficulty in this area.
Retrieve item from floor	Benjamin has no difficulty in this area.
Screw lid on jar	Benjamin has no difficulty in this area.
Comb back of head	Benjamin has no difficulty in this area.
Writing	Benjamin can write his name and address using a pen. He has difficulty locating the needed keys on a standard keyboard. Benjamin can operate the computer, using both the keyboard and the mouse.
Lift grocery bag	Benjamin has no difficulty in this area.
Coordination	Poor. Benjamin can to move limbs independently and engage in both simple and more complex tasks that are familiar, but he is easily distracted, and his lack of attention impairs his coordination.
Manipulation	Benjamin consistently prefers his right hand for skilled activity. He has good grip strength.
Comments:	None.
	Process Skills
Energy for task	Benjamin is physically able to do most tasks but seems detached and does not exert himself or have interest in the quality of his performance.
Knowledge/organization of task	Benjamin can function within familiar environments and historically would appropriately work on tasks once he started them. His skills in this area have decreased, and he often needs direct supervision to initiate and perform tasks.
Adaptation/praxis	Benjamin's praxis is adequate, but he is poor at recognizing and adapting to errors in his performance.
Comments:	None.

(Continued)

CASE EXAMPLE 4.1. BENJAMIN: USING THE PSYCHODYNAMIC FRAME OF REFERENCE IN OCCUPATIONAL THERAPY INTERVENTION *(Cont.)*

EXHIBIT 4.2.	**Benjamin's Occupational Profile** *(Cont.)*
Behavioral and Cognitive Skills	
Communication and following social conventions	Benjamin's receptive and expressive language are within normal limits.
Cognitive and emotional regulation skills	Benjamin is easily frustrated and responds with cursing and angry outbursts when frustrated.
Level of arousal/attention	Benjamin is easily distracted, even in 1:1 settings.
Orientation	Benjamin is alert and oriented to person, place, time, and events.
Energy and drive	Benjamin is motivated to "make things better" but lacks the ability to plan or form a strategy for change because he "doesn't see the point in trying because things always turn out badly."
Memory and understanding	Benjamin can understand and follow a series of 2 or more related instructions but does not anticipate problems and does not problem solve solutions when familiar strategies do not work. He does not ask for help if he does not understand instructions and instead relies on random guessing. Benjamin has difficulty with coworkers and is afraid that he will anger them if he asks questions. He often believes that his coworkers do not like him, causing him to avoid interacting with them.
Higher level cognition	Benjamin has difficulty with many executive function skills, including keeping track of time, making plans, ensuring work is finished on time, and looking for help or more information when it is needed.
Sensory–Perceptual Skills	
Sensory	Benjamin has no difficulty in this area.
Self-perception	Benjamin has poor self-awareness and a generally negative view of himself and situations.
Pain	Benjamin has no difficulty in this area.
Skin integrity	Benjamin's skin is intact.
Comments:	None.

Note. Occupational profile template from American Occupational Therapy Association (2017). Analysis of participation format adapted from Skubik-Peplaski, Paris, Boyle, & Culpert (2009). ADLs = activities of daily living; IADLs = instrumental activities of daily living; SES = socioeconomic status.

his intense fear of failure and felt that society was against him.

Because the journaling suggested he liked writing, the occupational therapist suggested that Benjamin write a story for his children. He was very interested in writing the children's story, because he seldom saw his children and it could help him stay connected to them. With the help of his occupational therapist, he wrote a short story suitable for young children. In doing this he was able to express both his fears and the things that made him happy. He also felt that he had a way to interact with his children. He enjoyed this activity and began to write other stories that were

interesting to him and focused on positive outcomes to situations and challenged his distorted thinking patterns.

Over time and with support from his therapist, Benjamin was able to assimilate the positive skills he wrote about into positive personal coping skills and this fostered a more functional relationship with his children and ex-wife. Following his intervention using expressive writing, Benjamin has returned to his own apartment, is working in the grocery business on a part-time basis, and continues to work with his therapist. With the help of social services, he now has supervised visitations with his children.

APPLYING THE PSYCHODYNAMIC FRAME OF REFERENCE IN CLINICAL REASONING

The psychodynamic frame of reference offers a tool to consider the inner workings of the mind and of feelings. It has always been widely used by occupational therapy practitioners in mental health settings. Aspects associated with this frame of reference (e.g., imagery, visualization, creative expression) are now often incorporated into pain management and supportive care settings (Williamson, 2016). Importantly, the psychodynamic frame of reference provides a clinical reasoning path that uses nonlinear thinking.

An important aspect of effective clinical reasoning is the incorporation of nonlinear thinking. *Linear thinking* is a process of thought that follows a step-by-step progression where a response to a step must be elicited before another step is taken. It is the type of thinking most often used in science and medicine. The clinical pathways described earlier are a result of linear thinking. *Nonlinear thinking* is reasoning characterized by expansion of thought in multiple directions rather than in a single, stepwise direction. Nonlinear thinking is inherently creative, very much like brainstorming, allowing unhindered thought to flow in an attempt to discover something special in the process.

Time and growing scientific evidence has shown that most of Freud's original assumptions were false. As the scientific field of psychology grew from Freud's early work, psychoanalytic theory evolved with a focus narrowed to the supportable aspects of psychodynamic theory. Its application in the field of occupational therapy mirrors this evolution. The contemporary psychodynamic frame of reference focuses almost exclusively on ego functions and emotional expression. As the body of science grows in the area of expressive therapies and nonlinear thinking, we may see the emergence of a new frame of reference that is science based but has its origins in psychodynamic theory.

The *half-life of knowledge* is the amount of time that has to elapse before half of the knowledge in a particular area is superseded, refined to exclude errors, or shown to be untrue (Arbesman, 2012). As explained by Arbesman, this means that if scientific knowledge is growing by a factor of 10 every 50 years, half of what scientists may have known about a particular subject will be wrong or obsolete in 45 years. As we move forward in our consideration of frames of reference, it is important to understand that

- Knowledge is not static,
- Maintaining expertise requires an active and curious mind, and
- Theories that are not studied or refined are likely to fall into disuse.

Theory can be a good foundation for clinical reasoning, but it is best if supported by science. Psychodynamic theory has persisted in usefulness in occupational therapy because it offers an explanation and framework to consider something that has not been reliably captured by scientific research: an understanding of emotions and personality. The practitioner's thinking that is triggered through consideration of the psychodynamic model remains important to occupational therapy clinical reasoning, but other more empirically supported approaches informed by cognitive neuroscience and behavioral science theories are preferred in the context of evidence-based practice.

In Chapter 3, the neurodevelopmental therapy (NDT) frame of reference was introduced. Like the psychodynamic, the NDT frame of reference offers something distinctive, even though the supporting science is not there. NDT has largely been supplanted by the science-driven motor learning frame of reference. Current NDT practitioners usually use a combination of traditional NDT approaches with science-driven motor learning approaches. Similarly, practitioners using the psychodynamic frame of reference tend to pair it with a scientifically rigorous additional frame of reference, such as a combination of psychodynamic with the developmental systems frame of reference.

DEVELOPMENTAL SYSTEMS FRAME OF REFERENCE

An aspect of Freud's original theory that is not addressed in the occupational therapy psychodynamic frame of reference is his consideration of the individual's developmental life course. Freud considered developmental differences in his discussion of psychosexual stages and was one of the first scientists to identify developmental stages as important, but Freud's psychosexual stages have been replaced by more contemporary science and are seldom considered in contemporary practice in any health field. Although Freud's psychosexual stage model is no longer used, extensive study and data collection in human development has taken place.

Study of human development considers 2 essential processes:

1. *Maturation:* process of the individual's biological, social, and emotional change from a simple to a more complex level of function, and
2. *Development:* changes in performance that are learned but heavily influenced by maturational processes.

Developmental systems theory (DST) is a collection of models of maturation and development that incorporate contemporary science as a tool to explain human development, reflecting the contributions of genes, environment, and factors within the individual that affect the emergence of a more mature individual (Crain, 2010). It is from DST that the developmental systems frame of reference is derived. The elements of the developmental systems frame of reference are presented in Exhibit 4.3.

EXHIBIT 4.3. **Elements of the Developmental Systems Frame of Reference**

- **Focus:** The developmental systems frame of reference is the knowledge of human maturation and development, including the contributions of genes, environment, and factors within the individual that affect participation in daily occupations.
- **Basic assumptions:**
  - Individual development occurs over changing times and places within an individual's lifespan that can be assessed in terms of health trajectories—predicted pattern of health or disablement that is likely given the internal and external influences on the individual as they develop and mature.
  - Individual development occurs within a specific point in history that affects the developmental process. Health trajectories may start or change over the life course on the basis of individual, social, and economic influences.
  - Early experiences can "program" an individual's future health and development in a positive or negative manner. Although adverse events can negatively affect any point in a person's life course, the impact will be greatest if the adverse event occurs during a sensitive period of development.
  - Individual choice and personal motivations are essential influencers on development throughout the lifespan.
- **Function–disability continuum:** This frame of reference considers function to be successful physical maturation and acquisition of skills to allow performance of skills and community participation at the level expected on the basis of the individual's chronological age. Dysfunction is reflected in patterns of developmental delay or atypical developmental trajectories that do not support age-appropriate performance and participation.
- **Postulates of change:** Change can occur by offering contextual supports to maturation and development, including actions that improve or restore health and function, improve or restore supportive aspects of the individual's environment (including family support), and increase opportunities for learning needed skills.

Like the psychodynamic frame of reference, the developmental systems frame of reference is widely used in all areas of occupational therapy practice. The developmental systems frame of reference differs from the psychodynamic frame of reference because it is supported by substantial scientific evidence. Human maturation and development result in observable changes that can be easily observed and scientifically measured. This frame of reference is sometimes used as stand-alone frame of reference, but it is as often used as an adjunct to other frames of reference to embed a longitudinal context of the person's age, level of maturation, and occupational performance trajectory of change over time.

In Chapter 1, "Overview of the Clinical Reasoning Process," the humorous concept of *knobology,* a lazy approach to clinical practice where the "why" of a modality is ignored, was introduced. Knobology is seldom a concern with the 2 frames of reference presented in this chaper because there is no rote path to intervention offered by either frame of reference. With these 2 frames of reference we are more likely to see hasty generalization as described in Practice Wisdom 4.1. *Hasty generalization* occurs in clinical reasoning when decisions are made on the basis of superficial information. The generalization that an intervention is justified is impulsively assumed rather than reflectively considered.

For example, the psychodynamic and the developmental systems frames of reference are foundational and widely used in occupational therapy practice, but it would be a hasty generalization to assume that every arts and crafts activity automatically is supported by the psychodynamic frame of reference or that use of toys in therapy with children automatically assures that a developmentally appropriate intervention is occurring.

As noted earlier, it is acceptable to use more than a single frame of reference to support clinical reasoning as long as the elements of the frames of reference used are compatible. In the case of Benjamin (Case Example 4.1), the developmental systems frame of reference would help to highlight the expected social performance levels to guide goal setting and would still be consistent with the elements of the psychodynamic frame of reference. Another example of combining these 2 approaches is presented Case Example 4.2.

The approach to intervention in Julia's case is developmentally appropriate, respecting the typical fears and cognitive development of a 2-year-old while encouraging active participation and offering a tool to express emotions for which she will not have words. Even typically developing 2-year-old children are challenged to express their feelings and fears through language, and the complex experiences Julia must face makes expression even more challenging. The psychodynamic frame of reference was used when choosing art and imagery to offer Julia an avenue to express her fears and frustrations. The case also demonstrates the cohesion between the psychodynamic and developmental systems frames of reference. Through engagement in play activities that encourage both movement and emotional expression, Julia's recovery should be optimized.

PRACTICE WISDOM 4.1. **Hasty Generalization**

"Hasty generalization is a term used in the study of logic that describes what occurs when the contents of an argument's stated premises fail to adequately support its proposed conclusion. In other words, the logical error of hasty generalization occurs when the individual reaches an inductive generalization based on insufficient evidence."

CASE EXAMPLE 4.2. JULIA: INTEGRATING DEVELOPMENTAL SYSTEMS AND PSYCHODYNAMIC FRAMES OF REFERENCE IN OCCUPATIONAL THERAPY INTERVENTION

Julia is age 2 years, 4 months. Her mom decided to take her to the doctor on Monday morning to have her examined, assuming Julia just had a sore chest from coughing and an earache. Julia's pediatrician was suspicious and ordered several diagnostic tests, and within the day the family learned that she had a tumor in the left upper-chest cavity, and within the next weeks she was given the diagnosis of Stage 4, Group 4, high-risk embryonal rhabdomyosarcoma, a type of soft-tissue malignant tumor that accounts for approximately 3.5% of the cases of cancer among children ages 0–14 years (National Cancer Institute, 2017). Julia had 6 weeks of chemotherapy and radiation treatment with supportive occupational therapy during the cancer treatment and currently during Julia's recovery from cancer treatment. Exhibit 4.4 provides her occupational profile.

Julia's physicians and parents want her to work to regain full active left arm movement. Her fearfulness has limited her progress in therapy, and she has resisted play and social opportunities that her parents have offered. Julia has many developmentally typical patterns, including fears of pain and being separated from her parents, which have been compounded by the negative experience associated with her cancer treatment. Julia knows she had cancer and that the painful things she disliked had to happen to "kill the cancer." Julia likes to play "kill the cancer" games as part of her therapy.

Julia's occupational therapist is careful to talk to Julia about what she is doing, especially during the range of motion (ROM) exercises for her left arm. Today they have an easel and paintbrush. While the

EXHIBIT 4.4.	Julia's Occupational Profile		
Client	**Reason the client is seeking service and concerns related to engagement in occupations**	Referral for family support for ADL training, parent education, and child developmental support.	
	Occupations in which the client is successful	Julia has age-appropriate occupational performance in basic ADLs, social participation, play, sleep and rest, and education prior to cancer treatment.	
	Personal interests and values	Julia likes to be read to and to watch videos. Julia likes princesses.	
	Occupational history (i.e., life experiences)	Julia is a survivor of Stage 4, Group 4, high-risk embryonal rhabdomyosarcoma. Julia had 6 weeks of chemotherapy and radiation treatment with supportive OT during cancer treatment and is currently in remission. She has been immune suppressed with very limited access to other children since her cancer diagnosis. Julia is an only child and very dependent on her mother. *Impact on occupation:* Julia is limited in her ability to develop skills due to limited ROM in left shoulder and upper limb.	
	Performance patterns (routines, roles, habits, & rituals)	*Occupational roles:* Daughter, niece, granddaughter, cancer survivor. As a preschool child, Julia's routines and habits are managed by the adults in her life.	
Environment		*Supports to occupational engagement*	*Barriers to occupational engagement*
	Physical (e.g., buildings, furniture, pets)	Julia has no difficulty accessing her environment.	Julia fatigues easily.
	Social (e.g., spouse, friends, caregivers)	Julia lives with her parents.	Julia has had very little exposure to other children her age due to her suppressed immune system.

(Continued)

CASE EXAMPLE 4.2. JULIA: INTEGRATING DEVELOPMENTAL SYSTEMS AND PSYCHODYNAMIC FRAMES OF REFERENCE IN OCCUPATIONAL THERAPY INTERVENTION (Cont.)

EXHIBIT 4.4.	**Julia's Occupational Profile (Cont.)**	
Context	**Cultural** (e.g., customs, beliefs)	No issues related to culture or beliefs were identified during assessment.
	Personal (e.g., age, gender, SES, education)	Age 2 years, 4 months. Female.
	Temporal (e.g., stage of life, time, year)	Julia is in early childhood and depends on others for organizing her daily occupations.
	Virtual (e.g., chat, email, remote monitoring)	Not applicable in this case.
Client goals	**Client's priorities and desired targeted outcomes**	To return to daily activities in a manner that is pain-free and includes the full use of her right arm.
ANALYSIS OF PARTICIPATION		
Basic ADLs		
Eating/oral–motor	Julia finger-feeds herself and can use a spoon.	
Grooming	Julia washes her hands with supervision. She cooperates with face washing, hair care, and toothbrushing.	
Bathing/transfer	Julia can get in and out of the bathtub with parent supervision. She is age appropriate in bathing performance.	
Dressing upper body	Julia cooperates with dressing by pushing her right arm through a sleeve. She has limited left trunk and shoulder mobility and relies on others to assist with dressing the left side of body.	
Dressing lower body	Julia likes to wear dresses and skirts and is age appropriate in her ability to put them on. She assists with putting on pants.	
Toileting	Julia's family has not yet started toilet training with her. She wears diapers and is dependent in diaper management.	
Problem solving/memory	Julia has typical problem-solving and memory skills for his age.	
Comments:	Julia still complains of pain with weight bearing in the left arm and limits use of this arm.	
IADLs		
Community mobility	Julia depends on her family for all aspects of community mobility.	
Health management/prevention	Julia is age appropriate in being dependent on adults in this area.	
Home management	Julia is age appropriate in being dependent on adults in this area.	
Financial management	Julia is age appropriate in being dependent on adults in this area.	
Leisure	Julia is a quiet child who enjoys princess movies and her tablet computer. She is fearful and anxious and prefers to stay near a parent.	
Safety	Julia is age appropriate in being dependent on adults in this area.	
Comments:	Julia is afraid of being separated from her parents.	

(Continued)

CASE EXAMPLE 4.2. JULIA: INTEGRATING DEVELOPMENTAL SYSTEMS AND PSYCHODYNAMIC FRAMES OF REFERENCE IN OCCUPATIONAL THERAPY INTERVENTION (Cont.)

EXHIBIT 4.4.	Julia's Occupational Profile (Cont.)
Motor and Praxis Skills	
Sitting: Static/dynamic	Julia is able to sit well independently. Her static sitting is adequate. She can maintain her posture during dynamic sitting, but she tires easily.
Standing: Static/dynamic	Julia's static standing is adequate. She can adjust her standing posture to activity demands but does not have good dynamic balance.
Joint stability and skeletal mobility	Julia has moderate limitations in active left shoulder flexion, external rotation, and internal rotation. She had some tightness in the left axillary region and complains of pain during PROM. Julia has full PROM in all joints.
Place can on shelf	Test was adapted to have her stack 3 1-in. cubes on a table. She was able to perform the task with her right hand using a controlled release pattern.
Retrieve item from floor	Julia is mobile and can move to and from the floor effectively.
Screw lid on jar	Julia is unable to do this. It is not a developmentally appropriate task for her.
Comb back of head	Julia is unable to do this. It is not a developmentally appropriate task for her.
Write name	Julia is unable to do this. It is not a developmentally appropriate task for her.
Lift grocery bag	Julia is unable to do this. It is not a developmentally appropriate task for her.
Coordination	Julia uses her arms in a unilateral pattern and is unable to perform bimanual tasks (e.g., buttoning, cutting). She can run and hop, but she does this only for a short period of time.
Manipulation	Julia can hold an object distally with the fingers of either hand.
Comments:	Julia has age-appropriate motor movements but has limited strength, coordination, and endurance.
Process Skills	
Energy for task	Julia is below average in this area. She is hesitant to try new things and does not persist at tasks that require physical effort.
Knowledge/organization of task	Julia can perform cognitive tasks at an age-appropriate level.
Communication and social skills	Julia is able to understand and follow discussions. Her verbal communication is age appropriate.
Cognitive and emotional regulation skills	Julia is anxious and fearful.
Level of arousal/attention	Julia attends well for her age.
Orientation	Julia is age appropriate in this area.
Energy and drive	Julia is below average in this area.
Higher level cognition	Julia is age appropriate in this area.
Comments:	Julia scored at the 24-month level for social–emotional skills on the developmental assessment. She understands the concept of sharing, family rules, and routines. She enjoys simple make believe and laughs at incongruous events. This score is within the typical range for her age.
Sensory–Perceptual Skills	
General sensory	Julia has intact basic sensory function.
Hearing and Vision	Julia has normal vision and hearing.

(Continued)

CASE EXAMPLE 4.2. JULIA: INTEGRATING DEVELOPMENTAL SYSTEMS AND PSYCHODYNAMIC FRAMES OF REFERENCE IN OCCUPATIONAL THERAPY INTERVENTION *(Cont.)*

EXHIBIT 4.4.   Julia's Occupational Profile *(Cont.)*

Self-perception	Julia is age appropriate in this area.
Pain	Julia complains of left trunk and shoulder pain. She is fearful and limits her activity because of her experience with painful medical procedures.
Skin integrity	Julia's skin is intact.
Comments:	None.

Note. Occupational profile template from American Occupational Therapy Association (2017). Analysis of participation format adapted from Skubik-Peplaski, Paris, Boyle, & Culpert (2009). ADLs = activities of daily living; IADLs = instrumental activities of daily living; OT = occupational therapy; PROM = passive range of motion; ROM = range of motion.

therapist does the painful ROM exercises, he asks Julia what she thinks the cancer "bugs" look like. After completing the exercises he draws cartoon bugs on the easel, following Julia's guidance. Julia then gets to hold the paintbrush in her left hand, and with big arm movements paints over the "bugs" so they can no longer be seen. Julia is also encouraged to do exercises on her stuffed animals and to explain to them that if they are brave they can paint a picture, too.

SUMMARY

This chapter provided an in-depth exploration of widely used frames of reference in the field of occupational therapy. The psychodynamic frame of reference was introduced first because of its importance, widespread applicability, and frequent confusion with older Freudian views taught in general psychology courses. The psychodynamic frame of reference is still more theory based than driven by scientific evidence, but it persists because there is a need for guidance in the assessment and goal setting that does not focus on physical ability but on mental and emotional functions.

The psychodynamic frame of reference is an invaluable resource for occupational therapy practitioners as either a stand-alone frame of reference, as it is typically used in mental health settings, or as an adjunct to frames of reference that focus on physical functions in other practice areas. This frame of reference potentially offers clinical reasoning support in all 5 of the broad categories of occupational therapy services: (1) remediation, (2) maintenance, (3) compensation, (4) development, and (5) education.

Practitioners should consider evidence from the scientific literature in clinical reasoning as well as from client needs and goals. In the cases of Benjamin and Julia, motivation was a key concern that affected their ability to achieve desired goals. The psychodynamic frame of reference supported functional performance through use of creative expression to build on strengths and develop the needed internal confidence and motivation to move toward goals.

The developmental systems frame of reference is more science driven than theory driven, but like the psychodynamic approach, it is not likely to be specifically cited in research and scholarly work as a specific frame of reference. Like the psychodynamic frame of reference, the developmental systems frame of reference offers clinical reasoning support as either a stand-alone frame of reference, because it is typically used in early childhood settings or as an adjunct to frames of reference. This frame of reference also potentially offers clinical reasoning support in all 5 of the broad categories of occupational therapy services.

This chapter introduced the idea of the half-life of facts to offer a rationale for the critical analysis of frames of reference and the need for continuous consideration of new information in clinical reasoning. In both of the frames of reference presented in this chapter, new knowledge has supplanted older beliefs and has altered our understanding of human functioning. For example, it is now known that early exposure to extremely fearful events affects the developing brain, particularly in those areas involved in emotions and learning (National Scientific Council on the Developing Child, 2010). Failure to address Julia's fears as part of her therapy could lead to ongoing activity and social limitations as she matures. Both frames of reference described in this chapter would guide the practitioner to focus on Julia's emotional needs and offer her the best possible recovery experience.

Flexibility and adaptability in application of the psychodynamic and developmental systems frames of reference are partly why they are so widely used in occupational therapy practice. As we will see in later in this text, many of the frames of reference with strong scientific support are more narrowly focused and more specific to only some of categories of occupational therapy service.

LEARNING ACTIVITIES

1. Evidence-based practice typically centers on a clinical question rather than about a frame of reference. This is the main reason that it is hard to find scholarly evidence on specific frames of reference. Develop a clinical question for the cases of Benjamin and Julia that would address aspects of ego functioning described in this chapter.

2. Building on your work from Question 1, make a table with 2 columns and identify the support you find that uses scientific reasoning in the first column and support gained through narrative reasoning in the second column to answer the clinical question.

3. Read Gunnarsson, Wagman, Håkansson, and Hedin, (2015). Is the Tree Theme Method consistent with occupational therapy's psychodynamic frame of reference? Why or why not?

4. In this chapter, 2 examples of expressive interventions were offered: (1) art activity and (2) creative writing. Think of another expressive activity that you enjoy. Look in your favorite search engine and see if that activity has been used in a clinical setting. Discuss what you think are the potential advantages and drawbacks of the activity you chose.

5. The NDT frame of reference was introduced in Chapter 3. This is another frame of reference that, like the psychodynamic frame of reference, has a historical foundation and little recent research to support its use. Write a short paper expressing your opinion about why these approaches continue to be used and whether you support their continued use in occupational therapy practice.

REFERENCES

Ainsworth, M. (1973). The development of infant–mother attachment. In B. Cardwell & H. Ricciuti (Eds.), *Review of child development research* (Vol. 3, pp. 1–94) Chicago: University of Chicago Press.

American Occupational Therapy Association. (2017). AOTA occupational profile template. *American Journal of Occupational Therapy, 71*(Suppl. 2), 7112420030. https://doi.org/10.5014/ajot.716S12

Arbesman, S. (2012). Q & A: Samuel Arbesman. The half life of facts. *The Economist* [Blog post]. Retrieved from http://www.economist.com/blogs/babbage/2012/11/qa-samuel-arbesman

Beck, A., & Hurvich, M. (1959). Psychological correlates of depression: Frequency of masochistic dream content in a private practice sample. *Psychosomatic Medicine.* https://doi.org/10.1097/00006842-195901000-00007

Beck, A., & Ward, C. (1961). Dreams of depressed patients characteristic themes in manifest content. *Archives of General Psychiatry, 5,* 462–467. https://doi.org/10.1001/archpsyc.1961.01710170040004

Bellak, L., Hurvich, M., & Gediman, H. (1973). *Ego functions in schizophrenics, neurotics, and normal: A systematic study of the conceptual, diagnostic, and therapeutic aspects.* New York: Wiley.

Bowlby, J. (1969). *Attachment. Attachment and loss: Vol. 1—Loss.* New York: Basic Books.

Brown, C., Stoffel, V., & Muñoz, J. P. (Eds.). (2011). *Occupational therapy in mental health: A vision for participation.* Philadelphia: F. A. Davis.

Bruce, M., & Borg, B. (2002). *Psychosocial frames of reference: Core for occupation-based practice* (3rd ed.) Thorofare, NJ: Slack.

Cole, M. (2012). *Group dynamics in occupational therapy* (4th ed.). Thorofare, NJ: Slack.

Cole, M., & Tufano, R. (2008). *Applied theories in occupational therapy: A practical approach.* Thorofare, NJ: Slack.

Cooper, P. R., & Davis, D. A. (2016). Using writing as therapy: Finding identity—An evaluation of its effects upon clinical outcomes and service. *International Journal of Therapy and Rehabilitation, 23,* 64–74. https://doi.org/10.12968/ijtr.2016.23.2.64

Crain, W. (2010). *Theories of development: Concepts and applications* (6th ed.). Florence, KY: Taylor & Francis.

Danzer, G. (2012). Integrating ego psychology and strengths-based social work. *Journal of Theory Construction and Testing, 16,* 9–15. Retrieved from https://www.researchgate.net/profile/Graham_Danzer/publication/259744067_Integrating_Ego_Psychology_and_Strengths-Based_Social_Work/links/00b4952d8ca56d9f5a000000/Integrating-Ego-Psychology-and-Strengths-Based-Social-Work.pdf

Fidler, G., & Fidler, J. (1963). *Occupational therapy.* Los Angeles: University of California Press.

Freud, S. (1923). *The ego and the id.* Retrieved from https://www.sigmundfreud.net/the-ego-and-the-id-pdf-ebook.jsp

Gunnarsson, A. B., Wagman, P., Håkansson, C., & Hedin, K. (2015). The Tree Theme Method® (TTM): An occupational therapy intervention for treating depression and anxiety: Study protocol of a randomized controlled trial. *BMC Psychology, 3,* 1–7. https://doi.org/10.1186/s40359-015-0097-9

Mandich, M. (2015). Classic theories of human development. In A. Cronin & M. Mandich (Eds.), *Human development and performance throughout the lifespan* (2nd ed., pp. 38–59). Boston: Cengage Learning.

National Cancer Institute. (2017). *Childhood rhabdomyosarcoma treatment: (PDQ®)—Health professional version.* Retrieved from https://www.cancer.gov/types/soft-tissue-sarcoma/hp/rhabdomyosarcoma-treatment-pdq

National Scientific Council on the Developing Child. (2010). *Persistent fear and anxiety can affect young children's learning and development.* Retrieved from https://developingchild.harvard.edu/resources/persistent-fear-and-anxiety-can-affect-young-childrens-learning-and-development/

Rholes, W. S., & Simpson, J. A. (2004). Attachment theory: Basic concepts and contemporary questions. In W. S. Rholes & J. A. Simpson (Eds.), *Adult attachment: Theory, research, and clinical implications* (pp. 3–14). New York: Guilford.

Skubik-Peplaski, C., Paris, C., Collins Boyle, D., & Culpert, A. (Eds.). (2009). *Applying the* Occupational Therapy Practice Framework: *Using the Cardinal Hill Occupational Participation Process in client-centered care* (2nd ed.). Bethesda, MD: AOTA Press.

Slayton, S., D'Archer, J., & Kaplan, F. (2010). Outcome studies on the efficacy of art therapy: A review of findings. *Art Therapy: Journal of the American Art Therapy Association, 27,* 108–118.

Sleight, A. G., & Stein Duker, L. I. (2016). Toward a broader role for occupational therapy in supportive oncology care. *American Journal of Occupational Therapy, 70,* 7004360030. https://doi.org/10.5014/ajot.2016.018101

Theory. (2016). In *Merriam Webster's dictionary.* Retrieved from http://www.merriam-webster.com/dictionary/theory.

Thomas, Y., Gray, M., McGinty, S., & Ebringer, S. (2011). Homeless adults engagement in art: First steps towards identity, recovery and social inclusion. *Australian Occupational Therapy Journal, 58,* 429–436. https://doi.org/10.1111/j.1440-1630.2011.00977.x

Wendland, L. V. (1956). Psychodynamic aspects of occupational therapy. *American Journal of Occupational Therapy,* 10244–10247.

Williamson, A. (2016). Brief psychological and hypnotic interventions in chronic pain management. *Journal of Contemporary Psychotherapy, 46,* 179–186. https://doi.org/10.1007/s10879-016-9327-6

Behavioral Science Frames of Reference

5

Anne Cronin, PhD, OTR/L, ATP, FAOTA, and Garth Graebe, MOT, OTR/L

CHAPTER HIGHLIGHTS

- Considers the behavioral science frames of reference as tools to illustrate theory development and organization.
- Explores the elements of the behavioral science frames of reference in a clinical reasoning context.
- Describes the function–dysfunction continuum within the behavioral science frames of reference.
- Reviews the state of the science supporting specific behavioral science frames of reference: social learning, applied behavior analysis, and cognitive–behavioral therapy.
- Introduces a hierarchy for considering level of evidence in clinical practice settings.
- Illustrates the use of a behavioral science frame of reference in occupational therapy intervention and in clinical reasoning through a case example.

KEY TERMS AND CONCEPTS

Applied behavior analysis	Early and intensive behavioral	Operant conditioning
Behavioral change	intervention	Positive reinforcement
Behavioral science	Emerging practice	Promising practice
Behavioral science frames of	Evidence-based practice	Science
reference	Evidence-informed practice	Self-regulation
Classical conditioning	Habit	Social learning theory
Cognitive–behavioral therapy	Learning	Theories
Cognitive strategy training	Modeling	Unsupported practice
Discrete trial training	Narrative reasoning	

In this chapter, readers will learn about the behavioral science frames of reference within the scope of occupational therapy's domain and process and consider the integration of science into clinical reasoning. The behavioral science frames of reference are good tools to illustrate this integration because they are built using the scientific method. These approaches all have a long history of rigorous research and data that have been used to refine them over time. Contemporary frames of reference that are discussed in this chapter include social learning, applied behavior analysis (ABA), and cognitive–behavioral therapy (CBT).

The psychodynamic frame of reference, presented in Chapter 4, "Psychodynamic and Developmental Systems Frames of Reference," is supported by theory but has limited support in the form of scientific evidence. The behavioral frames of reference in this chapter contrast with the psychodynamic frame of reference because they are all highly science driven, with their historical theory narrowed and refined to reflect science.

USE OF SCIENCE IN CLINICAL REASONING

The term *science* refers to "knowledge or a system of knowledge covering general truths or the operation of general laws especially as obtained and tested through scientific method" ("Science," 2016). This definition of *science* suggests not only an idea (i.e., theory) of how things work but also a systematic approach to testing the theory to ascertain facts. Theory and science are distinct but interrelated. *Theories* generate hypotheses that can be proved or disproved through scientific methods. Over time, as understanding changes, the originating theories guiding the science must also change. The evolution of behavioral science into distinct researchable frames of reference illustrates the growth of knowledge and of how knowledge leads to refinement and evolution within scientific theories.

The scientific literature on behavioral approaches to human performance is vast, and the reference to this literature in occupational therapy contexts is sometimes confusing. This confusion is because specific clinical behavioral frames of reference that are very distinct from each another all draw from the same early foundational work and, as in this chapter, are often presented together.

Behavioral science is "a branch of science (as psychology, sociology, or anthropology) that deals primarily with human action and often seeks to generalize about human behavior in society" ("Behavioral Science," 2016). Within the behavioral sciences, there are 2 distinct research pathways to exploring human behavior: (1) research grounded in neural function (i.e., information processing) and (2) research grounded in observable behavior (i.e., social and relational sciences). This chapter focuses on the latter.

In this text, *behavioral science frames of reference* include several distinct approaches to intervention, including social learning, cognitive–behavioral approaches, and ABA. They are often useful with clients who have difficulty learning needed behaviors, who lack structure in their lives, and who may need reinforcement from their environment or others to participate productively in occupations (Brown, Stoffel, & Muñoz, 2011). The behavioral science frames of reference rely heavily on the idea of conditioning through reinforcement and the support of positive habit formation.

The behavioral science frames of reference have given occupational therapy practitioners such valuable tools as reinforcement and modeling to shape new, more functional or desirable behaviors. For example, consider a person living in a group home who may need positive reinforcement to motivate the completion of a daily task. This reinforcement may be in the form of a tangible reward such as a favorite food or a token reward. A token reward may be stickers with a tangible reward given after

a certain number of stickers have been accumulated. Ideally, the reward is eventually removed when the new behavior has become ingrained, but the possibility exists that the old maladaptive behavior will return once the reward is no longer offered.

BEHAVIORAL THEORY HISTORY

The science of understanding overt human behavior started when Ivan Pavlov (1927), a Russian psychologist, demonstrated that a visual stimulus could produce a physiological response even when a tangible item was not present. When a favorite food enters the mouth, it produces a response such as increased saliva. Pavlov showed that through conditioning using reinforcement (now called *classical conditioning*), simply ringing a bell could produce the same response (Mandich, 2016).

Psychologist B. F. Skinner (1953), building on Pavlov's work, showed that behavior that was reinforced by the environment would produce a repetition of that behavior. He called these phenomena *operant conditioning.* Operant conditioning is thought to be responsible for the formation of habits. Behavior that is continuously reinforced will become habitual, and once a *habit* is formed, reinforcement is no longer needed to perpetuate that behavior. Both adaptive and maladaptive habits can be formed in this way.

The use of *positive reinforcement* is thus an effective technique used by therapists to establish a habitual adaptive response to environmental stimuli. Psychologist Albert Bandura was also a student of the early behaviorists, but he looked at interpersonal aspects of and influences on behavior. As we move forward in this chapter, you will see clear distinctions between the

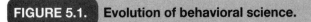

FIGURE 5.1.   Evolution of behavioral science.

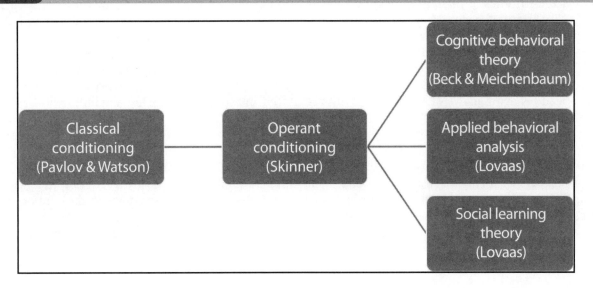

behavioral approaches. Bandura's work provides a historical bridge between behaviorist and cognitive learning theories.

Bandura's (1986) social learning theories expand on the principles of reinforcement and motivation by suggesting that behaviors are supported through observation, imitation, and modeling and that these behaviors form the basis of learning to function socially. Bandura explained that people form an idea of how new behaviors are performed by observing the behavior of others and through social exchanges. When people later apply the ideas gained through observation to guide their own behavior, the process is called *modeling.*

Necessary conditions for the effective modeling of a behavior include the individual's ability to attend to the behavior, cognitive ability to remember the behavior, physical capacity to reproduce the behavior, and motivation to engage in the behavior. Bandura suggested that individuals were motivated to be part of their environment and therefore engaged in behavior consistent with the behavior of others for intrinsic reasons. This intrinsic motivation contrasts with Skinner, who believed that extrinsic rewards from people's environment cause their behavior. The evolution of behavioral science and the specific behavioral frames of reference considered in this chapter are shown in Figure 5.1.

BEHAVIORAL FRAMES OF REFERENCE FOR OCCUPATIONAL THERAPY

In Chapter 1, "Overview of the Clinical Reasoning Process," *assumptions* were defined as the guiding beliefs that lead the clinical reasoning process within a particular frame of reference. These guiding beliefs are the ideas and concepts that provide possible explanations for observed patterns of performance. The term *assumptions* has been widely used in the analysis of frames of reference, but the term is misleading when the frame of reference is drawn from a science rather than a theory. The foundations of the behavioral frames of reference are scientifically tested and are considered to be fact rather than assumption. This chapter considers the behavioral sciences as a broad, science-driven foundation for several distinct behavioral science–derived frames of reference that are important to occupational therapy practice.

Exhibit 5.1 presents the basic overview of some elements of the behavioral science frames of reference commonly used in occupational therapy. The behavioral science frames of reference also have unique terminology (see Table 5.1).

In the occupational therapy practice setting, the behavioral science frames of reference offer the understanding that by reinforcing desired behaviors or patterns of behavior, people will develop skills that support positive

---

> **EXHIBIT 5.1.** General Elements of Behavioral Science Frames of Reference as Used in Occupational Therapy
>
> - **Focus:** The focus of this frame of reference is the building of desired behaviors to support occupational participation, which may include the establishment of new behaviors, the modification of existing behaviors, and the extinction of maladaptive behaviors.
> - **Basic assumptions:** Human behavior is deterministic, occurring as a result of intrinsic or extrinsic influences. Because behavior is deterministic, prediction of behavior is possible, and behavior can be changed by changing the influences on it.
> - **Function–disability continuum:** Function is reflected in socially and developmentally supportive learning that results in effective behavior to support occupation. Dysfunction includes both failure to learn needed behaviors and faulty learning that leads to the development of ineffective or maladaptive behavior.
> - **Postulates of change:** Behavioral change occurs through learning that is supported by the reinforcement of desired behaviors and the reduction in unwanted behavior by reducing the reinforcement derived from it. It is in defining the behavior of focus and the strategy for delivering supportive reinforcement that the factions within the behavioral frame of reference differ.

---

learning and habit development. ***Behavioral change,*** in this context, occurs through learning that is supported by the reinforcement of desired behaviors and the reduction in unwanted behavior by reducing the reinforcement derived from it. (*Punishment* is also described as a tool to elicit behavior change, but punishment is not a recommended tool in the clinical setting.)

How a specific behavior is defined and the strategy for delivering supportive reinforcement is what differentiates the behavioral frames of reference. As illustrated in Figure 5.1, 3 distinct approaches to behavior change—social learning theory, ABA, and CBT—draw from these basic postulates of change. We consider each as a distinct frame of reference for occupational therapy practitioners.

Social Learning Theory Frame of Reference

Social learning theory, as introduced by Bandura (1986), focuses on learning because human behavior is determined by a 3-way relationship among cognitive factors, environmental influences, and behavior. *Learning* is described as involving observation, extraction of information from those observations, and intentional choice in the performance of the behavior. Bandura explored the role of motivation more broadly than Skinner (1953), considering not only past reinforcement and promised reinforcements but also reinforcement that is intrinsic to the individual such as the vicarious reinforcement of seeing and recalling the model being reinforced.

TABLE 5.1.	Definitions of Terms Common to Behavioral Science Frames of Reference
APPROACH	**DEFINITION**
Classical conditioning	Process that enables learning to occur from repeatedly pairing some neutral stimulus with one that evokes a response.
Operant conditioning	Type of behavioral conditioning in which the behavioral response is strengthened in the presence of reinforcement.
Shaping	Strategy used with operant conditioning that involves a deliberate and gradual plan to change behavior.
Chaining	Method of teaching a behavior using sequences of individual behaviors that, when linked together, form a terminal behavior.
Reinforcement	Consequence to an action that increases or decreases the likelihood of the action being repeated. Reinforcement can be both positive and negative.
Modeling	Form of learning in which individuals develop skill in performance through the observation of how others perform in the same situation.

Bandura's (1986) work also considers *self-regulation,* which is people's ability to control their own behavior. His work on self-regulation is widely used by occupational therapy practitioners in all domains of practice. It is from the social learning frame of reference that we draw the clinical teaching skills of self-regulation, including

- *Self-observation:* teaching clients to notice and consider their own behavior in performance contexts;
- *Judgment:* teaching clients to compare their own behavior (or the behavior of others) with a standard of expected performance; and
- *Self-response:* teaching clients to affirm their own successes as approaching the standard of expected performance and teaching them to change their behavior if they do not approach the desired standard.

Social learning theory also assumes that with modeling and self-regulation of performance, people's ability to imitate and comply with social expectations improves. The social learning frame of reference links effective social learning to the development of positive self-esteem and views it as supporting healthy personality development. The social learning frame of reference, like the biomechanical, the psychodynamic, and the developmental systems frames of reference, is very broad and is widely incorporated into occupational therapy practice.

Social learning theory is a broad approach with widespread applications, and it is highly supportive of interventions to teach and practice self-regulation. Social learning theory offers clinical reasoning support in all 5 of the broad categories of occupational therapy services. For example, general behavioral support programs, such as positive behavior support (PBS), use social learning theory as a foundation and provide an example of an evidence-based practice tool often used as a school or institution-wide strategy to supported desired behaviors by means of reinforcement in the environment.

Social learning theory is so widely applied that it is seldom labeled by practitioners or researchers as a frame of reference. The social learning frame of reference does not require intensive 1:1 intervention or extensive training of service providers. Of all the behavioral approaches, social learning strategies are the ones most widely used in occupational therapy (Perez, Carlson, Ziviani, & Cuskelly, 2012).

ABA

ABA is a frame of reference originally described by clinical psychologist Ole Ivar Lovaas (1987) that is devoted to developing interventions that will lead to changes in observed behavior. The clinical focus of Lovaas's work was young children with autism spectrum disorder (ASD). Occupational therapy practitioners trained in ABA focus on the observable relationship of behavior to the environment, including antecedents and consequences, without resorting to what they term *hypothetical constructs,* such as thoughts, emotions, and other cognitive activity that do not manifest in observable behaviors. ABA focuses on understanding behavior and how the environment affects it. This approach uses reinforcement and conditioning as extrinsic influences to support desired actions and responses.

Occupational therapy practitioners are most likely to encounter ABA interventions in their classic form in early childhood and school settings. This approach begins with an analysis of a specific problematic behavior so it can be determined why the individual is engaging in the behavior. The occupational therapy practitioner then defines behavior sequences of individual actions that, when linked together, form a terminal behavior (behavioral chains).

In the ABA frame of reference, the individual behaviors that make up the desired behavioral chain are usually taught individually as discrete tasks through drill-based repetition. This approach is called *discrete trial training,* and it is a method of teaching in simplified and structured steps. In these discrete trials, the new learning is supported through systematic and repeated trials of antecedent–behavior–consequence chains to shape the desired behavior (Mohammadzaheri, Koegel, Rezaee, & Rafiee, 2014). This approach is characterized by the use of adult-selected materials that are presented repeatedly to promote success. The interventions are highly structured to control the antecedent stimuli, the prompts used, and the consequences of identified behaviors. Structured ABA procedures have been very effective in producing behavioral changes, especially in young children with ASD (Welch & Polatajko, 2016).

ABA is not just a collection of intervention strategies but a "professional decision-making framework that draws on the best available evidence, client values and context, and clinical expertise" (Slocum et al., 2014, p. 53). This understanding of ABA as a decision-making framework helps illustrate the use of science-derived knowledge in clinical decision making. Although ABA strategies are most often associated with ASD, they have been effectively used with a variety of other client populations, including persons with traumatic brain injuries (Heinicke & Carr, 2014), dementia (Noguchi, Kawano, & Yamanaka, 2013), neurogenetic conditions (Will & Hepburn, 2015), and intellectual disabilities (Hassiotis et al., 2012).

This frame of reference potentially offers clinical reasoning support in 3 of the broad categories of occupational therapy services: (1) remediation, (2) compensation, and (3) development. Its demonstrated strength is in the development of highly structured task performance, especially in early childhood. The ABA frame of reference is not a maintenance approach, but repeated trials of a needed task can be introduced to retrain a skill that was previously mastered that has deteriorated over time. It is also not an approach aimed at education in health-promoting habits and routines. (Sometimes distinctions such as these become cloudy because although routines can be taught through the ABA frame of reference, their more qualitative consideration as an individual decision to support personal health is not explicitly considered in this frame of reference.) A common concern about the ABA frame of reference and its utility within the occupational therapy domain of practice is its focus on isolated behaviors without consistently considering self-awareness, internal environmental, and personal factors.

CBT

The **CBT** frame of reference is also grounded in an understanding of conditioning, shaping, modeling, and reinforcement. Unlike ABA, which focuses on specific learning of skills, the CBT frame of reference focuses on addressing faulty learning. This approach aims to help people challenge their beliefs and replace errors in thinking (e.g., overgeneralizing, catastrophizing) with more balanced thoughts that are grounded in fact. As with ABA, this frame of reference supports positive behavioral change, but CBT's focus is on improved self-awareness that leads to a decrease in self-defeating behavior (Hassett & Gevirtz, 2009).

Classical CBT is a talk-based therapy that may involve a discussion of specific events to help people change the way they thinks about a trigger or challenging event. This approach was originally developed by psychiatrist Aaron Beck as a treatment for depression and by psychologist Albert Ellis to build skills in adults with anxiety disorders (Brown et al., 2011). CBT can include many diverse, but related, techniques such as relaxation training, mindfulness- and acceptance-based behavioral techniques, and cognitive restructuring (Shepardson, Funderburk, & Weisberg, 2016).

The CBT frame of reference assumes that changing maladaptive thinking leads to change in affect and behavior. This approach has been widely used by psychologists to support people with anxiety-related problems, but it has also been used in the treatment of schizophrenia (Nowak, Sabariego, Switaj, & Anczewska, 2016), post-stroke depression (Kootker et al., 2015), work-related stress (Gardner, Rose, Mason, Tyler, & Cushway, 2005), Parkinson's disease (Foster, Bedekar, & Tickle-Degnen, 2014), and chronic pain management (van Huet, Innes, & Stancliffe, 2013). Occupational therapy practitioners using a CBT frame of reference apply its theoretical foundations to activity performance. Rather than using a talk therapy approach, occupational therapy practitioners apply CBT in task-based psychoeducational interventions with clients.

A good example of such an intervention is the Cognitive Orientation to daily Occupational Performance (CO–OP) Approach,™ which has been successfully used with a wide range of clinical populations (Dawson, McEwen, & Polatajko, 2017; Scammell, Bates, Houldin, & Polatajko, 2016). This approach has been most effective with clients who can problem solve and reflect on their own performance. Variants of this approach have also been used effectively to support the development of self-regulation skills in children (Mac Cobb, Fitzgerald, & Lanigan-O'Keeffe, 2014) and adults (Stein & Cutler, 2002). The CBT frame of reference offers clinical reasoning support in all 5 of the broad categories of occupational therapy services: (1) remediation, (2) compensation, (3) maintenance, (4) education, and (5) development.

EVIDENCE CONSIDERATIONS

Strong scientific evidence supports each of the 3 behavioral frames of reference presented in this chapter. In considering these approaches, it important to understand that the treatment-specific guidance offered by each behavioral frame of reference is very distinct to that specific frame of reference.

Each of the behavioral science approaches presented in this chapter emerged outside of the field of occupational therapy, but they are all important tools in the planning

FIGURE 5.2.   Continuum of evidence-based practice.

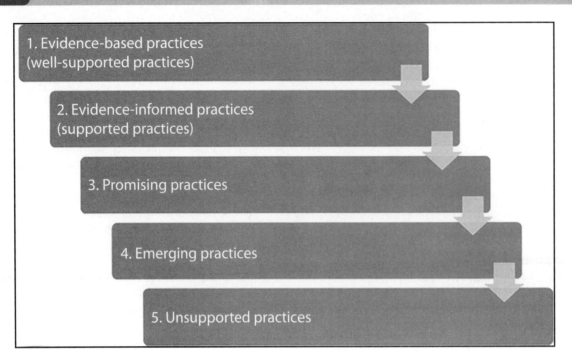

of effective occupational therapy goals and intervention. They are supported by evidence, but the evidence for their use is in the field of psychology and for use by specialist practitioners. Occupational therapy practitioners using these approaches will rely on evidence-informed practice. As we consider scientific evidence in the reasoning process, we look at it in terms of the continuum of practice (Figure 5.2).

Evidence-Based and Evidence-Informed Practice

Evidence-based practice is the conscientious use of current best evidence to identify the potential benefits, harms, and costs of any intervention while acknowledging that what works in one context may not be appropriate or feasible in another. Some authors prefer the term *evidence-informed practice* because it implies openness to more than empirically validated practices. As used in this text, the 2 terms are largely interchangeable, but evidence-informed practice may include strategies that have no empirical evidence but are logically consistent with established and well-supported practices.

The top tier of evidence-based practice includes published peer-reviewed literature reporting multiple-site replication of the practice in usual-care practice settings or at least 2 rigorous randomized controlled trials (RCTs) in different usual-care practice settings that have found the practice to be superior to an appropriate comparison practice. In addition, to be included in this top tier there must be no clinical or empirical evidence or theoretical

basis indicating that the practice constitutes a substantial risk of harm to those receiving it, compared with its likely benefits. These practices should have been shown to have a sustained effect at least 1 year beyond the end of treatment.

In evidence-informed practice, there is no clinical or empirical evidence or theoretical basis indicating that the practice constitutes a substantial risk of harm to those receiving it, compared with its likely benefits. There must be published peer-reviewed literature reporting research supporting the effectiveness of the practice in producing positive outcomes associated with improved participation in daily occupations, or at least 2 rigorous RCTs in highly controlled settings (rather than usual-practice settings) must have found the practice to be superior to an appropriate comparison practice.

Practice is also considered to be evidence informed when at least 2 studies with a between-groups design have found the practice to be equivalent (or superior) to another practice that is supported or well supported. Strong evidence supporting the practice in a highly controlled environment or by skilled practitioners working outside of the occupational therapy domain demotes an evidence-based practice to this level when the practice is altered to support an occupational therapy context.

Promising Practice

A practice is considered a *promising practice* when little or no clinical evidence or theoretical basis has indicated that the practice constitutes a substantial risk of harm to those receiving it, compared with its likely benefits. At least 1 study using some form of control or comparison group must have established the practice's efficacy over placebo or found it to be comparable to or better than an appropriate comparison practice, and that study must have been published in a peer-reviewed journal. Using expressive media (e.g., creative writing) as a tool to support motivation and behavior change is a promising practice.

Emerging Practice

An *emerging practice* has no clinical or empirical evidence or theoretical basis indicating that the practice constitutes a substantial risk of harm to those receiving it, compared with its likely benefits. Emerging practices have often been recently developed, and they may have been evaluated using less rigorous evaluation designs. These practices may not have been presented in a peer-reviewed publication. The use of mobile devices such as smartphones to support the CBT approach is an emerging practice. The category of emerging practice is intended to capture new ideas and developments. A practice should move to another category within 5–6 years of its emergence as studies are conducted and published.

Unsupported Practice

Finally, an *unsupported practice* has no clinical or empirical evidence or theoretical basis indicating that the practice constitutes a substantial risk of harm to those receiving it, compared with its likely benefits. This category includes recently developed practices with no scientific evaluation and long-standing practices that are popular but not supported as effective by scientific evidence.

APPLYING BEHAVIORAL SCIENCE–BASED FRAMES OF REFERENCE

The foundations of the behavioral frames of reference are soundly enough grounded in scientific evidence to be considered evidence based in the contexts for which they were originally developed. Applications of the social learning approach are widespread in occupational therapy literature and have been inclusive of all practice areas. In general, applications based on this approach are considered either evidence based or evidence informed. Some selected samples of intervention approaches are described to help readers learn the scope of influence that the behavioral science frames of reference have had in occupational therapy practice.

Applying Social Learning

The social learning frame of reference assumes that humans are intrinsically social and able to learn from observing and modeling the social behaviors of others. Occupational therapy practitioners often structure occupations and activity settings that support social inclusion and structured activity participation with avenues to model and practice social behaviors. For example, Whatley, Fortune, and Williams (2015) studied aspects of social inclusion in a community garden. In this study the community garden was the environmental context of the interactions, but the focus of the intervention was social inclusion.

Similarly, Copley, Turpin, Gordon, and McLaren (2011) developed and evaluated an occupational therapy program aimed at learning and social competence for refugee high school students. Finally, Mthembu et al. (2014) explored the use of social networking sites among adolescents. Social learning approaches have been replicated and studied in usual-care practice settings, and there is no evidence or theoretical basis indicating that the practice constitutes a substantial risk of harm to those receiving it, compared with its likely benefits.

Applying ABA

ABA is a highly evidence-based approach for supporting behavior change in young children. This approach is a specific application of the behavioral frames of reference that is most commonly used in early intervention in children with ASD. Although widely used by psychologists and teachers, ABA is often not the primary frame of reference used by occupational therapy practitioners. Welch and Polatajko (2016) explored this conundrum and reported that ABA has widespread reputational problems that are caused by misperceptions held by a variety of professionals, including occupational therapy practitioners. The ABA community is aware of the stigma associated with it and has identified 3 primary problems with ABA's reputation:

1. Many professionals working outside the field of ABA misunderstand it as being limited to discrete trial training,
2. It is perceived to fail to consider generalization, and
3. It is perceived to fail to consider client desires and interests (Welch & Polatajko, 2016, p. 2).

ABA is actually a broad approach that requires a high degree of training to implement. It is strength based and based on developing specific skills for learning. This approach is highly individualized and can assimilate and respond to client desires and interests. The relative paucity of its use in occupational therapy may be in part because it is misunderstood. Also, its use may be limited by the need for training beyond entry-level occupational therapy education. Finally, it is worth considering that for children with ASD to make the most meaningful gains, *early and intensive behavioral intervention (EIBI)* using the ABA approach is required (Leaf et al., 2016). EIBI is most effective when the following parameters are in place:

- The intervention must be implemented intensively, with the current consensus being that formal intervention should occur 25–40 hours per week (Reichow, 2012);
- Treatment must be comprehensive, encompassing all aspects of child development; and
- Staff providing the intervention must be adequately trained to implement the procedures with a high degree of fidelity and quality (Leaf et al., 2016).

Interprofessional conflicts sometimes occur when families must choose how to spend their limited resources in terms of time, physical demands, and money. A family committed to 40 hours of EIBI per week will be less likely to seek occupational therapy support in addition to EIBI, especially because proponents of EIBI report that their approach is comprehensive and no additional specialists are needed. Also, ABA applied beyond the early childhood period is less effective and has not been found to reduce caregiver burden (Hassiotis et al., 2012).

Occupational therapy practitioners are trained in many frames of reference and tend to blend other frames into their interventions. Conflict over the strict application of the ABA frame of reference has been the source of some negative professional exchanges. This is unfortunate because, as Welch and Polatajko (2016) argued, the ABA approach and the tenets of the occupational therapy practice domain have many points of agreement.

Applying CBT

Several meta-analyses have demonstrated that CBT is effective for common mental health difficulties such as anxiety and depression in a wide range of client populations (Butler, Chapman, Forman, & Beck, 2006). In classical CBT, the trained CBT therapist and the client work together as a team to identify and solve problems by changing the client's thinking, behavior, and emotional responses using a talk therapy approach (Beck Institute for Cognitive Behavior Therapy, 2016).

In occupational therapy, this approach is used to support performance of activities and includes both talk and active participation in tasks related to the client's goals. Cole and Tufano (2008) described the occupational therapy variant of this approach as offering useful techniques to teach clients self-management skills. CBT also lends itself well to group interventions and is widely used by occupational therapy practitioners in mental health settings.

In evaluating scholarly evidence, readers must consider the evidence in terms of its relevance to their practice of occupational therapy. The fact that a great deal of evidence exists for talk therapy–based approaches such as CBT does not mean that using CBT concepts in an occupational therapy activity-based program will have the same results, although the evidence suggests that there is a likelihood that positive results may occur. *Evidence-based practice* does not mean that practitioners must adopt every approach that has been confirmed by

science or that they must reject approaches that have less support.

Behavioral approaches in general have been highly influential and are well suited to support occupational therapy interventions across practice areas. Highly specific approaches such as ABA and CBT can also be valuable but require that practitioners have additional training with them. Although there is relatively little evidence that specifically considers occupational therapy adaptations to either ABA or CBT, occupational therapy practitioners using these approaches in a nonstandard manner should consider them to be evidence-informed practices.

The occupational therapy literature contains 3 recent studies applying CBT. Alcorn and Broome (2014) described the effective use of behavioral strategies in an occupational performance coaching model to support people with chronic conditions. Perez et al. (2012) explored the perceived contributions of occupational therapy practitioners in PBS programs. Kootker et al. (2015) involved occupational therapy practitioners in a CBT approach to address poststroke depression in a rehabilitation hospital.

Cognitive Strategy Training Used as a Cognitive–Behavioral Intervention in Occupational Therapy

Cognitive strategy training is a treatment approach with its roots in behavioral science. It focuses on teaching the client strategies that support early and mid-phase skill acquisition of the target task through the teaching and support of executive function abilities, such as sequencing, planning, error detection, problem solving, and organizing behavior. They can be either general or domain specific.

An example of a general cognitive strategy is Meichenbaum's Goal–Plan–Do–Check, which was adapted for use in the occupational therapist–developed CO–OP Approach (Dawson et al., 2017). The CO–OP Approach was introduced as an intervention to improve occupational performance in children with developmental coordination disorder. This intervention has 3 basic objectives:

1. Skill acquisition;
2. Development of a global problem-solving strategy to help solve additional performance problems; and
3. Generalization of newly learned skills to the person's everyday life (Polatajko et al., 2001).

This approach has a strong evidence base with this population and has since been adopted for use with a variety of populations, including people with ASD, cerebral palsy, and cerebrovascular accident. In a review of this approach by Scammel et al. (2016), the approach was deemed useful in the 8 clinical conditions reviewed, although adaptations to the CO–OP Approach were sometimes recommended. Case Example 5.1 applies the behavioral frame of reference in adult rehabilitation illustrates some of its basic features.

CASE EXAMPLE 5.1. JEREMY: USING THE BEHAVIORAL FRAME OF REFERENCE IN OCCUPATIONAL THERAPY INTERVENTION

Jeremy, age 30 years, was referred to occupational therapy because of recent behavioral problems. He suffered a traumatic brain injury (TBI) when he was age 10 years and has had functional difficulties at various times as he developed into adulthood. Jeremy's case is typical of the ongoing needs and challenges experienced in brain injury as roles and occupations change over time. Exhibit 5.2 describes Jeremy's occupational profile.

Jeremy's occupational therapy practitioner decides to build a PBS plan and use a token system to encourage behavioral change. Jeremy's mother will remind him to shower each morning. If he completes his shower, he will be given a poker chip. He will be allowed to cash in every 7 chips he accumulates for a favorite dessert. If he is able to accumulate 20 chips, he can cash them in for a new video game.

In the beginning, Jeremy was excited at the prospect of earning a new game and showered for the first 2 days but not the 3rd or 4th. He was reminded that he needed 7 chips for a dessert and 20 for a new game.

EXHIBIT 5.2.	Jeremy's Occupational Profile		
Client	**Reason the client is seeking service and concerns related to engagement in occupations**	Referred to OT for impairments in basic organizational skills, self-care, and behavioral issues after TBI. *Impact on occupation:* Lately, he has been refusing to shower and attend to personal hygiene, which has greatly frustrated his mother. He will agree to his mother's requests to bathe, but he does not follow through.	
	Occupations in which the client is successful	Jeremy helps around the house by taking care of the lawn when his brother comes over to supervise. He requires considerable prompting by his brother to start mowing the grass, but once he starts the task he tends to complete it.	
	Personal interests and values	Jeremy enjoys watching television.	
	Occupational history (i.e., life experiences)	Jeremy was hit by a car at age 10 years and incurred a significant TBI resulting in cognitive impairment. He was able to complete his education through high school with extensive support and SE. He has had various odd jobs, although he has not been able to maintain a job for any length of time because of his poor organizational and social skills. He stopped working 5 years ago and is now on total disability. Jeremy demonstrates significantly impaired cognition as a result of his TBI. Lately, his behavior has been deteriorating. His mother does not know what to do so she either takes it or avoids the situation by not asking for his participation.	
	Performance patterns (routines, roles, habits, & rituals)	Jeremy claims to have no valued roles. He does not understand role obligations and views his mother as someone who "just tells me what to do all of the time." Jeremy's days are largely spent watching television and playing video games.	
Environment		***Supports to occupational engagement***	***Barriers to occupational engagement***
	Physical (e.g., buildings, furniture, pets)	Jeremy has no difficulties with physical accessibility.	
	Social (e.g., spouse, friends, caregivers)	Jeremy lives with his mother and grandmother.	Jeremy's mother does not like to upset him because he can be very impulsive, and she has been allowing him to do mostly what he pleases. Jeremy's cooperation has lessened and his negative behaviors (e.g., whining, yelling, cursing) have increased.

(Continued)

CASE EXAMPLE 5.1. JEREMY: USING THE BEHAVIORAL FRAME OF REFERENCE IN OCCUPATIONAL THERAPY INTERVENTION (Cont.)

EXHIBIT 5.2.	Jeremy's Occupational Profile (Cont.)	
Context	Cultural (e.g., customs, beliefs)	No issues related to culture or beliefs were identified during assessment.
	Personal (e.g., age, gender, SES, education)	Age 30 years. Male. Completed high school.
	Temporal (e.g., stage of life, time, year)	Jeremy is a young adult but is unable to independently function in society.
	Virtual (e.g., chat, email, remote monitoring)	Jeremey is able to use a telephone and social media.
Client goals	Client's priorities and desired targeted outcomes	Jeremy has been living with his mother, but if he does not regain the ability to regulate his actions and does not assist with household chores, he may need to find somewhere else to live. Both Jeremy and his mother want him to be able to stay in his mother's home.

ANALYSIS OF PARTICIPATION	
Basic ADLs	
Eating/oral–motor	Jeremy has no difficulty in this area.
Grooming	Jeremy has no physical limitations in this area, although he often neglects to shave or comb his hair.
Bathing/transfer	Jeremy has no physical limitation in this area, but he does not see any value to be gained by bathing.
Dressing upper body	Jeremy has no physical limitations in this area.
Dressing lower body	Jeremy has no physical limitations in this area.
Toileting	Jeremy has no physical limitations in this area.
Problem solving/memory	Jeremy tends to ignore problems or ask his mother and grandmother for help with even the most basic problems. His memory is very impaired, and he requires frequent reminders and constant supervision for safety.
Comments:	Jeremy likes the way he is living and does not understand why he should change his behavior. As long as he has access to his video game system and television, he is content.
IADLs	
Community mobility	Jeremy does not drive or own a vehicle and relies on his mother for transportation. He rarely leaves the house except for doctor's appointments.
Health management/prevention	Jeremy relies on his mother for health maintenance. He does not understand that poor hygiene will lead to health problems because he is unable to understand the possible future consequences of his actions.
Home management	Other than taking care of the lawn, Jeremy does not engage in any other homemaking activity.
Financial management	Jeremy has no financial management skills. Finances are managed by his family.
Leisure	Jeremy's leisure activities are sedentary; television and video games are his only source of leisure activities.

(Continued)

CASE EXAMPLE 5.1. JEREMY: USING THE BEHAVIORAL FRAME OF REFERENCE IN OCCUPATIONAL THERAPY INTERVENTION *(Cont.)*

EXHIBIT 5.2.	**Jeremy's Occupational Profile** *(Cont.)*
Safety	Jeremy requires 24-hour supervision because of his poor safety awareness, impulsiveness, and significant deficits in attention.
Comments:	Jeremy relies on his mother and grandmother for all of his basic needs. His occupational participation is extremely limited. He has no age-appropriate friends and rarely ventures into the community.
Motor and Praxis Skills	
Sitting—static/dynamic	Jeremy is able to maintain static sitting on a regular chair or stool. He has good dynamic sitting.
Standing—static/dynamic	Jeremy has no difficulty in this area.
Joint stability and skeletal mobility	Jeremy has no difficulty in this area.
Place can on shelf	Jeremy has no difficulty in this area.
Retrieve item from floor	Jeremy has no difficulty in this area.
Screw lid on jar	Jeremy has no difficulty in this area.
Comb back of head	Jeremy has no difficulty in this area.
Writing	Jeremy has no difficulty in this area.
Lift grocery bag	Jeremy has no difficulty in this area.
Coordination	Jeremy has no difficulty in this area.
Manipulation	Jeremy has no difficulty in this area.
Comments:	Jeremy's negative outbursts have been verbal rather than physical. Because the negative behavior has been escalating, his mother is concerned that he may become physically aggressive in the future.
Process Skills	
Energy for task	Jeremy has no difficulty in this area for preferred tasks.
Knowledge/organization of task	Jeremy has difficulty learning tasks, but his knowledge of familiar tasks is adequate.
Adaptation/praxis	Jeremy has no difficulty in this area.
Comments:	None.
Behavioral and Cognitive Skills	
Communication and following social conventions	Jeremy's receptive and expressive language is within normal limits. Jeremy is able to communicate and understand verbal communication. He has been more difficult to manage because of his lack of understanding of social conventions. He is often impolite and does not interact respectfully with other adults.
Cognitive and emotional regulation skills	Jeremy is alert and oriented to time and place. He has difficulty regulating his emotions and is easy to anger when he becomes frustrated. Although he has never physically hurt anyone, his mother is concerned that he may, if pushed too far.
Level of arousal/attention	Jeremy is easily distracted, even in 1:1 settings. He likes fast-moving images and prefers cartoons on television and fast-moving video games.
Orientation	Jeremy is alert and oriented ×4.*
Energy and drive	Jeremy is not motivated to change his behavior because he sees nothing wrong with the way he chooses to live.

(Continued)

CASE EXAMPLE 5.1. JEREMY: USING THE BEHAVIORAL FRAME OF REFERENCE IN OCCUPATIONAL THERAPY INTERVENTION *(Cont.)*

EXHIBIT 5.2.	**Jeremy's Occupational Profile *(Cont.)***
Memory and understanding	Jeremy is able to understand and follow a series of 2 or more related instructions but does not anticipate problems and does not problem solve solutions when familiar strategies do not work. He will ask for help with even the most basic of problems. He requires frequent cueing and redirection because of memory impairments.
Higher level cognition	Jeremy has significant difficulty with most EF skills.
	Sensory–Perceptual Skills
Sensory	Jeremy has no difficulty in this area.
Self-perception	Jeremy has poor self-awareness and truly does not care about himself and situations outside his immediate gratification needs.
Pain	Jeremy does not complain of pain.
Skin integrity	Jeremy's skin is intact.

Note. Occupational profile template from American Occupational Therapy Association (2017). Analysis of participation format adapted from Skubik-Peplaski, Paris, Boyle, & Culpert (2009). * (1) Who are you? (2) Where are you? (3) What are the date and time? (4) What just happened to you? ADLs = activities of daily living; EF = executive function; IADLs = instrumental activities of daily living; OT = occupational therapy; SE = special education; SES = socioeconomic status; TBI = traumatic brain injury.

His therapist taped the 2 chips he had earned to the wall near his bed as a visual reminder of his goal. This stimulated him to again engage in daily showering, and he soon had enough chips to earn a dessert, which he accepted. He was then encouraged to try and earn enough for a new video game. He was able to eventually earn enough chips for the video game and was showering daily. At this point, his mother decided that he had changed his behavior and stopped awarding him chips when he showered. He soon began to refuse to shower, reverting to his old maladaptive behavior. The token system was restarted, and his behavior improved.

Although the token system worked to change Jeremy's behavior, he was unable to habituate to showering without the token system. His mother was satisfied with the system, however, because she no longer worried about him getting upset because he was more cooperative. She also instituted subtle changes by beginning to require additional self-care tasks in addition to showering to earn a chip, such as earning a chip when he showered and brushed his teeth. Although the use of the token system was effective with Jeremy, the limits of this approach required ongoing use because habituation, in this case, was elusive.

SCIENTIFIC AND NARRATIVE REASONING USING THE BEHAVIORAL FRAMES OF REFERENCE

Narrative reasoning is as a central mode of clinical reasoning in occupational therapy (Mattingly, 1991). It is an inductive strategy used to understand a person's experiences with disability, impairment, illness, or challenges to occupational performance. Therapists reason narratively when they engage dynamically with their clients to understand the experience of that person rather than having an exclusive focus on science-driven constructs such as disability and illness. Being able to empathize with clients helps practitioners establish rapport and a relationship that facilitates effective communication.

The case of Jeremy illustrates some common behavioral issues seen by occupational therapy practitioners. In many instances, social and behavioral deficits occur in conjunction with physical impairments. Next, consider the case of Amanda, which uses both scientific and narrative reasoning (Case Example 5.2).

SUMMARY

This chapter examined 3 distinct behavioral frames of reference that are important in occupational therapy practice. In reviewing the text to this point, readers have been introduced to 3 important frames of reference that are described as *historical:* the (1) psychodynamic, (2) developmental systems, and (3) social learning frames of reference. Because these approaches were developed in the early 20th century, they have been scrutinized, tested,

CASE EXAMPLE 5.2. AMANDA: USING SCIENTIFIC AND NARRATIVE REASONING

Amanda, age 41 years, has deficits in language comprehension and visual perception that make using traditional behavioral interventions more challenging. She was referred to occupational therapy after a self-inflicted gunshot wound that caused left temporal damage. She also abuses several substances. Amanda's occupational profile is shown in Exhibit 5.3.

Both the social learning frame of reference and the CBT frame of reference could support Amanda

in developing needed skills. As you further explore the science underlying these 2 approaches, you may feel more strongly drawn to one or the other of them. Amanda's difficulties fall well within the scope of the behavioral frames of reference but might also be addressed in other ways. Clinical reasoning requires serious consideration of the client's occupational profile and the use of narrative reasoning to help focus and guide the application of scientific reasoning.

EXHIBIT 5.3.	Amanda's Occupational Profile		
Client	**Reason the client is seeking service and concerns related to engagement in occupations**	Referred to OT for intervention and treatment after a gunshot wound (self-inflicted) that caused left temporal lobe damage, with polysubstance abuse disorder. *Impact on occupation:* Amanda is currently in a rehabilitation hospital after her discharge from acute care. She hopes to be discharged to a transitional apartment with mental health support.	
	Occupations in which the client is successful	Prior to her injury Amanda had impoverished habits and roles as a result of her substance abuse.	
	Personal interests and values	Amanda values the idea of rebuilding her role as a mother. She also hopes to return to her work as a waitress.	
	Occupational history (i.e., life experiences)	Amanda is estranged from her husband and children and has not been in touch with them for more than 3 years. She regrets this and regrets the loss of her maternal role. Before her injury, Amanda worked as a waitress at a truck stop. Amanda is a participant in a MAT program for polysubstance abuse of opioids and alcohol use disorder.	
	Performance patterns (routines, roles, habits, & rituals)	Amanda could not identify any other desired roles. Amanda requires assistance with both ADLs and IADLs.	
Environment		***Supports to occupational engagement***	***Barriers to occupational engagement***
	Physical (e.g., buildings, furniture, pets)	Amanda has no difficulties with physical accessibility.	
	Social (e.g., spouse, friends, caregivers)	Amanda has a support group through the MAT program for polysubstance abuse.	She indicates that she has no friends or family support.
Context	**Cultural (e.g., customs, beliefs)**	Amanda has been living in poverty and has a sense of fatalism that is often associated with chronic poverty.	
	Personal (e.g., age, gender, SES, education)	Age 41 years. Female. Lower income.	
	Temporal (e.g., stage of life, time, year)	Amanda is in middle adulthood.	
	Virtual (e.g., chat, email, remote monitoring)	Amanda is able to use the telephone, email, and social media.	

(Continued)

CASE EXAMPLE 5.2. AMANDA: USING SCIENTIFIC AND NARRATIVE REASONING *(Cont.)*

EXHIBIT 5.3.	Amanda's Occupational Profile *(Cont.)*	
Client goals	**Client's priorities and desired targeted outcomes**	Amanda has a very negative view of her recent life choices and described herself as a user. She wants to regain her independence in ADLs and IADLs and wants to be able to return to work. She has been told that social services will help her try to re-establish contact with her children when she has been drug free and working for 6 months.
ANALYSIS OF PARTICIPATION		
Basic ADLs		
Eating/oral–motor		Amanda requires total assist and receives tube feeding.
Grooming		Modified independent. Amanda needs extra time and to perform tasks while seated.
Bathing/transfer		Modified independent. Amanda needs extra time and to perform tasks while seated. Does sit/pivot transfer to bath seat.
Dressing upper body		Amanda needs maximum assistance with a pullover shirt.
Dressing lower body		Amanda needs maximum assistance when in supine on bed. She is unable to dress herself in other positions.
Toileting		Modified independent with side rails/grab bars to aid stability. Amanda does sit/pivot transfer to toilet.
Problem solving/memory		Amanda has both long-term and short-term memory loss secondary to her injury. She requires frequent reminders and constant supervision for safety. She is unable to execute tasks with 2 or more steps and does not detect obvious errors in her performance.
Comments:		None.
IADLs		
Community mobility		Amanda does not drive or own a vehicle. She currently uses a wheelchair for transportation in the community.
Health management/prevention		She has a history of poor health judgment and poor nutrition. Medications currently are managed by health care team. Amanda had been living with a boyfriend who was sometimes physically abusive.
Home management		Amanda had managed basic homemaking, including cooking and laundry, before her injury.
Financial management		Amanda was able to manage her own finances before her injury.
Leisure		Amanda reports no leisure interests. In the past, much of her free time involved getting high and recovering from getting high.
Safety		Amanda requires 24-hour supervision because of poor safety awareness, impulsiveness, and significant deficits in attention.
Comments:		Amanda does not plan to return to her previous living arrangement.
Motor and Praxis Skills		
Sitting—static/dynamic		Amanda has fair sitting balance at edge of bed.
Standing—static/dynamic		Amanda requires maximal assistance in the sit-to-stand movement. In standing, she needs minimal assist to maintain the position.
Joint stability and skeletal mobility		Amanda has no difficulty in this area.
Place can on shelf		Amanda requires demonstration and maximal verbal cues with hand over hand to initiate task performance.

(Continued)

CASE EXAMPLE 5.2. AMANDA: USING SCIENTIFIC AND NARRATIVE REASONING *(Cont.)*

EXHIBIT 5.3. Amanda's Occupational Profile *(Cont.)*	
Retrieve item from floor	Amanda requires moderate assistance due to limited sitting balance.
Screw lid on jar	Amanda requires demonstration and moderate verbal cues with hand over hand to initiate task performance.
Comb back of head	Amanda requires demonstration and moderate verbal cues with hand over hand to initiate task performance.
Writing	Amanda is able to write her name legibly. She has difficulty writing lists, but these difficulties seem to be related to cognitive processing rather than a motor problem.
Lift grocery bag	Amanda has difficulty because of poor balance and generalized weakness.
Coordination	Amanda has impairments with uneven timing and jerkiness of movement. Poor attention and endurance further limit performance in this area.
Manipulation	Amanda's grip strength and manipulation skills are adequate to the demands in this setting.
Comments:	None.
Process Skills	
Energy for task	Amanda has no difficulty in this area.
Knowledge/organization of task	Amanda has impaired judgment and problem solving. She needs prompting to initiate each step of a multistep task and needs cueing to select appropriate items for task completion.
Adaptation/praxis	Amanda requires maximal verbal cues to anticipate and respond to environmental cues. She has difficulty learning new tasks.
Comments:	None.
Behavioral and Cognitive Skills	
Communication and following social conventions	Amanda's expressive language is within normal limits She has impaired recall of verbal and visual content, including speech perception. She has much difficulty recognizing written words and following written instructions. Amanda's social interactions are within functional limits.
Cognitive and emotional regulation skills	Amanda has been very emotional and was quickly frustrated during the initial assessment.
Level of arousal/attention	Amanda is easily distracted, even in 1:1 settings.
Orientation	Amanda is alert and oriented ×4.*
Energy and drive	Amanda says that she is motivated to change her behavior but has little personal insight and needs prompting to initiate most tasks.
Memory and understanding	Amanda is able to follow a series of 1–2 related instructions when they are physically demonstrated to her. She does not consistently follow verbal instruction and has poor selective attention to auditory and visual input. Amanda has a disturbance of language comprehension and impaired long-term memory.
Higher level cognition	Amanda has significant difficulty with most executive function skills.
Sensory–Perceptual Skills	
Sensory	Amanda has inconsistent responses to auditory sensation and has poor visual perception of spatial relations, visual sequences, visual closure, and visual figure–ground.
Self-perception	Amanda is very self-critical and describes herself as a loser.

(Continued)

CASE EXAMPLE 5.2. AMANDA: USING SCIENTIFIC AND NARRATIVE REASONING *(Cont.)*

EXHIBIT 5.3.	Amanda's Occupational Profile *(Cont.)*
Pain	Amanda does not complain of pain.
Skin integrity	Amanda's skin is intact.
Comments:	None.

Note. Occupational profile template from American Occupational Therapy Association (2017). Analysis of participation format adapted from Skubik-Peplaski, Paris, Boyle, & Culpert (2009). *(1) Who are you? (2) Where are you? (3) What are the date and time? (4) What just happened to you? ADLs = activities of daily living; IADLs = instrumental activities of daily living; MAT = medication-assisted treatment; OT = occupational therapy; SES = socioeconomic status.

and refined over time. The evidence-supported aspects of these approaches are now seen as common knowledge and are not often specifically labeled in the scientific literature as a guiding *frame of reference*. This can be confusing, because it is easiest to understand clinical reasoning driven by frames of reference when those frames of reference are clearly labeled. Also, it is easy to assume that no guiding frame of reference was used when none has been articulated.

The 3 behavioral science frames of reference presented here were all developed on the basis of research that initially focused on a specific clinical population. The frame of reference with the broadest scope of the 3 is the social learning frame of reference. Both the ABA and the CBT frames of reference are very intervention focused. The more specific the focus of a frame of reference, the easier it is to develop specific research to help refine it. Compared with the psychodynamic frame of reference, the evidential support for all 3 behavioral science frames of reference is strong.

In another comparison with the psychodynamic frame of reference, each of 3 frames of reference have a discrete focus and were developed with a specific clinical issue in mind. This focus is reflected in the more limited utility of these frames of reference in the 5 categories of occupational therapy service: remediation, maintenance, compensation, development, and education. All 3 of the frames of reference presented—social learning, ABA, and CBT—are supportive of remediation and maintenance approaches but less directly supportive of compensation, development, or education approaches.

The 2 remaining frames of reference presented in this section of the text, the motor learning frame of reference and the sensory processing frame of reference, were both highly influenced by the behavioral science frames of reference and have been intensively researched. The continuum of evidence-based practice introduced in this chapter is an important tool when considering these newer frames of reference.

LEARNING ACTIVITIES

1. The overall elements of behavioral science as a frame of reference were presented in Table 5.1. Using this table format and your textbooks or other sources, gain the knowledge that you need to develop frame-of-reference tables for social learning theory, ABA, and CBT.
2. The clinical intervention approach described for Jeremy is a token economy. Choose and describe another behavioral science–based intervention strategy that could be used to support Jeremy's task performance. What frame of reference is your intervention strategy intended to reflect?
3. Look up *functional behavioral assessment* online. Use this framework to identify what purpose Jeremy's negative behaviors serve.
4. Using the case of Amanda, choose 1 of the 3 behavioral science frames of reference as a guide and use that frame to guide your identification of 3 priority problem areas for intervention.
5. Choose any sort of behavioral intervention strategy of interest to you in your occupational therapy practice. Search the available scientific evidence on this intervention both in general and in occupational therapy intervention–specific contexts. Write a short essay that describes the intervention strategy, the existing evidence, and your assessment of the strategy as evidence based, evidence informed, promising, emerging, or unsupported.

REFERENCES

Alcorn, K., & Broome, K. (2014). Occupational performance coaching for chronic conditions: A review of literature. *New Zealand Journal of Occupational Therapy, 61,* 49–56.

American Occupational Therapy Association. (2017). AOTA occupational profile template. *American Journal of Occupational Therapy, 71*(Suppl. 2), 7112420030. https://doi.org/10.5014/ajot.2017.716S12

Bandura, A. (1986). *Social foundations of thought and action.* Englewood Cliffs, NJ: Prentice-Hall.

Beck Institute for Cognitive Behavior Therapy. (2016). *What is cognitive behavior therapy?* Retrieved from https://beckinstitute.org/get-informed/what-is-cognitive-behavior-therapy

Behavioral science. (2016). In *Merriam Webster's online dictionary.* Retrieved from http://www.merriam-webster.com/dictionary/behavioral%20science

Brown, C., Stoffel, V., & Muñoz, J. P. (2011). *Occupational therapy in mental health: A vision for participation.* Philadelphia: F. A. Davis.

Butler, A., Chapman, J., Forman, E., & Beck, A. (2006). The empirical status of cognitive–behavioral therapy: A review of meta-analyses. *Clinical Psychology Review, 26,* 17–31. https://doi.org/10.1016/j.cpr.2005.07.003

Cole, M., & Tufano, R. (2008). *Applied theories in occupational therapy: A practical approach.* Thorofare, NJ: Slack.

Copley, J., Turpin, M., Gordon, S., & McLaren, C. (2011). Development and evaluation of an occupational therapy program for refugee high school students. *Australian Occupational Therapy Journal, 58,* 310–316. https://doi.org/10.1111/j.1440-1630.2011.00933.x

Dawson, D. R., McEwen, S. E., & Polatajko, H. J. (Eds.). (2017). *Cognitive Orientation to daily Occupational Performance in occupational therapy: Using the CO–OP Approach™ to enable participation across the lifespan.* Bethesda, MD: AOTA Press.

Foster, E. R., Bedekar, M., & Tickle-Degnen, L. (2014). Systematic review of the effectiveness of occupational therapy–related interventions for people with Parkinson's disease. *American Journal of Occupational Therapy, 68,* 39–49. https://doi.org/10.5014/ajot.2014.008706

Gardner, B., Rose, J., Mason, O., Tyler, P., & Cushway, D. (2005). Cognitive therapy and behavioural coping in the management of work-related stress: An intervention study. *Work and Stress, 19,* 137–152. https://doi.org/10.1080/02678370500157346

Hassett, A., & Gevirtz, R. (2009). Nonpharmacologic treatment for fibromyalgia: Patient education, cognitive–behavioral therapy, relaxation techniques, and complementary and alternative medicine. *Rheumatic Disease Clinics of North America, 35,* 393–407. https://doi.org/10.1016/j.rdc.2009.05.003

Hassiotis, A., Robotham, D., Canagasabey, A., Marston, L., Thomas, B., & King, M. (2012). Brief Report: Impact of applied behavior analysis (ABA) on carer burden and community participation in challenging behavior: Results from a randomized controlled trial. *Journal of Intellectual Disability Research, 56,* 285–290. https://doi.org/10.1111/j.1365-2788.2011.01467.x

Heinicke, M. R., & Carr, J. E. (2014). Applied behavior analysis in acquired brain injury rehabilitation: A meta-analysis of single-case design intervention research. *Behavioral Interventions, 29,* 77–105. https://doi.org/10.1002/bin.1380

Kootker, J. A., Rasquin, S. C., Smits, P., Geurts, A. C., van Heugten, C. M., & Fasotti, L. (2015). An augmented cognitive behavioral therapy for treating post-stroke depression: Description of a treatment protocol. *Clinical Rehabilitation, 29,* 833–843. https://doi.org/10.1177/0269215514559987

Leaf, J. B., Leaf, R., McEachin, J., Taubman, M., Ala'i-Rosales, S., Ross, R. K., & Weiss, M. J. (2016). Applied behavior analysis is a science and, therefore, progressive. *Journal of Autism and Developmental Disorders, 46,* 720–731. https://doi.org/10.1007/s10803-015-2591-6

Lovaas, O. (1987). Behavioral treatment and normal educational and intellectual functioning in young children with autism. *Journal of Consulting and Clinical Psychology, 55,* 3–9. https://doi.org/10.1037/0022-006X.55.1.3

Mac Cobb, S., Fitzgerald, B., & Lanigan-O'Keeffe, C. (2014). The Alert Program for self-management of behaviour in second level schools: Results of Phase 1 of a pilot study. *Emotional and Behavioural Difficulties, 19,* 410–425. https://doi.org/10.1080/13632752.2014.903593

Mandich, M. (2016). Classic theories of human development. In A. Cronin & M. Mandich (Eds.), *Human development and performance throughout the lifespan* (2nd ed., pp. 38–59). Boston: Cengage Learning.

Mattingly, C. (1991). The narrative nature of clinical reasoning. *American Journal of Occupational Therapy, 45,* 998–1005. https://doi.org/10.5014/ajot.45.11.998

Mohammadzaheri, F., Koegel, L., Rezaee, M., & Rafiee, S. (2014). A randomized clinical trial comparison between pivotal response treatment (PRT) and structured applied behavior analysis (ABA) intervention for children with autism. *Journal of Autism and Developmental Disorders, 44,* 2769–2777. https://doi.org/10.1007/s10803-014-2137-3

Mthembu, T. G., Beets, C., Davids, G., Malyon, K., Pekeur, M., & Rabinowitz, A. (2014). Influences of social network sites on the occupational performance of adolescents in a secondary school in Cape Town, South Africa: A phenomenological study. *Australian Occupational Therapy Journal, 61,* 132–139. https://doi.org/10.1111/1440-1630.12085

Noguchi, D., Kawano, Y., & Yamanaka, K. (2013). Care staff training in residential homes for managing behavioural and psychological symptoms of dementia based on differential reinforcement procedures of applied behaviour analysis: A process research. *Psychogeriatrics, 13,* 108–117. https://doi.org/10.1111/psyg.12006

Nowak, I., Sabariego, C., Świtaj, P., & Anczewska, M. (2016). Disability and recovery in schizophrenia: A systematic review of cognitive behavioral therapy interventions. *BMC Psychiatry, 16,* 228. https://doi.org/10.1186/s12888-016-0912-8

Pavlov, I. (1927). *Conditioned reflexes: An investigation of the physiological activity of the cerebral cortex* (G. V. Anrep, Ed. & Trans.). London: Oxford University Press.

Perez, M., Carlson, G., Ziviani, J., & Cuskelly, M. (2012). Contribution of occupational therapists in positive behaviour support. *Australian Occupational Therapy Journal, 59,* 428–436. https://doi.org/10.1111/j.1440-1630.2012.01036.x

Polatajko, H. J., Mandich, A. D., Missiuna, C., Miller, L. T., Macnab, J. J., Malloy-Miller, T., & Kinsella, E. A. (2001). Cognitive Orientation to daily Occupational Performance (CO–OP): Part III—The protocol in brief. *Physical and Occupational Therapy in Pediatrics, 20,* 107–123. https://doi.org/10.1080/J006v20n02_07

Reichow, B. (2012). Overview of meta-analyses on early intensive behavioral intervention for young children with autism spectrum disorders. *Journal of Autism and Developmental Disorders, 42*, 512–520. https://doi.org/10.1007/s10803-011-1218-9

Scammell, E. M., Bates, S. V., Houldin, A., & Polatajko, H. J. (2016). The Cognitive Orientation to daily Occupational Performance (CO–OP): A scoping review. *Canadian Journal of Occupational Therapy, 83*, 216–225. https://doi.org/10.1177/0008417416651277

Science. (2016). In *Merriam-Webster's dictionary.* Retrieved from http://www.merriam-webster.com/dictionary/science

Shepardson, R. L., Funderburk, J. S., & Weisberg, R. B. (2016). Adapting evidence-based, cognitive–behavioral interventions for anxiety for use with adults in integrated primary care settings. *Families, Systems, and Health, 34*, 114–127. https://doi.org/10.1037/fsh0000175

Skinner, B. F. (1953). *Science and human behavior.* New York: Macmillan.

Skubik-Peplaski, C., Paris, C., Boyle, D., & Culpert, A. (Eds.). (2009). *Applying the* Occupational Therapy Practice Framework: *Using the Cardinal Hill Participation Process in client-centered care* (2nd ed.). Bethesda, MD: AOTA Press.

Slocum, T. A., Detrich, R., Wilczynski, S. M., Spencer, T. D., Lewis, T., & Wolfe, K. (2014). The evidence-based practice of applied behavior analysis. *Behavior Analyst, 37*, 41–56. https://doi.org/10.1007/s40614-014-0005-2.

Stein, F., & Cutler, S. (2002). *Psychosocial occupational therapy: A holistic approach* (2nd ed.). Albany, NY: Delmar/Thomson Learning.

van Huet, H., Innes, E., & Stancliffe, R. (2013). Occupational therapists perspectives of factors influencing chronic pain management. *Australian Occupational Therapy Journal, 60*, 56–65. https://doi.org/10.1111/1440-1630.12011

Welch, C. D., & Polatajko, H. J. (2016). Applied behavior analysis, autism, and occupational therapy: A search for understanding. *American Journal of Occupational Therapy, 70*, 700460020. https://doi.org/10.5014/ajot.2016.018689

Whatley, E., Fortune, T., & Williams, A. E. (2015). Enabling occupational participation and social inclusion for people recovering from mental ill-health through community gardening. *Australian Occupational Therapy Journal, 62*, 428–437. https://doi.org/10.1111/1440-1630.12240

Will, E., & Hepburn, S. (2015). Applied behavior analysis for children with neurogenetic disorders. *International Review of Research in Developmental Disabilities, 49*, 229–259. https://doi.org/10.1016/bs.irrdd.2015.06.004

Motor Learning Frame of Reference

Anne Cronin, PhD, OTR/L, ATP, FAOTA, and Garth Graebe, MOT, OTR/L

6

CHAPTER HIGHLIGHTS

- Provides an example of the process of theory development in science through motor learning science.
- Differentiates among the concepts of *motor development*, *motor control*, *systems theory*, and *motor learning theory*.
- Defines the key elements of the motor learning frame of reference within the occupational therapy domain.
- Explores the elements of the motor learning frame of reference in a clinical reasoning context.
- Describes the function–dysfunction continuum within the motor learning frame of reference.
- Provides case examples illustrating the use of the motor learning frame of reference in occupational therapy intervention and as a problem-solving tool in clinical reasoning.
- Delineates a basic structure for evidence-based data collection in occupational therapy practice.

KEY TERMS AND CONCEPTS

Associative stage	Mastery climate	Paradigm
Autonomous stage	Motor abilities	Part practice
Cognitive stage	Motor control science	Practice
Constant practice	Motor development science	Scientific method
Distributed practice	Motor learning	Self-organization
Dynamical system theory	Motor learning frame of reference	Systems theory
Learning	Motor program	Variable practice
Learning theories	Motor skill	Whole practice
Massed practice	Open-loop motor control	

In this chapter, readers will learn about the motor learning frame of reference within the scope of occupational therapy's domain and process. The chapter focuses on frames of reference that are grounded in scientific theory, which is supported with strong scientific knowledge gathered by means of the scientific method. Because the motor learning frame of reference is a newer approach built on both science and theory, this chapter uses it to clarify the interrelated roles of science, theory, and theory development in clinical reasoning.

THEORY DEVELOPMENT AND CLINICAL REASONING

The distinction between *everyday theories* and *scientific theories* is the scientific commitment to systematic observation of the phenomenon in question that strives to be objective, logical, and critical. The critical process of formulating, testing, and modifying hypotheses through observation, measurement, and experimentation in the consideration of scientific theory is called the **scientific method** (see Figure 6.1). Every scientist, regardless of discipline, enters into the scientific method with a background of foundational knowledge in their field of specialization. This foundational knowledge colors the ideas of and types of questions that scientists ask, much as a pair of sunglasses changes the view of the wearer.

For the purpose of our discussion, we call this collective background knowledge the *paradigm of the scientist*. A **paradigm** is a philosophical and theoretical framework within which theories, laws, and generalizations, and the experiments performed in a discipline or area of science, are formulated ("Paradigm," 2016).

Occupational therapy also has a paradigm, and the scientific method both uses and is a component of that paradigm. The occupational therapy paradigm is the collective knowledge and beliefs upon which occupational science and the profession of occupational therapy are based. Consider Figure 6.1 as depicting the entire occupational therapy paradigm, including the scientific method but not exclusive to it. The paradigm is important to understand because, when faced with the same clinical

FIGURE 6.1.	Scientific method.

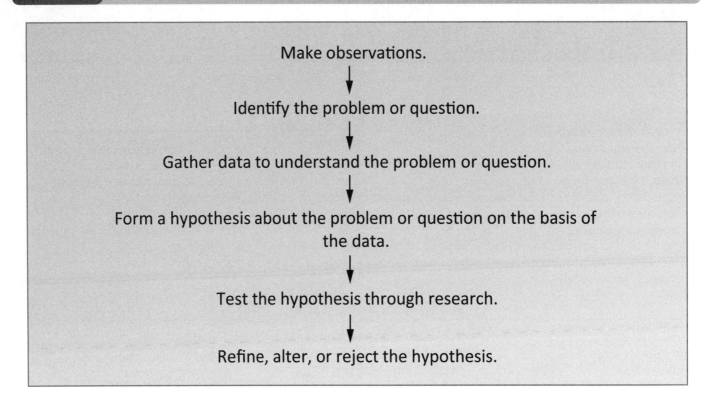

Make observations.

↓

Identify the problem or question.

↓

Gather data to understand the problem or question.

↓

Form a hypothesis about the problem or question on the basis of the data.

↓

Test the hypothesis through research.

↓

Refine, alter, or reject the hypothesis.

presentation, practitioners from different fields with different professional paradigms will ask different questions and follow a different clinical reasoning pathway.

The *scientific method is* often described as starting with observations that, through the lens of the person's paradigm, lead to interesting questions. Through this method, scientific theories emerge, are studied, and are refined. The process is iterative, meaning that it is ongoing, and all steps of the process inform future steps. Aspects of scientific theories that are tested extensively and over time are accepted as knowledge rather than theory. An example of this is the biomechanical frame of reference presented earlier in this text. Although theory may be generated within this frame of reference, the assumptions and postulates of change are grounded in scientifically supported knowledge.

MOTOR CONTROL SCIENCE

Motor control science is a focused field of scientific inquiry that informs the understanding of human movement and provides a research foundation for the motor learning frame of reference. Motor control research typically focuses on the role of the central nervous system (CNS) in the control of posture and movement. Specific aspects of motor performance, especially sports performance, also have an extensive scientific research basis. The motor learning frame of reference draws from motor control

science. Examples include information about establishing of motor programs within the CNS, the sensory system's contributions to motor function, and task constraints on movement. The distinction between a science and a frame of reference is that the frame of reference emphasizes clinical application of the information, and it may also include theory as well as science.

Motor development science is the study of skill acquisition over time as a result of physical maturation and environmental supports. From this area, the motor learning frame of reference draws a systems perspective on emerging behavioral motor milestones, the ability to anticipate and adapt actions to a changing environment, reflexive modulations in movement skills, and the supporting systems for specific motor behaviors, such as postural control (Shumway-Cook & Woollacott, 2012).

Systems theory originated in mathematics but has been applied to many areas of science, including motor control science. *Systems theory* defines a specific type of system, a dynamical system, which is an open system that exchanges energy and influences with the environment and results in a process of change over time. *Dynamical systems theory (DST)* proposes that the body is a complex system composed of millions of interacting parts. This theory argues that the coordination of these interacting parts is not located in a single organ (e.g., brain) but rather emerges from the complex interactions of all the different parts. DST focuses on self-organization and emergent motor actions. In *self-organization,* the various forces operating within and upon the system interact in such a way as to create an emergent set of properties that is organizing to the system as a whole. Movement, in the form of motor activity, is an emergent property from the interaction of multiple influences on the system that require a response or reaction. In this context the human open system is continuously exposed to factors that challenge the equilibrium of the system and may result in a state of disequilibrium. Disequilibrium is a near constant in everyday motor function and, in this theory, is a catalyst for reorganizing movement into new (or different) and increasingly complex behavior. DST has been incorporated into many of the frames of reference used by occupational therapy practitioners, including the developmental systems and the motor learning frames of reference.

Learning theories are conceptual frameworks that describe assumptions about how information is received, processed, and retained in a manner that allows it to be retrieved and used in new situations. For our purposes, *learning* is the process of acquiring the capacity for skilled action that results from practice. Learning cannot be observed directly but must be inferred from behavior (i.e., performance), and it produces a permanent change in behavior. This view of learning is widely accepted scientifically and provides the foundation for the frames of reference presented in this text.

MOTOR LEARNING FRAME OF REFERENCE

Understanding the *motor learning frame of reference* continues the discussion of clinical reasoning because it combines the foundational sciences of motor control and motor development with applications of systems theory and learning theory. Systems theory and learning theory consider internalized mental processes that influence human performance but cannot be measured directly; rather, they can only be inferred from the observation of performance. Both of these theories have continued to evolve and be refined in light of new scientific knowledge.

As noted when we presented the psychodynamic frame of reference, when theory addresses internalized mental processes, research findings are inferred or interpreted in terms of the theory rather than by specifically testing it. This distinction between what can be observed and what is internal to the person may be confusing to readers. This chapter discusses theory vs. science because it is common for textbooks and other scholarly sources to lump motor control and motor learning theory together instead of differentiating theory from science. Combining these is reasonable; the theory and science are closely linked and consistent with one another. The distinction is made here to help support the clinical reasoning process, especially as we move into later chapters where there is less congruence between theory and science.

The motor learning frame of reference has profoundly affected occupational therapy clinical practice in part because it so effectively translates basic science into concrete clinical applications. Table 6.1 describes major contributors to the modern motor learning frame of reference.

Early Motor Learning Theory

Early motor learning theory was informed by hierarchical models of motor control and motor development that emphasized the role of higher centers of the brain in regulating movement. Although older literature described the influences of motor development science as a hierarchical model, contemporary research shows that motor

TABLE 6.1.	Contributions to Motor Learning Frame of Reference			
CONTRIBUTIONS	MOTOR CONTROL SCIENCE	MOTOR DEVELOPMENT SCIENCE	SYSTEMS THEORY	LEARNING THEORY
Measurement	It is measured through scientific tools such as electromyography and *f*MRI.	It is measured qualitatively and quantitatively through direct observation of performance.	It is measured in terms of system organization and increasing complexity over time.	It is measured across time; learning must be inferred from behavior and degrees of skill acquisition.
Concepts	Generalized motor programs are pre-structured sets of commands from the CNS.	It is characterized by a predictable sequence of acquisition that is heterarchical rather than hierarchical.	Output depends on the control parameters acting on the system at the time.	Learning produces a permanent change in behavior.
Applications	Control of a single muscle can be adequately described with changes in the threshold of motor unit recruitment.	Contextual factors from the environment can influence the pattern and quality of skill acquisition.	An attractor is a preferred pattern that leads to a consistent pattern of performance.	Effective learning can be generalized to new challenges and contexts.

Note. CNS = central nervous system; *f*MRI = functional magnetic resonance imaging.

development does not perfectly reflect CNS maturation, and the exclusive focus on higher centers of the brain in regulating movement has been disproved. Many independent studies have established that the coordination of the interacting parts of the human system is not exclusively controlled by the brain (which was the older hierarchical model) but rather emerges from the complex interactions of all the different parts.

One prominent early researcher of motor learning was psychologist Esther Thelen. She was interested in infant movement development and in one study explored the changes in the stepping behavior of infants during development (Boudreau, 2009). Basic to early development is the observation that when young infants are held upright, they will start stepping, as if they want to walk. This is called the *stepping response* and is a common item on infant developmental screening tools. This response is interesting because it is present near birth and then disappears at around 2 months of development, only to reemerge as true stepping later in infancy.

The older, hierarchical explanation for the emergence–disappearance–re-emergence of the stepping reaction was based on an assumption about the development of the CNS. According to this older view, infants lose the motor control programs required for stepping as primitive postural reflexes are inhibited and various protective extension and equilibrium reactions develop to replace the more primitive patterns. Although aspects of this older explanation are sound, through her experiments Thelen was able to create the stepping behavior in children who were thought to be lacking the necessary CNS maturity. She did this by partially submerging their legs in water, effectively making the legs lighter, and this caused children to start spontaneously stepping. Thelen's study showed that it was not simply CNS maturity that caused the change in movement patterns but also the physical weight of the infant's legs in relation to the infant's motor strength.

Thelen's study shows that the older hierarchical model does not completely explain motor behavior, but it also illustrates the DST concepts of *self-organization* and *emergent motor actions*. When the weight of the growing infant's legs required more strength to move than the infant had, the movement stopped. Through exploring a single aspect of human motor development, Thelen effectively "disproved" the hierarchical model of change in the brain as the sole explanation for motor skill acquisition. When infants experienced the buoyancy of water, thus reducing the strength needed to step, the stepping reaction (thought to have disappeared) proved to be present (Boudreau, 2009). The hierarchical model continues to be essential to the understanding of human motor control, but Thelen and other colleagues have shown that there are additional influences within the human motor control system that affect the emergence of motor skill.

Expansion of Motor Learning Theory

Thelen's research expanded the explanation for motor skill acquisition and emergent motor behavior, illustrating the process of theory development and refinement in science. A good idea (i.e., the hierarchical pattern of motor skill acquisition) was built into a theory, this theory was explored, and scientific experiments were developed to test aspects of the original theory.

From this early scientific process many frames of reference used in occupational therapy emerged, including both neurodevelopmental therapy (NDT) and sensory integration (SI). Research on human movement has continued and researchers, including Thelen, studied "exceptions" to the foundational theory. From these studies additional data were gathered, some of which supported the theory and some of which refuted it.

Today's accepted model of motor control development is heterarchical—its elements are unranked (i.e., nonhierarchical) or can potentially be ranked in different ways. Expanding theory from an exclusively top-down hierarchical model is consistent with contemporary motor control science, which views motor control in terms of several systems acting in parallel with elaborate multidirectional communication between neural centers (Mandich, 2016).

Clinical frames of reference such as NDT and SI will be discarded as unscientific if they do not update and alter assessment and intervention strategies to incorporate the refined understanding of human movement grounded in contemporary science. This is why NDT practitioners actively integrate strategies derived from motor control science into their practice. Although aspects of the original NDT theory are not supported by modern science, the frame of reference still has much clinical utility. Retaining the useful and replacing the "disproven" aspects with scientifically supported clinical interventions reflect expert clinical reasoning and support best practice principles.

Motor Learning: Occupational Therapy Considerations

Motor learning is the acquisition, retention, and transfer of specific movement patterns to a motor solution. It emerges from the individual's interaction with the task and the environment and results from practice. Motor learning results in a relatively permanent change in movement behavior measured after a retention period. The motor learning frame of reference is part of the occupational therapy paradigm but has been used and studied by many other professional disciplines. Occupational therapy's conceptualization of the motor learning frame of reference focuses on aspects of its extensive literature that support function and client outcomes within the domain of occupational therapy. The general elements of the motor learning frame of reference as used in occupational therapy are presented in Exhibit 6.1.

> **EXHIBIT 6.1.** **Elements of Motor Learning Frame of Reference**
>
> - **Focus:** The focus of this frame of reference is on the actual movement itself and the functional end goal of the movement—in other words, not just moving to move but moving with a purpose, because that is what will allow the person to learn (Li, 2013).
> - **Basic assumptions:** Motor learning results from practice and is supported by active movement, error detection, and error correction. Motor learning may be enhanced through visual imagery along with active practice. In addition to motor capability, motor learning requires attention, memory, and motivation to support learning.
> - **Function–disability continuum:** Optimal functional movements are efficient and support the performance of daily occupations. Inefficient or impaired movement can be improved through the use of feedback and practice.
> - **Postulates of change:** Through the use of repetitive movements, the body builds a memory of that movement and is then able to refine movement patterns to greater efficiency. Movement can be learned and practiced by using different degrees of freedom to create a more efficient movement pattern. Uncoordinated or inefficient movements can be relearned and changed to develop into coordinated functional movements (Li, 2013). Practice can be performed in various ways: massed, distributed, whole or part practice, mental, variable, or scheduled. Feedback, either intrinsic or extrinsic, is another important component of success.

The motor learning frame of reference distinguishes between *motor abilities,* which are genetically or physiologically predetermined and provide a foundation for skilled performance, and *motor skill,* which is the capability to produce a performance result reliably and efficiently (Schmidt & Lee, 2013). Attaining motor abilities involves a process of learning that is reflected in progress from novice to skilled motor performance throughout the lifespan. Motor learning occurs in all persons, both those with typical motor patterns and those with atypical motor patterns. Motor abilities may be a limiting factor in the level of skill a person is able to achieve. These abilities may be perceptual–motor abilities (e.g., multilimb coordination, finger dexterity, rate control) or physical proficiency (e.g., strength, flexibility, endurance). In addition, people with neurological conditions may need to relearn previously acquired motor skills.

A *motor program* is a set of motor commands that has been established through learning at the executive level and defines the essential details of a skilled action (Schmidt & Lee, 2013). Motor programs emerge through learning and limit the person's movement patterns to make actions efficient and effective. Some motor programs are triggered and performed with little input from the environment during the performance of the action, such as the quick retraction of one's arm when one touches a hot object. This

type of movement involves *open-loop motor control.* The motion is triggered on the basis of environmental cues, but once triggered it is fairly stereotypical and not easy to change while the action is occurring. Open-loop motor programs are typically used to control rapid, discrete movements in stable, predictable environments (Schmidt & Lee, 2013).

Other motor programs are more flexible and responsive to variable environmental conditions. These actions are controlled by the use of a feedback, error detection, and error correction process during the performance of the movement. The possible potential combinations of muscle and joint activities that the person is capable of producing are nearly infinite. This vast flexibility in possible movements would be nearly impossible for people to manage without some way to regulate the movements into patterns.

Shumway-Cook and Woollacott (2012) identify 3 stages of motor learning: (1) cognitive, (2) associative, and (3) autonomous. These stages are widely used in occupational therapy practice when designing supports for clients engaged in motor learning tasks and when designing specific motor interventions (see Figure 6.2).

Cognitive stage

The first stage of motor learning, the *cognitive stage,* is characterized by the establishment of task goals. At this stage, learning generally involves the use of explicit knowledge about the task and often involves the use of language. Verbal rehearsal, in which the person recites, often audibly, the steps to a task, is a common learning strategy in the cognitive stage. This early cognitive stage of learning requires that the learner initiate the movement; too much feedback or coaching in this stage can be disruptive (Mandich, 2016). Learners at this stage are getting the idea of the task, which includes assessing their own abilities, developing strategies, learning regulatory constraints, and formulating (and refining) a motor program to successively approximate a task. Individuals at this stage of learning are often halting, inefficient, and inaccurate in their movements. During this stage, extrinsic feedback offering knowledge of results is most important. In the cognitive stage, there is a rapid improvement in performance.

Associative stage

The second stage, the *associative stage,* is characterized by a more gradual improvement in performance. In this stage, individuals practice the movement or pattern of movements. With practice, the spatial and temporal aspects of movement become well organized, and movement errors decrease. As compared with the cognitive stage, learners in this stage are more relaxed and more accurate. Less working memory is involved in the performance of the new skill, resulting in lowered cognitive

FIGURE 6.2. **3 stages of learning a motor program.**

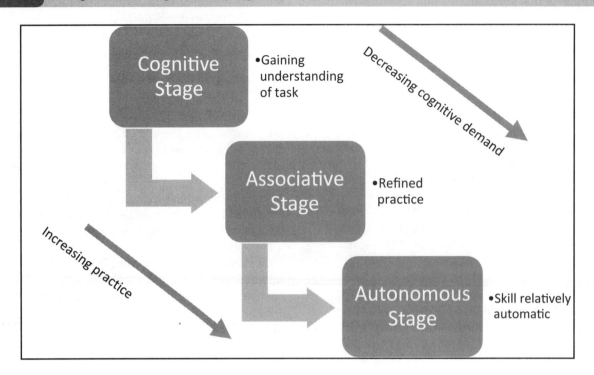

demand. Learners still make errors, but the errors are more minor and fewer than before. As learners progress, the need for extrinsic feedback decreases, and there is a greater reliance on intrinsic (especially proprioceptive) feedback. During the associative stage, feedback and coaching are helpful in correcting and improving motor skill.

Autonomous stage

In the third, *autonomous stage*, the movement proceeds automatically, and people no longer need to explicitly think about task performance. At this stage, learners' motor performance is consistent, fluid, and efficient. People recognize their own errors and are able to adapt to variables in the environment. When the initial skill becomes automatic in a particular learning environment, for instance when young adults learn to drive the family car, motor learning may be extended to different performance environments, such as different cars. In this stage, excessive attention to the skill can result in the phenomenon known as *paralysis from analysis,* wherein the more attention that is paid to the skill, the more its performance worsens (Mandich, 2016).

STATE OF SCIENCE AND EVIDENCE CONSIDERATIONS

Strong scientific evidence from motor control science and specific studies of motor learning supports the motor learning frame of reference. Of the frames of reference

presented in this text, motor control science is one of the most evidence based. The motor learning frame of reference collects and integrates information from diverse sources to understand the acquisition of movement patterns. This frame of reference provides a good model for occupational therapy practitioners for considering and assimilating scientific innovation. Expert practitioners, in the area of motor learning and other areas of practice continually explore new information and consider it against their prevailing knowledge to inform practice decisions.

Small changes in understanding can have a big clinical impact. For example, the older, hierarchical view of human motor development assumed that people must have effective proximal motor control before they could develop effective distal motor control. In other words, one should not work on fine motor skills until the large shoulder muscles were well controlled. This view has, however, been discounted in current. It is well established that "control over proximal body segments is not a necessary precursor to distal hand function" (Shumway-Cook & Woollacott, 2012, p. 585). Therefore, interventions should not be exclusively hierarchical but designed to be functional and task specific in addressing client needs.

NDT and Motor Learning

As noted earlier, the NDT frame of reference is still influential, although its original form is based on a hierarchical model of development. Although NDT theory has not changed substantially, current practice within the NDT frame of reference assimilates aspects of motor control science and motor learning into NDT strategies. Particularly for pediatric practitioners, NDT tools for analyzing atypical movements and establishing optimal positioning and alignment uniquely support the occupational therapy practitioner in problem-solving complex motor and positioning needs. Using NDT principles informed by motor control science and a motor learning frame of reference elevate the NDT frame of reference from unsupported to emerging practice. Evidence-based practice permits contextual and client-specific influences and allows room for alternative and innovative approaches. Although strong scientific evidence is highly valued, there is justification through robust clinical reasoning for making alternative choices.

Tango Dancing as a Motor Learning Intervention

The motor control frame of reference focuses on the fact that the body can move in various ways, allowing individuals many different movement options at any given point in time (Li, 2013). This frame of reference focuses on the actual movement and the functional end goal of the movement (Li, 2013)—in other words, not just moving to move but moving with a goal beyond the movement.

The motor learning frame of reference considers not just practice parameters but also the impact of the learning environment and motivation in supporting the learning of movements. Motor learning supports development of skills to achieve a desired movement in the most effective and efficient way within a mastery climate. A *mastery climate* encourages individuals to judge success in terms of a positive change in one's performance, not in comparison to others (Schmidt & Lee, 2013). Guided practice of desired movements and movement sequences in a mastery climate allows poorly coordinated movements to be changed and developed into coordinated functional movements (Li, 2013).

A person with Parkinson's disease (PD) can experience many of types of motor dysfunction, including tremors, rigidity, lack of postural control, bradykinesia, akinesia, and overall instability (Foster, Golden, Duncan, & Earhart, 2013). Using cognitive strategies to support learning dance steps, paired with music to aid in maintaining the rhythm and pace of motions, people with PD can practice postural control and fluid movement patterns in an enjoyable and meaningful manner.

In a study by Hackney and Earhart (2009), tango dance classes were structured so that the dance students learned only a small portion of the dance and practiced it for a whole class period. This allowed for learning of repetitive movements and prepared participants for more complex motor actions. The dance is ideally done by partnering a person with PD with a physically able person to allow demonstration of accurate movements and feedback. Specific feedback on aspects of performance is important in this intervention approach (Kilduski & Rice, 2003). Practitioners using tango dance as a tool to support participation in daily occupations could either teach or assist in the dance class.

A weakness of traditional repetitive exercise approaches is that practicing movements outside of a functional context can become meaningless to the person. Providing opportunities for movement that is functional and social offers a rewarding and naturalistic context for intervention.

Motor Learning Frame of Reference in Occupational Therapy Intervention

The motor learning frame of reference is the most widely used frame of reference in addressing impairments of movement across all practice settings. Its strong scientific foundation makes it a preferred approach and one that is used extensively by practitioners in many disciplines. The challenge for occupational therapy practitioners is to apply this frame of reference as a tool to support occupation rather than as a stand-alone intervention for motor impairment. Case Example 6.1 illustrates applying this frame of reference in a way that supports occupational therapy's domain.

Noah's case illustrates the importance of the learning environment. The learning environment should be structured with both the demands of the activity and the individual's motivation in mind. Incorporating activities valued by Noah and his family in the natural environment of his home was an essential support to this intervention. A motivating learning environment supports the persistent practice of the skill to achieve autonomous skilled movements.

To be considered skilled, movement patterns should demonstrate consistency, flexibility, and efficiency (Muratori, Lamberg, Quinn, & Duff, 2013). *Motor skill consistency* refers to the repeatability of performance, that is, the ability to perform the task consistently during a period of trials conducted over several sessions. *Flexibility in motor skill performance* refers to the ability to adapt and modify task performance on the basis of changing environments or conditions. Finally, *efficiency* refers to the lack of need to recruit additional muscle groups and to minimize the demand on the cardiovascular and musculoskeletal systems.

PRACTICE STRATEGIES

Practice is an essential aspect of teaching and supporting motor skills. *Practice* involves repetition, feedback, error detection, and error correction. Error warrants special consideration because it is a critically important part of the learning process. Lee et al. (2016) found that efforts to minimize errors during practice consistently resulted in the least effective condition for learning. This wisdom

CASE EXAMPLE 6.1. NOAH: CP

Noah, age 3.5 years, has a diagnosis of spastic hemiplegia-type cerebral palsy (CP) and has weakness on the left side of his body. He has been seen by occupational therapy and physical therapy practitioners since he was 9 months old and was selected to participate in a program of constraint-induced movement therapy (CIMT) to help teach him to use his weaker arm more often (see Exhibit 6.2).

CIMT is a short-term, intensive intervention that involves constraint of the noninvolved arm and intensive movement practice with the involved arm (Case-Smith, DeLuca, Stevenson, & Ramey, 2012; Ramey, Coker-Bolt, & DeLuca, 2013). It is an evidence-based intervention

that is built on the motor learning frame of reference. The use of teaching and skill practice of targeted movement is the basis of this intervention approach.

Noah's CIMT program involved 2 occupational therapy home visits of 50–60 minutes weekly for a period of 6 weeks. In these visits, functional goals were set with the family, and the family was taught to immobilize his right arm. The parents and Noah's nanny were taught how to prompt use of the left hand in activities and in play. Specific activities, such as playing with modeling compound and assisting with ADL activities, were taught and repeated over the 3-week period. Initially, Noah was in the cognitive stage of

EXHIBIT 6.2.	Noah's Occupational Profile		
Client	**Reason the client is seeking service and concerns related to engagement in occupations**	Occupational therapy program of CIMT to support function left upper-limb use. *Impact on occupation:* Noah has significant delays in physical, communication, and adaptive skills.	
	Occupations in which the client is successful	Noah has some developmentally appropriate early ADL skills.	
	Personal interests and values	Noah loves being held and being read to. He enjoys using touchscreen devices to play games. Noah enjoys being around other children.	
	Occupational history (i.e., life experiences)	Noah has a diagnosis of spastic hemiplegia-type CP and has weakness on the left side of his body. He was selected to participate in a program of CIMT to train him to use his weaker arm more often. Noah has moderate spasticity in both extremities on his left side and low tone in his trunk muscle groups. Noah is the smallest of triplets born at 30 weeks' gestation. He was in the NICU for 3 months after birth. He has been seen for EI by OT and PT since birth. Both of Noah's brothers are typically developing and very active.	
	Performance patterns (routines, roles, habits, & rituals)	Noah's routines are currently managed by the adults in his life.	
Environment		*Supports to occupational engagement*	*Barriers to occupational engagement*
	Physical (e.g., buildings, furniture, pets)	Noah's family has a large home and a large playroom for the boys.	Noah is usually kept in a playpen or on an adult's lap to keep his brothers from trampling him.
	Social (e.g., spouse, friends, caregivers)	Noah and his 2 brothers are cared for at home. Noah's parents share the caregiving in the evening and on weekends, and they have hired a nanny for the daytime. Both parents work but have cut their work hours to 35 hours per week.	

(Continued)

CASE EXAMPLE 6.1. NOAH: CP *(Cont.)*

EXHIBIT 6.2.	Noah's Occupational Profile *(Cont.)*	
Context	**Cultural** (e.g., customs, beliefs)	No issues related to culture, customs, or beliefs were identified during assessment.
	Personal (e.g., age, gender, SES, education)	3.5-year-old male. Noah's family has been assertive in seeking services for him and have good financial and family resources to help meet his needs.
	Temporal (e.g., stage of life, time, year)	Noah is a preschooler whose primary interactions are with his family.
	Virtual (e.g., chat, email, remote monitoring)	Not applicable to Noah at this time.
Client goals	**Client's priorities and desired targeted outcomes**	Noah's goal is to improve participation in developmental play activities and ADLs. Noah also has the goal of improving functional use of left upper limb.
ANALYSIS OF PARTICIPATION		
Basic ADLs		
Eating/oral–motor		Noah finger-feeds using his right hand. He is able to hold and use a lidded sippy cup with his right hand. For meals and snacks, he is positioned in a regular high chair. Noah has no oral–motor impairments. He does have difficulty with bimanual tasks during meals, such as opening containers and using utensils (without the assistance of a scoop dish).
Grooming		Noah requires more assistance than his brothers. He is able to hold a toothbrush and brush his teeth, but he has difficult washing and drying his hands.
Bathing/transfer		Noah is able to climb into and out of the bathtub by himself.
Dressing upper body		Noah assists by extending his neck and his arms but is otherwise dependent in this task. He is unable to manage any type of fastener.
Dressing lower body		Noah assists with weight shifts and by extending his legs. He does use his right arm to pull up and adjust pants, but he requires moderate assistance to complete lower body dressing.
Toileting		Noah is developmentally appropriate in basic toileting. He is able to manage a child-sized potty seat. He has occasional accidents but is largely potty-trained.
Problem solving/memory		Noah is developmentally appropriate in this area.
Comments:		None.
IADLs		
Community mobility		Noah is developmentally appropriate in this area. He rides in a stroller and complies with car seat positioning during transportation.
Health management/prevention		Not applicable developmentally.
Home management		Noah does not have chores around the house. His brothers are required to pick up their toys, put their clothes in the hamper, and help with small tasks around the house such as sorting laundry.
Financial management		Not applicable developmentally.

(Continued)

CASE EXAMPLE 6.1. NOAH: CP *(Cont.)*

EXHIBIT 6.2.	**Noah's Occupational Profile *(Cont.)***
Leisure/play	Noah enjoys functional and imitation play. He enjoys the company of other children, but his mobility and upper-limb limitations restrict his ability to participate with the group.
Safety	Noah is developmentally appropriate in this area.
Comments:	None.
	Motor and Praxis Skills
Sitting—static/dynamic	Noah is able to sit on a stool without support for a developmentally appropriate period of 10 minutes. He has limited dynamic balance and often needs to catch himself when his arms are actively engaged.
Standing—static/dynamic	Noah is able to stand without support briefly. His ability is enough to assist with transfers. He uses a rear-facing pediatric walker and has poor dynamic balance in standing.
Joint stability and skeletal mobility	Noah has full PROM in all limbs. He has moderately limited AROM in both his left arm and left leg. Noah rolls on the floor and tries to belly crawl. He can take steps with support and is able to move in a gait trainer, but his movements in this walker are asymmetrical and largely unilateral.
Place can on shelf	Noah is unable to do this without postural supports.
Retrieve item from floor	Noah is unable to do this without postural supports.
Screw lid on jar	Noah is unable to do this without external stabilization of the jar.
Comb back of head	Noah is developmentally appropriate in this area.
Writing	Noah is developmentally appropriate in this area.
Lift grocery bag	Noah is unable to do this.
Coordination	Noah has difficulty in all bilateral and bimanual activities. Does not have adequate stability (without external support) for most coordinated tasks. On the QUEST (DeMatteo et al., 1992), Noah demonstrated some functional grasp–release patterns with his left hand, but he was significantly impaired by associated movements.
Manipulation	Noah is developmentally appropriate with his right hand. He scored a 25 on the AHA (Holmefur, Aarts, Hoare, & Krumlinde-Sundholm, 2009), indicating that his left hand is not used functionally.
Comments:	Noah has been prompted to use his left arm in all therapy sessions, but without 1:1 supervision, he seldom uses the limb.
	Process Skills
Energy for task	Noah is developmentally appropriate in this area.
Knowledge/organization of task	Noah is developmentally appropriate in this area.
Adaptation/praxis	Noah's hemiplegia and developmental level makes this area difficult to assess.
Comments:	None.
	Behavioral and Cognitive Skills
Communication and following social conventions	Noah is developmentally appropriate in this area.
Cognitive and emotional regulation skills	Noah is developmentally appropriate in this area.
Level of arousal/attention	Noah is developmentally appropriate in this area.

(Continued)

CASE EXAMPLE 6.1. NOAH: CP *(Cont.)*

EXHIBIT 6.2.   Noah's Occupational Profile *(Cont.)*

Orientation	Noah is developmentally appropriate in this area.
Energy and drive	Noah is developmentally appropriate in this area.
Memory and understanding	Noah is developmentally appropriate in this area.
Higher level cognition	Noah is developmentally appropriate in this area.
Sensory–Perceptual Skills	
Sensory	Noah is developmentally appropriate in this area.
Self-perception	Noah is developmentally appropriate in this area.
Pain	Noah has no problems in this area.
Skin integrity	Noah has no problems in this area.
Comments:	None.

Note. Occupational profile template from American Occupational Therapy Association (2017). Analysis of participation format adapted from Skubik-Peplaski, Paris, Boyle, & Culpert (2009). ADLs = activities of daily living; AHA = Assisting Hand Assessment; AROM = active range of motion; CIMT = constraint-induced movement therapy; CP = cerebral palsy; EI = early intervention; IADLs = instrumental activities of daily living; NICU = neonatal intensive care unit; OT = occupational therapy; PROM = passive range of motion; PT = physical therapy; QUEST = Quality of Upper-Extremity Skills Test.

learning, and use of his left arm required focused cognitive effort.

By the end of the 6-week period, Noah demonstrated significant improvements on all of the measures of hand function. He was spontaneously using his left hand in bimanual activities about 60% of the time and with adult prompting 100% of the time. His left-hand use was still far less dexterous than his right-hand use, but his active participation in play and ADL activities was greatly improved. Noah's left-hand use

still varied between the associative and cognitive stages of motor learning for practiced tasks, and he relied on the cognitive stage in new activities. He seemed more aware of his left arm and more inclined to try to use it, but he was not yet autonomous in its use. To maintain these gains and to continue to support bimanual upper-limb use, Noah will continue to need support and to be taught to use the limb in meaningful and motivating activities. Without continued practice, the new skills may fall out of use.

---

about error, although newly affirmed by Lee et al., has been around for a long time. Although the term *errorless learning* is often used in clinical settings, Lee et al. found no support for this approach in the acquisition of motor skills.

Regardless of the skill in question, more time spent in practice creates more opportunity for people to improve their capabilities. In the context of motor rehabilitation in general and CIMT in particular, it is clear that more practice is better (Muratori et al., 2013). Some of the research supporting the motor learning frame of reference has explored how to practice to gain the greatest impact. Several distinct supports to learning and specific practice patterns have been identified and are easily integrated into occupational therapy interventions.

In the learning environment it is important to promote a climate of mastery focusing on a positive change in targeted motor performance. A motivating learning environment also provides choice. The choice can be in the activity that is selected as the foundation for skill

practice, or it can be aspects of the activity (e.g., modeling dough color, song you sing while picking up toys).

Whole vs. Part Practice

Whole practice is a strategy that involves practicing a skill in its entirety. For example, clinicians may find that some tasks (e.g., transfers from wheelchair to toilet seat) are best practiced in their entirety (i.e., whole) because they are difficult to break into steps and once initiated one is committed to a follow through. Other tasks (e.g., putting on a shirt) are best learned when broken into separate parts. This is *part practice* and is a strategy that involves practicing components of a skill separately before putting the components together to practice the whole skill.

Muratori et al. (2013) reported that "to decide if part practice may be beneficial the task must be analyzed based on the number of segments as well as the degree that those segments are interdependent on one another"

(p. 100). A transfer is usually a continuous motor task that, once initiated, is difficult to stop. This type of task is best taught in whole practice. When a task is made up of discrete movements that are chained together into a sequence, such as putting on a shirt, part practice is more effective.

Distributed vs. Massed Practice

Once you have decided how to present the task to be learned, the next decision is how to structure practice sessions to optimize motor learning. Should a lot of practice be performed at once, such as doing 20–30 transfers in a day (i.e., *massed practice*), or would it be better to break up the practice, doing 1–2 transfers twice a day for 1 week (i.e., *distributed practice*)? Muratori et al. (2013) reported that

> massed practice requires all the trials to be performed in a manner that minimizes the amount of rest between trials so there is more time on task than there is spent during rest. Distributed practice divides repetitions into smaller chunks to allow for rest between trials (e.g., 5 trials now, 5 in 10 minutes).

Massed practice is generally considered to lead to faster acquisition of specific movement patterns, but the person may lack the flexibility to alter the movement to meet unexpected demands (Shumway-Cook & Woollacott, 2012). Learning may be slower in distributed practice, but this form of practice is more responsive to the cognitive and physical limitations of people in occupational therapy clinical settings, and this approach to practice may better support learning flexibility in task performance.

Constant vs. Variable Practice

Performance of only one motor task, performed exactly the same way time after time, is termed *constant practice* (Muratori et al., 2013). For Noah, constant practice might include using wrist and finger extension to roll out the same amount of modeling compound using the same start position on every practice trial. Although this may improve Noah's ability to perform this particular task, his ability to retain and transfer a skill is likely to be reduced after this type of constant practice (Kruisselbrink & Van Gyn, 2011).

Variable practice involves performing variations of the task or completely different tasks throughout a treatment session (Muratori et al., 2013). In the example of Noah, this would mean engaging in a variety of activities using modeling compound, emphasizing play that incorporates varying setup of the task and involves a variety of demands in terms of muscle force and activity duration. The literature has consistently corroborated that variable practice is the superior approach to support functional skill development.

Specificity and Location of Practice

Task-specific or task-oriented practice is an approach to rehabilitation that focuses on performance of functional tasks that are meaningful to the person (Lang & Birkenmeier, 2014; Muratori et al., 2013). This approach to practice is widely used in occupational therapy clinical settings across population types. It is heavily dependent on effective activity analysis and the occupational therapy practitioner's ability to arrange the environment to provide the proper affordances so that the task, or a modified version of the task, can successfully be completed.

In Noah's case, the occupational therapy practitioner may teach him a one-handed dressing technique to develop independence in self-dressing. Having assessed his functional capabilities, the occupational therapy practitioner may specifically choose a t-shirt to begin with because it is stretchy, has short sleeves, and lacks fasteners. This type of shirt would simplify the dressing task and increase Noah's probability of successful performance as he is learning.

MOTOR LEARNING RESEARCH AND CLINICAL PRACTICE

The motor learning frame of reference is widely used in research because it clearly applies to the rehabilitation needs of clinical populations and is highly measurable. The original exploration of motor practice as a tool to support motor learning emerged out of the field of physical education. Understanding implementation of motor practice strategies and considering exercise dosage is an area of emerging knowledge. Sakzewski, Ziviani, and Boyd (2016) commented that

> essential elements of (upper limb) therapies include: (1) intensive structured task repetition; (2) progressive incremental increase in difficulty; and (3) goal directed approach to enhance motivation and engagement in therapy. Despite evidence for contemporary (upper limb) therapies, many occupational therapists . . . fail to use a goal directed approach, persist in using traditional interventions with limited evidence and ineffective models of therapy provision (e.g., short duration blocks of weekly therapy without a structured home program). (p. 306)

Sakzewski et al. (2016) explored the barriers to translating evidence into clinical practice and found that occupational therapy practitioners were confident in delivering traditional bimanual occupational therapy interventions but were less knowledgeable, skilled, and confident in providing modified CIMT. Respondents in their study reported that achieving an adequate dose of therapy (>30 hours) was perceived as difficult to adopt, although therapists identified greater use of occupational

TABLE 6.2.	Structure for Evidence-Based Data Collection	
STRATEGY	**ACTION**	**CLINICAL REASONING**
Collect information, not interpretations.	Report facts.	Use evidence-based clinical reasoning to make hypotheses about the facts.
Measure something that matters.	Report performance, not details of structure or function.	Maintain a client-centered focus; measurement should relate to client-identified priorities.
Measure participation, not interventions.	Measure what the client does rather than what you do to and for the client.	Keep interventions occupationally based and measure the change in the occupation.
Measure during everyday living, not during therapy.	Performance in clinical settings can prepare clients for performance in their natural settings, but it is not the same as performing in those settings. Measure performance in real-life situations whenever possible.	Contextual factors greatly affect performance and participation; consideration of these factors should be part of the clinical reasoning process.
Record what you are measuring.	Keep a record of what does and does not work. Records can consist of bullet-point lists, graphs, photographs, videos, or notes.	Communication and collaboration are essential aspects of clinical reasoning. Consistent recording plans serve as a communication tool for all involved.

therapy home programs and group-based models of therapy as potential strategies to increase therapy dose.

Sakzewski et al. (2016) developed a year-long program of instruction and support for occupational therapy practitioners to measure the potential for change in clinical practice and the client outcomes associated with implementation of a more evidence-based approach to occupational therapy intervention. They were able to document a change toward more evidence-based approaches but found that respondents had been correct in identifying therapy dose as the most difficult evidence criterion to fulfill.

They found that only modest gains in the amount or dose of occupational therapy were possible through an increase in direct service provision. This suggests that increasing direct 1:1 therapy was not as useful in long-term training as embedding practice into individuals' natural activity contexts. The occupational therapy practitioners in this study learned to build more measurable home programs to help increase the dosage of the intervention to conform to the best evidence, but the inconsistent completion of home practice logs made the assessment of home program supports difficult to quantify. Many challenges are associated with studying clinical populations, such as children with CP, because of the inherent challenges of both dosage and documentation of indirect interventions in the real world.

Occupational therapy practitioners must be able to examine the evidence in the professional literature, and they must be able to collect objective data in their own practice. The client-specific data should guide clinical reasoning about what is effective for that particular client, and the data should be critically reviewed continuously during the evaluation and intervention process.

Dunn (2008) offered a basic structure for evidence-based data collection in one's practice. These collection strategies are summarized in Table 6.2.

MOTOR LEARNING AND COGNITION

There is a logical fit between the motor learning frame of reference and aspects of occupational therapy practice. This frame of reference is specific to the learning of movements and is applied equally well to elite athletes and to persons recovering from a spinal cord injury. The frame of reference itself is not focused on occupation, but it is effective in helping gain the motor skills needed to support occupational performance. When considering this, it is easy to forget that learning itself is a cognitive process. In fact, most purposeful movement requires cognitive direction. This is why motor delay is seen in persons with intellectual impairments and dementia, even when they have no dysfunction in their motor systems. It is also why acquiring a specific movement pattern, such as a dynamic tripod grasp, does not ensure that the individual will improve handwriting performance. There are complex aspects to many tasks such as handwriting that warrant a broader intervention approach that addresses the complexity of the occupation.

In reviewing the steps to learning a motor program presented in Figure 6.2, note that motivation must underlie the whole process, from taking on the cognitive acquisition of the movement to persisting with practice. Finally, in the autonomous stage the client must be motivated to use the motor program that has been built. Consider the interrelationship between cognitive function and motor performance in the case of Debbie (Case Example 6.2).

CASE EXAMPLE 6.2. DEBBIE: ALZHEIMER'S DISEASE

The motor learning frame of reference is most typically applied in occupational therapy practice settings to address injury or impairment to the motor system, but it can be applied even more broadly to support building and retaining functional movement sequences that optimize performance and reduce the cognitive demand on the individual performing the movement. Tapping into previously established autonomous movement patterns can help some clients remain functional despite cognitive decline such as in case of **Debbie,** age 90 years. This case applies the motor learning frame of reference as a tool to help maintain functional engagement in daily occupations as she is challenged by a decline in her cognitive processing skills. Debbie's occupational profile is provided in Exhibit 6.3.

The occupational therapy practitioner evaluating Debbie observed her during meals because her decline in self-feeding was a significant concern. Immediately after a food tray was placed in front of Debbie, she reached for the coffee cup. She picked it up and took a sip. Debbie then grimaced and began searching her tray for the sugar and creamer packets. Sometimes she found them; sometimes she did not. When she did find the packets, she carefully lined them up together and tapped them on the table 3 times. She then tore off the tops and dumped them into her coffee. She had a well-established motor program for managing her coffee, lining up the packets, tapping them, tearing off one end, dumping them into the cup, and then stirring. Debbie always sipped her coffee before eating.

When Debbie did not find the creamer and sugar packets, the whole sequence was interrupted, and she did not eat. Similarly, if she could not find the spoon, the sequence would similarly be interrupted. By simply prompting the nursing care staff to set all of Debbie's coffee supplies in the same place where they were easy to find, the whole mealtime motor program for eating could proceed with only standby supervision. In this case, the occupational therapy practitioner was able to use previously learned autonomous motor performance to facilitate task performance, even when Debbie no longer had the cognitive ability to organize and direct complex sequenced tasks such as self-feeding.

EXHIBIT 6.3.	Debbie's Occupational Profile	
Client	**Reason the client is seeking service and concerns related to engagement in occupations**	Referred to occupational therapy to support performance of ADLs. *Impact on occupation:* She has recently begun to need help with many day-to-day activities. Debbie has recently lost weight because she does not always eat when her meal tray is placed in front of her.
	Occupations in which the client is successful	Debbie can still bathe and toilet independently and will dress when handed clothing items.
	Personal interests and values	Debbie has always been a very social person and will join most social activities in her living unit. Debbie has enjoyed crafts and sewing in the past but has not been able to do these activities for several years.
	Occupational history (i.e., life experiences)	Debbie is in Alzheimer's Stage 6, severe decline. She needs constant supervision and frequently requires professional care. She needs assistance with aspects of all ADLs. Debbie is generally in good physical health, although she is slightly underweight and is prone to UTIs. Debbie has, until recently, been managing meals independently. Her family's primary focus is to help Debbie maintain her function in this area so that she does not need to be transferred to a unit where she is more restricted and has less opportunity to interact with others.
	Performance patterns (routines, roles, habits, & rituals)	Debbie has been a mother, grandmother, spouse, homemaker, and community volunteer. At this time, she still recognizes her 4 children but mixes up the names of her grandchildren and great-grandchildren. At this time Debbie's routines are managed by other adults.

(Continued)

CASE EXAMPLE 6.2. DEBBIE: ALZHEIMER'S DISEASE *(Cont.)*

EXHIBIT 6.3. Debbie's Occupational Profile *(Cont.)*

Environment		**Supports to occupational engagement**	**Barriers to occupational engagement**
	Physical (e.g., buildings, furniture, pets)	Debbie lives in an special care unit for people with Alzheimer's disease.	
	Social (e.g., spouse, friends, caregivers)	Debbie has a supportive extended family.	
Context	**Cultural** (e.g., customs, beliefs)	Debbie attends Christian worship services offered in her living unit.	No cultural issues were identified in this assessment.
	Personal (e.g., age, gender, SES, education)	90-year-old woman. College graduate. Retired middle income.	
	Temporal (e.g., stage of life, time, year)	Debbie is in late adulthood.	
	Virtual (e.g., chat, email, remote monitoring)	Debbie will talk on the phone when it is handed to her but otherwise does not use any information or communication technologies.	
Client goals	**Client's priorities and desired targeted outcomes**	The family wants to help Debbie remain healthy and independent for as long as possible. They are concerned that her inattention to meals may lead to health problems.	

ANALYSIS OF PARTICIPATION

Basic ADLs

Eating/oral–motor	Debbie has adequate oral–motor skills to both eat and drink independently. She does not always initiate or persist in the motor task of self-feeding.
Grooming	Debbie manages basic hygiene tasks largely independently. She does need occasional prompts, but they can be as simple as handing her a hairbrush.
Bathing/transfer	Debbie has an adapted shower with a seat and grab bars. She always has an attendant within earshot when she showers, but she is otherwise independent.
Dressing upper body	Debbie has no difficulty in this area.
Dressing lower body	Debbie has no difficulty in this area.
Toileting	Debbie is able to perform toileting tasks independently. She does have some incontinence and wears incontinence pads.
Problem solving/memory	Debbie has significant impairments in problem solving and short-term memory. She has difficulty with multistep tasks.
Comments	When ADL tasks are set up for Debbie in a familiar way, she will use the materials provided in the expected manner. Although she does not organize or sequence these tasks herself, she is able to complete them with minimal prompting.

IADLs

Community mobility	Debbie has little awareness of place or direction. She is dependent in all aspects of community mobility.

(Continued)

CASE EXAMPLE 6.2. DEBBIE: ALZHEIMER'S DISEASE *(Cont.)*

EXHIBIT 6.3.	**Debbie's Occupational Profile** *(Cont.)*
Health management/ prevention	Debbie has no awareness of her health management needs. She is dependent in this area.
Home management	Debbie does straighten her bed and her toiletries, keeping her living space tidy, but she engages in no other home management tasks.
Financial management	Debbie is dependent in this area.
Leisure	Debbie attends available leisure programs but is otherwise dependent in this area.
Safety	Debbie is dependent in this area.
Comments:	Within the restricted environment of the Alzheimer's unit, Debbie functions reasonably well. When taken off the unit, she becomes very anxious and agitated.
	Debbie has only basic age-related motor decline. She does not learn new motor tasks and has difficulty planning movements under novel conditions.
	Motor and Praxis Skills
Sitting—static/dynamic	Debbie performs within age expectations.
Standing—static/dynamic	Debbie performs within age expectations.
Joint stability and skeletal mobility	Debbie performs within age expectations.
Place can on shelf	Debbie has adequate motor control to do this task.
Retrieve item from floor	Debbie has adequate motor control to do this task.
Screw lid on jar	Debbie has adequate motor control to do this task.
Comb back of head	Debbie has adequate motor control to do this task.
Writing	Given paper and a writing implement, Debbie will go through the motions of writing. Her actual handwriting is illegible and lacks content.
Lift grocery bag	Debbie has adequate motor control to do this task.
Coordination	Debbie has a very slow reaction time, and her movements are often jerky and inconsistent.
Manipulation	Debbie has adequate motor control to do routine manipulation tasks such as managing a toothbrush. She has difficulty with very fine tasks such as managing buttons or tying shoes.
Comments:	None.
	Process Skills
Energy for task	Debbie has little intrinsic motivation. She is compliant with prompts but does not persist in tasks without supervision.
Knowledge/organization of task	Debbie is able to perform many routine tasks that were learned earlier in life. She does not organize or sequence tasks well.
Adaptation/praxis	Debbie has very poor adaptation/praxis skills.
Comments:	None.
	Behavioral and Cognitive Skills
Communication and following social conventions	Debbie is able to perform social behaviors that were learned earlier in life. She is able to talk but does not reliably express needs or follow conversations.

(Continued)

CASE EXAMPLE 6.2. DEBBIE: ALZHEIMER'S DISEASE *(Cont.)*

EXHIBIT 6.3. Debbie's Occupational Profile *(Cont.)*

Cognitive and emotional regulation skills	Debbie is very impulsive and can be very labile with her emotions. She has very little self-regulatory skill.
Level of arousal/attention	Debbie is interested in her immediate environment, but her attention span is very short.
Orientation	Debbie knows her name and recognizes her children and some of the regular staff in the facility. She is not oriented to time or place.
Energy and drive	Debbie has very little intrinsic drive. She does move around a lot and has adequate physical energy for her current task demands.
Memory and understanding	Debbie has significant impairments in this area.
Higher level cognition	Debbie has significant impairments in this area.
Sensory–Perceptual Skills	
Sensory	Debbie has typical age-related declines in vision, hearing, and balance. She does not wear eyeglasses or a hearing aid.
Self-perception	Debbie has significant impairments in this area.
Pain	Debbie expresses pain with physical agitation and emotional liability.
Skin integrity	Debbie has typical age-related declines in skin integrity resulting in frequent bruising and skin irritation when toileting is not managed promptly.
Comments:	None.

Note. Occupational profile template from American Occupational Therapy Association (2017). Analysis of participation format from Skubik-Peplaski et al. (2009). AD = Alzheimer's disease; ADLs = activities of daily living; IADLs = instrumental activities of daily living; UTIs = urinary tract infections.

The motor learning frame of reference is science driven and supports the use of scientific reasoning in the process of forming a clinical hypothesis and in the testing of that hypothesis through data gathering during occupational therapy intervention. The case of Debbie introduces the inclusion of both scientific and narrative reasoning to offer a more holistic perspective of the client and her needs.

SUMMARY

The motor learning frame of reference emerged from sport and exercise science. The extensive body of science supporting this approach has largely been drawn from studies of athletes and the desire to optimize training for superior performance in sports. Many supporting studies have also focused on the clinical populations typically seen in occupational therapy practice, but this body of evidence is smaller.

It is absolutely essential for occupational therapy practitioners working with persons with movement disorders of any type to understand motor learning approaches, but care should be taken to consider the extenuating factors of overall physical deconditioning, pain, and fatigue, as well as the impact of medical interventions

when using this frame of reference. This frame of reference is highly prescriptive about exercise and practice, and occupational therapy practitioners could easily slip into *knobology* (the study of application without theory; see Chapter 1, "Overview of the Clinical Reasoning Process") rather than considering the challenging human factors commonly seen in rehabilitation settings. Similarly, evidence has shown that assuming that improvement in motor performance automatically results in improved functional performance is a hasty generalization that is not supported by the data.

Chapter 3, "Hypothesis Generation and Refinement," listed the broad categories of occupational therapy service as remediation, maintenance, compensation, development, and education. The motor learning frame of reference is primarily used in the remediation and the maintenance approaches.

Although strongly supported by scientific evidence, clinical implementation of the motor learning frame of reference in a manner consistent with the literature is often challenging. In considering frames of reference, the occupational therapy practitioner must carefully consider the environmental supports and constraints that will have an impact on the intervention. Sometimes these constraints are not obvious at the outset; therefore, carefully structured data collection systems can be essential clinical reasoning tools. With intervention and client-specific data, clinical decisions can be affirmed or reconsidered, supportive strategies can be developed to enhance the client's ability to adhere to recommended protocols, and occupational therapy practitioners will have a solid foundation for choosing interventions to meet client needs that may fall outside of established clinical pathways.

The motor learning frame of reference does not address compensation involving the use of alternative strategies or devices to allow a person to perform a highly valued task. This approach also does not support the education approach, which focuses on the promotion of positive behaviors. Although the occupational therapy practitioner may educate a client about health-promoting exercise routines, the education aspect is not a consideration in the motor learning frame of reference.

LEARNING ACTIVITIES

1. The motor learning intervention approach described for Noah is CIMT. Choose and describe another evidence-informed motor learning intervention strategy that could be used to support the development of Noah's motor performance.
2. Look up "mirror therapy" online. Describe this approach using the constructs of the motor learning frame of reference.
3. Review the NDT frame of reference presented earlier in this text. The NDT is a theoretical frame of reference that is not well supported by science but has persisted in clinical usage. Consider what you have learned to date about clinical reasoning, theory, and science, and write an essay that presents the modern use of the NDT approach as it is informed by motor control science. Take a personal stand on whether the continued use of the NDT approach is good for the profession.
4. Return to the case of Brody from Chapter 3 of this text. Using this case, develop a motor learning–based intervention strategy that is also developmentally supportive. Summarize how the motor learning postulates of change are applied in your example.
5. Read Fluet et al. (2017), or choose a similar article on a specific motor skill intervention of interest to you. Write up a take-home message from the study in this article as you would present it to professional colleagues. Include your reactions to any unexpected or anomalous findings presented.
6. In your clinical experiences with persons with cognitive loss, identify multistep motor tasks learned before the memory loss that they could still use (but not adapt) in their daily functions.

REFERENCES

American Occupational Therapy Association. (2017). AOTA occupational profile template. *American Journal of Occupational Therapy, 71*(Suppl. 2), 7112420030. https://doi.org/10.5014/ajot716S12

Boudreau, J.-P. (2009). Embodied mind and learning in infancy: A tribute to Esther Thelen. *Journal of Sport and Exercise Psychology, 31*(Suppl.), S8.

Case-Smith, J., DeLuca, S. C., Stevenson, R., & Ramey, S. L. (2012). Multicenter randomized controlled trial of pediatric constraint-induced movement therapy: 6-month follow-up. *American Journal of Occupational Therapy, 66,* 15–23. https://doi.org/10.5014/ajot.2012.002386

DeMatteo, C., Law, M., Russell, D., Pollock, N., Rosenbaum, P., & Walter, S. (1992). *QUEST: Quality of Upper Extremity Skills Test.* Hamilton, ON: McMaster University, CanChild Centre for Childhood Disability Research.

Dunn, W. (2008). *Bringing evidence into everyday practice: Practical strategies for healthcare professionals.* Thorofare, NJ: Slack.

Fluet, G. G., Patel, J., Qiu, Q., Yarossi, M., Massood, S., Adamovich, S. V., . . . Merians, A. S. (2017). Motor skill changes and neurophysiologic adaptation to recovery-oriented virtual rehabilitation of hand function in a person with subacute stroke: A case study. *Disability and Rehabilitation, 39,* 1524–1531. https://doi.org/10.1080/09638288.2016.1226421

Foster, E., Golden, L., Duncan, R., & Earhart, G. (2013). Community-based Argentine tango dance program is associated with increased activity participation among individuals with Parkinson's disease. *American Congress of Rehabilitation Medicine, 94,* 240–249. https://doi.org/10.1016/j.apmr.2012.07.028

Hackney, M., & Earhart, G. (2009). Short duration, intensive tango dancing for Parkinson disease: A controlled pilot study. *Complementary Therapies in Medicine, 17,* 203–207. https://doi.org/10.1016/j.ctim.2008.10.005

Holmefur, M., Aarts, P., Hoare, B., & Krumlinde-Sundholm, L. (2009). Retest and alternate forms reliability of the Assisting Hand Assessment. *Journal of Rehabilitation Medicine, 41,* 886–891.

Kilduski, N., & Rice, M. (2003). Qualitative and quantitative knowledge of results: Effects on motor learning. *American Journal of Occupational Therapy, 57,* 329–336. https://doi.org/10.5014/ajot.57.3.329

Kruisselbrink, L., & Van Gyn, G. (2011). Task characteristics and the contextual interference effect. *Perceptual and Motor Skills, 113,* 1, 19–37. https://doi.org/10.2466/22.PMS.113.4.19-37

Lang, C. E., & Birkenmeier, R. L. (2014). *Upper-extremity task-specific training after stroke or disability: A manual for occupational therapy and physical therapy.* Bethesda, MD: AOTA Press.

Lee, T., Eliasz, K., Gonzalez, D., Alguire, K., Ding, K., & Dhaliwal, C. (2016). On the role of error in motor learning. *Journal of Motor Behavior, 48,* 99–115. https://doi.org/10.1080/00222895.2015.1046545

Li, K. (2013). Examining contemporary motor control theories from the perspective of degrees of freedom. *Australian Occupational Therapy Journal, 60,* 138–143. https://doi.org/10.1111/1440-1630.12009

Mandich, M. (2016). Classic theories of human development. In A. Cronin & M. Mandich (Eds.), *Human development and performance throughout the lifespan* (2nd ed., pp. 38–59). Boston: Cengage Learning.

Muratori, L. M., Lamberg, E. M., Quinn, L., & Duff, S. V. (2013). Applying principles of motor learning and control to upper extremity rehabilitation. *Journal of Hand Therapy, 26,* 94–103. https://doi.org/10.1016/j.jht.2012.12.007

Paradigm. (2016). *Merriam-Webster's dictionary.* Retrieved from https://www.merriam-webster.com/dictionary/paradigm

Ramey, S. L., Coker-Bolt, P., & DeLuca, S. C. (Eds.). (2013). *Handbook of pediatric constraint-induced movement therapy (CIMT): A guide for occupational therapy and health care clinicians, researchers, and educators.* Bethesda, MD: AOTA Press.

Sakzewski, L., Ziviani, J., & Boyd, R. N. (2016). Translating evidence to increase quality and dose of upper limb therapy for children with unilateral cerebral palsy: A pilot study. *Physical and Occupational Therapy in Pediatrics, 36,* 305–329. https://doi.org/10.3109/01942638.2015.1127866

Schmidt, R., & Lee, T. (2013). *Motor learning and performance: From principles to application* (5th ed.). Champaign, IL: Human Kinetics.

Shumway-Cook, A., & Woollacott, M. (2012). *Motor control: Translating research into clinical practice* (4th ed.). Philadelphia: Lippincott Williams & Wilkins.

Skubik-Peplaski, C., Paris, C., Boyle, D., & Culpert, A. (Eds.). (2009*). Applying the* Occupational Therapy Practice Framework*: Using the Cardinal Hill Occupational Participation Process in client-centered care* (2nd ed.). Bethesda, MD: AOTA Press.

Sensory Integration and Sensory Processing Frames of Reference

7

Rondalyn Whitney, PhD, OTR/L, FAOTA

CHAPTER HIGHLIGHTS

- Introduces Ayres Sensory Integration® (ASI) theory.
- Defines the key elements of ASI theory and the ASI and sensory processing frames of reference.
- Describes the function–dysfunction continuum within the general sensory integration frame of reference and the distinct differences between the ASI and sensory processing frames of reference.
- Provides a case example illustrating the sensory processing frame of reference in occupational therapy intervention and in clinical reasoning as a problem-solving tool.
- Underscores the importance of fidelity in examining evidence and applying knowledge.
- Introduces the data-driven decision-making process.
- Discusses the use of deliberation and argument to advocate professionally and for clients in a clinical reasoning context.

KEY TERMS AND CONCEPTS

Ayres Sensory Integration®
Data-driven decision-making process
Fidelity

Plasticity
Senses
Sensory diet

Sensory integration
Sensory integration theory
Sensory processing

This chapter draws from the body of sensory integration (SI) and sensory processing theory and science that was initiated by A. Jean Ayres in the 1950s (Ayres, 1972). Nearly 60 years of study and refinement of Ayres's work is considered in this text as the SI and sensory processing frames of reference. These 2 frames of reference have been extensively explored and refined since Ayres's initial work, and they are the first frames of reference presented in this text that emerged from scholarship within the field of occupational therapy.

In this chapter, readers will develop an understanding of current terminology, core concepts of the SI approach, and the clinical reasoning guiding evidence-based interventions that align with Ayres Sensory Integration® (ASI) theory.

OVERVIEW OF SI FRAME OF REFERENCE

In the late 1950s, Ayres, a scientist and occupational therapy practitioner, combined theoretical principles from neuroscientific, motor, and developmental theory to explain her observations on maturation of the motor system among children as they played or worked at learning (Ayres, 1972). Her observations led to the realization that adaptive behavior seemed to be dependent on the way children perceived and processed sensation. Ayres appreciated that sensory systems did not develop independently but that each sensory system instead seemed to be dependent on the simultaneous development of other systems, and integration among systems was needed for occupational engagement. For example, in early infant development, as a baby looked at a nubby teether, brought it to the mouth, and experienced the toy with the lips and tongue (tactile systems), the visual system and the tactile system appeared to mutually reference and reinforce each other. Thus, integration occurred across several systems.

SI is the ability to integrate sensation at the cell level for day-to-day use—or, rather, the ability to use information from the sensory system to do what one wants to do. Ayres (1972) theorized that integration across multiple systems fostered purposeful play and adaptive behavior. Studies have supported a relationship between sensory processing and motor performance as well as overall participation in daily life (Dunn, Little, Dean, Robertson, & Evans, 2016). SI theory developed to explain the relationship between the brain and behavior; it explains why people behave in certain ways in response to sensory input. As a child's sensory–motor system responds adaptively to the challenges presented during the day, the child can do the things she or he wants to do—play, learn, and be a good friend.

Sensory processing, then, refers to the neurophysiological process of receiving and responding to information that comes in through the senses. Functionally, the term *sensory processing* is also used in the diagnosis of sensory-based processing challenges, distinguishing the function from the theory and establishing the function–dysfunction continuum used for intervention (i.e., Kramer & Hinojosa, 2015; Miller, Anzalone, Lane, Cermak, & Osten, 2007). A child who experiences pudding with his or her tactile system, eating the food with the hands, smearing the custard on the arms and face, sucking the fingers, and tasting the bitterness of chocolate while seated upright in a chair, interacting with a sibling, and enjoying the experience of family mealtime has demonstrated the integration of multiple sensations for the purpose of eating.

Ayres postulated that sitting, standing, and motor planning predictably and importantly depend on sensory input through the vestibular and proprioceptive systems. Higher level learning tasks, such as reading, writing, and aligning numbers in early arithmetic, seem to be affected by dysfunction in the tactile, vestibular, and visual systems. From these clinical and scientific observations, Ayres hypothesized that the attention required for academic performance is related to the nervous system's ability to respond adaptively to tactile and other sensory phenomena. This was the beginning of Ayres' **SI theory** and the foundation of the SI and sensory processing frames of reference presented in this text. *SI frame of reference* is an umbrella term that includes ASI, sensory processing, and other sensory strategies (Figure 7.1).

Increased knowledge and refinement of theory is essential to science. As interest in using sensory-based interventions has grown and SI is increasingly requested as an intervention, confusion within both the scientific and the practice communities has also increased. Not surprisingly, then, some studies have found that the intervention has positive effects (Case-Smith, Weaver, & Fristad, 2014; Schaaf et al., 2014; Watling & Hauer, 2015), and other studies have found little effect (Leong, Carter, & Stephenson, 2015). Puddy and Wilkins (2011) provided clarification for the Centers for Disease Control and Prevention's suggestion that interventions be rated as established, emerging, unestablished, or ineffective or harmful.

Using the Scientific Rating Scale (California Evidence-Based Clearinghouse, 2018), Puddy and Wilkins (2011) rated SI and processing as unestablished as an effective intervention for autism spectrum disorder (ASD). In contrast, Zimmer and Desch (2012) of the American Academy of Pediatrics (AAP) considered SI an alternative therapy, acceptable when occupational therapy practitioners use sensory-based therapies as a component of a comprehensive treatment plan and when they co-create specific measurable goals with the family to improve participation in daily occupations. SI, then, offers the opportunity to engage with clinical science, using theory to guide intervention, reflect on outcomes, and use clinical knowledge to inform and further evolve theory.

FIGURE 7.1.   **SI theory frame of reference.**

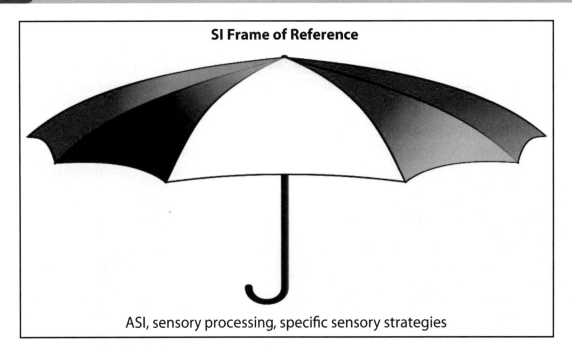

Note. ASI = Ayres Sensory Integration; SI = sensory integration.

EBP AND SI

Chapter 3, "Hypothesis Generation and Refinement," defined *evidence-based practice (EBP)* as the conscientious use of current best evidence to make decisions about client care and to expand the clinician's expertise through critical evaluation of the growing body of available research. As noted in that chapter, EBP requires practitioners to include a current review of research evidence, personal experience, policy influences, contextual influences, and information from the client and family in the clinical reasoning process. EBP integrates this information and considers it within the client's unique circumstances. To summarize, EBP, at a minimum, requires reflective consideration of 5 sources of information: (1) family and individual preferences, (2) empirically validated interventions, (3) professional judgment, (4) data-driven decision making, and (5) contextual evidence.

Practitioners' challenge is understanding the relative strength of the evidence for an actual client and clinical context and having the confidence that their selected treatment will improve the client's function and participation. Evidence-based reasoning must incorporate family and individual preferences and contextual evidence as well as empirical data to best meet the client's needs.

The body of literature, both scientific and lay, about SI and sensory processing is vast and has led to widely used clinical frames of reference. Parents rank occupational therapy as the most effective intervention for their child with ASD (39%), followed by speech therapy (27%), applied behavioral analysis (15%), and social skills classes (8%; Autism Speaks, 2012). Parents' view of occupational therapy is an important consideration because family preferences are a significant factor in evidence-based reasoning. Researchers have suggested that the outcomes predicted by the theory have been difficult to measure objectively, in part, because of methodological challenges, lack of agreement related to predicted outcomes, and poor treatment fidelity (Schaaf, 2015).

Early studies grounded in SI theory focused on change in level of impairment, which was difficult to operationalize as a neurological process (Schaaf, 2015). More recent studies have expanded the focus to participation and quality of life, and these studies seem to offer greater insight into the contributions of Ayres's approach (Schaaf Dumont, Arbesman, & May-Benson, 2018).

If practitioners strive to use only empirically validated interventions, they would not consider the 2 most prominent intervention approaches drawn from SI theory: ASI and sensory processing interventions. However, EBP allows additional client-centered factors to inform and drive the expansion of practice-based evidence. ASI is generally considered an evidence-informed, supported practice in occupational therapy. *Evidence-informed practice* includes the conscientious use of current best evidence to identify the potential benefits, harms, and costs of any intervention while acknowledging that what works in a certain context may not be appropriate or feasible in another.

Because the data have been conflicting and there have been few large-scale studies of ASI, the empirical validity has sometimes been challenged. Other intervention approaches that have emerged from this theory have lower levels of evidence and may be considered promising practices, emerging practices, or unsupported practices.

SI FRAME OF REFERENCE: FRAMING THE ARGUMENT

So, what's an occupational therapy practitioner to do? How do you critically evaluate interventions that seem promising but have not yet been empirically validated? In the presence of this controversy, how do practitioners defend their clinical reasoning and promising clinical practice innovations? An *argument* is "a coherent series of reasons, statements, or facts intended to support or establish a point of view" ("Argument," 2017). Effective occupational therapy practitioners must not only learn to critically evaluate the existing literature, they must also learn to communicate clearly and frame an argument to represent and reflect the clinical reasoning behind their choice of intervention. Exhibit 7.1 outlines the steps in framing an argument.

SI-based interventions are not the only interventions widely used in occupational therapy practice that lack empirical validation. In fact, the largest single body of research in the field of occupational therapy has been that pertaining to SI and sensory processing. Many commonly used interventions have less scientific evidence and also less controversy associated with them. The point of framing an argument is not to avoid controversy but to advocate for the best decision for the client. The ASI and sensory processing literature has had an enormous impact across professions, not just in occupational therapy. Table 7.1 summarizes some of the major contributors to the contemporary SI frame of reference.

UNDERLYING THEORY OF SI

The SI and sensory processing frames of reference are based in theory. Developing methodologies to test the theory underlying ASI is surprisingly complex. Remember that a *theory* is an idea, "a plausible or scientifically acceptable general principle or body of principles offered to explain phenomena" ("Theory," 2017). Also remember that both advances in science and anomalous data are used to challenge and advance theory. Since Ayres's early theorizing, there have been many advances in science and much data that have altered both the theoretical foundation of and practice within these frames of reference.

EXHIBIT 7.1.   Framing an Argument

Step 1. Be fair.
- Many clinical practices have yet to produce sufficient evidence (i.e., to establish) that the interventions are effective. *Deliberation* is the process of discussing contested issues by considering various perspectives in order to form opinions and guide judgment.
- Research is expensive and complicated, and clinical research is even more methodologically complex. Deliberating on research while acknowledging the strengths and weaknesses of an intervention and using the available evidence (including clinical observation) allows you to be fair in presenting your argument.

Step 2. Frame the argument.
- Researchers do not agree on SI's efficacy as a therapeutic intervention. The body of research on SI has shown that it has positive effects, but the literature has not supported SI's effectiveness. Still, what is known about neurological function suggests that the ability to accurately perceive sensory information and organize sensory input would affect a person's ability to interact within the environment and get work done (i.e., dressing, eating, bathing). Scientists agree on this part of the theory.
- Take the time to approach the controversy with care and serious consideration. People are more willing to consider your approach if you address the important reasons for their concern. The literature outlines 3 areas of controversy:
    1. Is there a distinct difference in the brain that can be identified as causing SPD?
    2. Does providing an intervention as outlined by the intervention protocol change sensory processing?
    3. Does the intervention improve overall occupational performance?
- Take each concern and prepare a critical assessment of the pros and cons for each approach to that concern.

Step 3. Use clinical reasoning.
- To decide when and whether to use SI intervention (or any intervention that is not empirically validated), use critical reasoning. *Unestablished* is not the same as *ineffective* or *harmful*. SI has been demonstrated to be safe. SI interventions will not harm a child so long as they are supervised. Chosen interventions are provided by an occupational therapist who may or may not use SI as the treatment strategy. Parents perceive SI to be effective in solving the problems that they highly value (Cohn, Kramer, Schub, & May-Benson, 2014). As long as the outcomes are met and costs are at or below what is expected, SI techniques should not be removed from consideration.
- Outcomes matter; identify outcomes that are above dispute. The evidence is consistent that families want outcomes related to occupational function (e.g., ADLs, family routines, social participation, academic success), not outcomes related to tolerance of the intervention itself (e.g., decreased tactile defensiveness, sensation tolerance, use of proprioceptive input; Pfeiffer, May-Benson, & Bodison, 2018).
- Gather evidence to support your ability to use clinical reasoning in selecting interventions that achieve desired outcomes and do not create nondesirable outcomes.

Note. ADLs = activities of daily living; SI = sensory integration; SPD = sensory processing disorder.

Senses

Even at a basic level, how many senses are there? As it turns out, the answer grows ever more complicated. Scientists categorize sensation in many ways. Depending on the way the sensory system and associated sensory receptors are subdivided, we could agree that the 5 traditional or common senses are those that children learn about in preschool: smell, taste, hearing, touch, and sight. Others think of the senses in terms of "special" senses or sensory information that comes into the nervous system through receptors that are located in very specialized areas of the body: olfactory, gustatory, auditory, visual, and vestibular (i.e., receptors in the inner ear).

General *senses* include sensations received by these categories of sensory receptors: mechanoreceptors (i.e., touch, pressure, vibration), nocioceptors (i.e., pain, tickle, itch), thermoreceptors (i.e., temperature), chemical balance (e.g., osmoreceptors), baroreceptors (which detect changes in pressure or flow in the blood vessels), and proprioceptors located in joints and muscles (which detect stretch and pressure to enable the cerebellum to conceptualize body position and movement). In addition to general proprioception

are the Pacinian corpuscles (which detect pressure on skin and an object's weight) and Meissner's corpuscles (i.e., fine touch perception; Bear, Connors, & Paradiso, 2015).

Ayres did not have all of this detail about senses when she formulated her early theory, but she did understand at an intuitive level what psychologist Esther Thelen later called *embodied learning* (Boudreau, 2009). SI theory focuses on the near senses of somatosensory or touch, proprioception or kinesthesia (i.e., receptors in the joints and muscles), gustation, and vestibular senses, as well as the better understood far (or distance) senses of vision, audition, and olfaction.

Because the frames of reference drawn from Ayres's theory look at the integration of sensation for use, input received via the senses is assessed, activities that provide strategic input are selected, and the outcome of SI is measured by the client's ability to adaptively integrate sensation to accomplish tasks and participate in life. Therefore, these approaches include motor output systems of praxis and kinesthesia, because they demonstrate adaptive integration of the sensory system. Table 7.2 presents the senses as they are considered in the SI and sensory processing frames of reference.

TABLE 7.1. Contributions to the SI Frame of Reference

CONSTRUCT	MEASUREMENT	CONCEPTS
ASI	Sensory processing is inferred from behavior and acquisition of performance.	<ul><li>Long-term neuronal function and behavioral response are synaptically mediated and can be altered by experience.</li><li>Optimal learning occurs when the client is engaged in self-directed activities that offer the "just-right" challenge.</li><li>Effective integration of sensory information produces increasingly adaptive responses.</li></ul>
Developmental theory	Measured through direct observation of actual performance and compared with age-dependent milestones.	<ul><li>Characterized by a predictable sequence of acquisition that is heterarchical rather than hierarchical.</li><li>Contextual factors from the environment can influence the pattern and quality of development.</li></ul>
Sensory–motor system	Measured with biomarkers or *f*MRI to quantitatively assess physiological responses to sensory input.	<ul><li>Neuronal function and behavioral responses are synaptically detected using biomarkers.</li><li>Unique patterns of sensory processing are detectible and reproducible under experimental conditions.</li></ul>
Social learning theory	Measured across occupations. Learning must be inferred from behavior and degree of skill acquisition.	<ul><li>Learning occurs through meaning making, and optimal learning occurs within the zone of proximal development.</li><li>Community plays a central role in development.</li></ul>

Note. ASI = Ayres Sensory Integration; *f*MRI = functional magnetic resonance imaging; SI = sensory integration.

TABLE 7.2. Senses Considered in the SI and Sensory Processing Frames of Reference

NAME	LOCATION	PURPOSE	ACTIVITY
		Sensory System (input)	
Auditory	Ear	Far sense; receives vibration from environment and translates it to sound.	<ul><li>Listening to music</li><li>Distinguishing bird calls</li><li>Attending to pitch and tone in voices</li></ul>
Gustatory	Tongue	Near sense; interprets different tastes (e.g., sweet, sour, salty, bitter).	<ul><li>Eating different foods</li><li>Licking salt off pretzels</li><li>Chewing on a lemon slice</li></ul>
Tactile	Skin and mouth	Near sense; protective, discriminative.	<ul><li>Rubbing</li><li>Temperature (tactile system)</li><li>Heavy blankets</li><li>Tickling</li></ul>
Visual	Eyes	Far sense; brings light and color into the nervous system.	<ul><li>Finding a fork in a cluttered utensil drawer</li><li>Reading</li><li>Identifying colors</li></ul>
Olfactory	Nose	Near sense; brings scents into the nervous system.	<ul><li>Identifying foods by smell</li><li>Distinguishing between spices</li><li>Inhaling calming (e.g., vanilla) or alerting (e.g., mint) scents</li></ul>

(Continued)

TABLE 7.2.	Senses Considered in the SI and Sensory Processing Frames of Reference *(Cont.)*		
NAME	**LOCATION**	**PURPOSE**	**ACTIVITY**
Proprioception	Muscles	Body scheme, including where body is in space and where body parts are relative to other body parts; balance (combined with vestibular); strength and endurance.	• Lifting heavy boxes • Tug of war • Grading force and direction (e.g., pouring water without spilling, throwing a ball and hitting a target)
Vestibular	Inner ear	Near sense; orient head in relation to the center of gravity.	• Swinging • Hanging upside down • Jumping • Twirling
Interoception	Inner organs	Near sense; pressure in organs indicating fullness or emptiness.	• Am I hungry? • Is my bladder full? • Is my heart pounding?
Motor System (output)			
Kinesthesia (motion)	Motor cortex	Motion	• Running and jumping over puddles
Praxis	Sensory–motor Ideation (prefrontal lobe) Motor planning (premotor cortex) Execution (motor cortex)	Smooth pursuit of motor tasks 3 phases of praxis: (1) Ideation (I have an idea), (2) motor planning (I know how), and (3) execution (I act).	• Having the idea you want to climb a tree; using the muscles of your arms, back, and legs to reach for the branches; and then climbing the tree.

Note. SI = sensory integration.

Distinguishing ASI and SI

ASI was the first and remains the most widespread intervention-based use of SI theory. Many researchers, both within and outside of occupational therapy, developed studies and adapted interventions based on their own ideas and understanding of the theory. This has led to a diversity of interventions and strategies being attributed to ASI that were not included in the original theory. In the roughly 60 years since Ayres's work was first published, there has been much controversy about SI's efficacy on the basis of studies that were called *SI studies* but did not adhere to the postulates of the theory. By the 1990s, it was common to hear statements such as "I do not believe in sensory integration" or "SI theory has been disproven."

To reduce controversy between intervention program outcomes that do and do not adhere to the principles of SI as outlined by Ayres and later researchers, the term *ASI* was explicitly defined (operationalized) and a trademark attained (Smith-Roley, Mailloux, Miller-Kuhaneck, & Glennon, 2007). *ASI* is an intervention approach that has a clear body of research specifically drawn from Ayres's theory. In this body of research, some interventions have been considered promising, but the data have not offered empirical validation of the approach.

ASI is a science-driven intervention process. The arena in which the greatest volume of new research is emerging is in the science underlying ASI—sensory processing. Sensory processing research typically focuses more on the neuroscience of sensory processing and the distinction among sensory processing differences, sensory profiles, and SPD (Tomchek, Little, & Dunn, 2015). Human behavior, neurological function, and learning are of interest to many different bodies of science.

As interest in Ayres's work has expanded over the years, greater clarification was needed to distinguish the principles of the SI framework consistent with Ayres's frame of reference and the efficacy of the evidence-based approaches used in intervention. The distinction between the scholarship related to ASI and sensory processing science is illustrated in Figure 7.2.

Measurement and Fidelity

As scientists began to focus on bridging the gap between what is observed (i.e., positive outcomes when using ASI) to what can be measured (i.e., outcomes indicating the efficacy of the intervention), several steps were identified, including the need to define (i.e., operationalize) the concepts of the theory so that they could be experimentally tested, create measurements that could identify whether sensory processing dysfunction did in fact occur, and create measurement tools that could accurately measure theoretically predicted outcomes. Because the outcomes originally described by Ayres were changes in brain function that remain difficult to measure, Schaaf and Davies (2010) developed a research protocol directed toward measures that systematically document clinical outcomes.

Fidelity, the extent to which an intervention follows the therapeutic principles of a theory, both supports clinical

FIGURE 7.2.   Ayres's theory as the foundation for occupational therapy intervention.

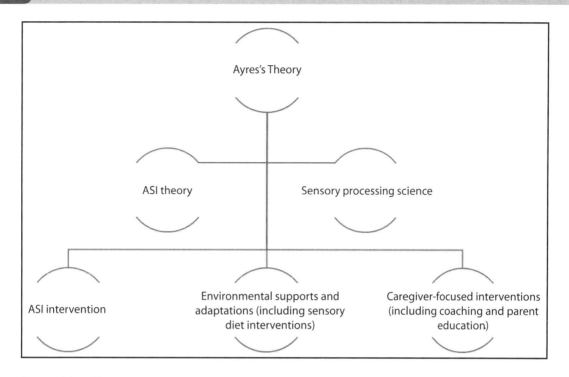

Note. ASI = Ayres Sensory Integration.

reasoning and helps to standardize treatment and measurement of outcomes. Occupational therapy practitioners and scientists have focused on fidelity in building the body of work to include SI theory, assessment, and treatment using the ASI approach. *Fidelity* in this context is the degree of exactness with which intervention ideals can be consistently reproduced, with the end result that different clinicians can consistently follow the same reasoning process during an intervention session and a clinician can consistently use the same reasoning process with different children.

In the study of SI, then, fidelity is the degree to which clinical practice (i.e., intervention) aligns with theory (i.e., follows the protocols) so that the practice can be predicted by theoretical principles. SI theory assumes that children have an innate drive to seek meaningful experiences from their environment. Interventions based on this theory aim to promote engagement in sensory-rich play, understand the meaning behind the play children engage in, and promote adaptive responses through the presentation and organization of sensation. Parham et al. (2011) developed the ASI Fidelity Measure to identify consistency in ASI intervention.

SI Approach

SI postulates that the nervous system has to first register information regarding sensation in response to a stimulus (i.e., the sensory receptor must be stimulated). After the initial registration of the sensation, people must process the information (intensity, judgment about the sensation) and, finally, organize the sensation for use—meaning organize it so it can be used to create an adaptive response in the environment.

For example, if a fly buzzes near my ear, I register the sensation (sound), process it (it's a fly, not a bee or wasp, but I still don't like it), and organize that sensory information for use (I decide to ignore the fly). If I perceive the sound to be that of a wasp, I am more likely to organize that information and use it to get away from the wasp. If I misperceive the buzzing sound as a threat, for example, and respond by screaming and running away, I have reacted to nonthreatening sensory input as though it was a threat. Atypical responses are not willful attempts to make life chaotic; they are instead "automatic, unconscious physiologic reactions to sensations" (Miller et al., 2007, p. 135).

In Ayres's theory, *SI* is a person's ability to respond adaptively to sensation over a broad range of intensities and durations. When sensory input is integrated, the person can use sensory information to support optimal arousal, attention, and activity level to meet the demands of the environment in a fluid, flexible manner or to respond in an adaptive way (Whitney & Pickren, 2014). When sensation is perceived and processed in a disordered way, response to that sensation is disordered as well (i.e., SPD). Figure 7.3 shows a conceptual model of SPD.

Researchers (Miller et al., 2007) have focused on integrating contemporary neuroscientific principles and have focused on the area of sensory processing. Sensory

FIGURE 7.3.   **Sensory processing disorder.**

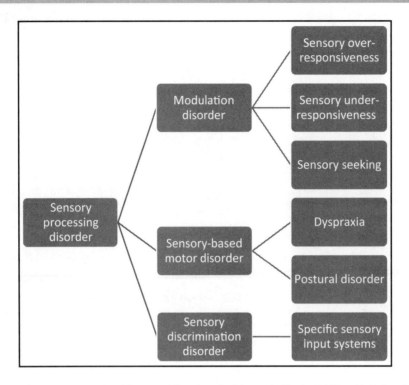

Source. From "Concept Evolution in Sensory Integration: A Proposed Nosology for Diagnosis," by L. J. Miller, M. E. Anzalone, S. J. Lane, S. A. Cermak, & E. T. Osten, 2007, *American Journal of Occupational Therapy, 61*, p. 137. Copyright © 2007 by the American Occupational Therapy Association. Adapted with permission.

processing is a part of the SI frame of reference, but a distinct body of research has also distinguished it from ASI. Miller and colleagues (2007) developed the classification of SPD presented here. The 3 subtypes, or patterns, of SPD are (1) disorders of modulation, (2) sensory-based motor disorders, and (3) sensory discriminatory disorders. Disorders of modulation have been shown to be heightened predictors of internalizing (e.g., anxiety, depression), externalizing (e.g., behavioral outbursts, kicking, hitting, fighting), and dysregulation problems (e.g., heightened emotional responses) that result in impaired quality of life, academic skills, and social participation (Kinnealey, Koenig, & Smith, 2011).

The SI frame of reference encompasses ASI, sensory processing interventions, and sensory strategies. This frame of reference proposes that delayed development of sensory processing systems can result in delayed development of ADLs (e.g., bathing, toileting, dressing, eating, functional mobility, personal hygiene and grooming), occupations (e.g., rest and sleep, education, work and play, social participation). Client factors such as performance patterns are also affected. Moreover, as misperceptions by the sensory systems continue, maladaptive responses to novel experiences in the environment and across contexts result in poor performance across those contexts and environments.

PRINCIPLES OF SI THEORY

The SI frame of reference includes ASI, sensory processing, and a variety of specific sensory strategies such as sensory diets and sensory-based environmental modifications. All of these distinct approaches have evolved from Ayres's original work and her SI theory. Here I describe core principles of Ayres's theory that are foundational to all of the approaches falling under the umbrella of the SI frame of reference.

Plasticity

Core principles of the SI frame of reference are based on the assumption of nervous system plasticity. *Plasticity,* the ability of the brain to change and reorganize in response to input, was an idea when Ayres started her work but is now accepted as scientific fact (Berlucchi, 2011). Ayres studied human development and noted that SI is a developmental process that mirrors human development. It is for this reason that ASI is considered a neurodevelopmental intervention approach. People learn through interaction with the environment and are motivated to engage in sensory-based activities.

Ayres's work focused on children, and she noted that as children are allowed to select various experiences and direct themselves through play, they become more flexible within a broader range of novel experiences. Children use new strategies to overcome perceived obstacles and, through play, they develop the ability to tolerate frustration, persist despite challenges, and modulate their response to a greater range of sensory information.

Sensory Experience

Providing intervention within the SI frame of reference focuses on enticing clients to engage in sensory-rich play to normalize development of the sensory–motor system. Therefore, interventions focus on promoting normal perception of tactile (or other sensory) input, reducing defensive behaviors, or avoiding behaviors that would delay development of the individual sensory system (Schaaf & Mailloux, 2015). Practitioners provide enticing ways for clients to experience sensation in safe, non-threatening activities. Vestibular input is used to facilitate or calm the nervous system—fast vestibular input (e.g., a swing) is alerting to the system, whereas slow vestibular input (rocking in a chair with a parent) is calming. Occupational therapy practitioners create multiple environments rich in sensory activities that, through engagement in play, enhance muscle tone, strength, and body scheme.

When sensory perception is faulty, the nervous system produces faulty motor responses. The goal of intervention, then, is to reduce the frequency, intensity, and duration of maladaptive strategies for coping with underlying sensory processing dysfunction. Socially disruptive behaviors can impair progress in academic skills, impede developmental milestones, and create impairment in family routines, social participation, and quality of life. Outcomes within the ASI frame of reference measure sensory discrimination, sensory modulation, and SI that result in organized, purposeful behavior. Thus, the measure of outcomes must be organized, purposeful behavior, and a change in a person's ability to do what is expected and desired, not improved tolerance of the intervention itself.

Participation and Occupation

Emerging evidence has supported the link between sensory processing and social participation, cognition, and engagement in valued occupations (Dunn et al., 2016; Schaaf et al., 2014). Posture, praxis, and bilateral motor coordination are observable, measurable outcomes of SI, so they are the best documented of the changes resulting from ASI. Changes in ADLs, IADLs, education, work, social participation, play, rest and sleep are more subjective, so they have less supporting evidence than ASI or other approaches within this frame of reference. However, these less-observable outcomes, which are measured through occupational engagement and participation, are among the most valued.

Outcome Measurement

As with the frames of reference presented earlier in this text, the SI frame of reference conceptualizes outcomes by focusing on those aspects of the literature that help support function and client outcomes within the domain of occupational therapy (Exhibit 7.2).

One of Ayres's important contributions was a focus on measurement. She developed standardized assessment tools consistent with her theory to identify and study SI dysfunction. As SI theory grew in popularity, there was a gradual drift away from the use of standardized measurement and an extension of the theory's principles beyond the scope proposed by Ayres. This drift led to some hasty generalizations promoting intervention practices that were not supported by evidence or functional outcomes.

The ***data-driven decision-making (DDDM) process*** was developed by Schaaf (2015) and colleagues (Schaaf & Mailloux, 2015) to assist occupational therapists in responding to the prevalence of interventions attributed to SI that had not been rigorously studied. The DDDM process was developed to promote better outcome measurement skills and systematic decision making and to document outcomes resulting from occupational therapy using ASI. The DDDM was designed to help ensure fidelity in compliance with ASI standards.

Using DDDM with ASI, clinicians
- Identify challenges experienced by the child,
- Identify environmental factors that might be affecting participation,
- Gather and interpret evaluation findings and create a clinical hypothesis,
- Develop and scale client-centered goals,
- Identify outcome measures,
- Create optimal space for intervention,
- Provide the intervention, and
- Evaluate whether the outcome of interest has been achieved (and, if not, revise the clinical hypothesis as needed and reinitiate intervention).

Types of Intervention That Have Evolved From Ayres's Theory

Of the intervention approaches presented in Figure 7.2, ASI is only at the supported practice level. Even this placement is generous, because other disciplines, including the AAP, rate it lower, as a promising practice.

Sensory processing interventions and sensory strategies are drawn from the same original theory developed by Ayres but differ significantly from the interventions she developed. These additional approaches within the SI frame of reference include environmental supports and adaptations that are usually caregiver-mediated interventions rather than child-focused ones (Reynolds et al., 2017). The empirical data supporting these 2 approaches are largely based on case reports and are widely considered to be empirically unsupported.

EXHIBIT 7.2.	SI Frame of Reference: General Elements
Focus	The focus of this frame of reference is the child's ability to discriminate, modulate, and integrate the sensory information needed for developmentally appropriate tasks (i.e., fully participate in daily life; Schaaf & Davies, 2010).
Basic assumptions	SI is an active developmental process that mirrors human development. The brain serves as an information processor that transforms sensory data into meaningful information that supports function and participation. Errors in sensory information processing can occur as errors of input, errors of encoding for memory, and errors of output. • Problems with the ability to process and modulate sensory input contribute to deficits in the ability to organize the behavior needed for developmentally appropriate tasks. • Problems with the ability to store the information for later use in the form of mental schema make it hard to retrieve the information and to support function. • Problems in how the brain decides what to do with the information and how it will react to the stimulus can lead to inappropriate or dysfunctional behavior. Children have an inborn drive toward higher development and are motivated to explore sensory challenges to advance their own development. Active engagement of the child is essential for developmental change. Using neurobiological and developmental science foundations to plan and engage the child in behaviors that provide organized sensory information tailored to the child's needs can lead to improved sensory processing and adaptive behaviors.
Function–disability continuum	Function occurs through adaptive responses that result from effective sensory modulation, discrimination, and integration. Dysfunction, in the form of sensory defensiveness, avoidance, underregistration of sensation, or poor modulation, manifests as maladaptive behaviors such as poor postural control, praxis or bilateral integration, and participation. Function–dysfunction continuums are relevant within each sensory system.
Postulates of change	• Active engagement in a sensory-rich environment entices the child to play and motivates adaptive responses. • Child-directed activity taps into the child's inner drive for developmental advancement. • If occupational therapy practitioners increase the complexity of challenge so that the child needs to exert some degree of effort, then the child will be more likely to master challenge and move to a higher level adaptive response. • If occupational therapy practitioners present or facilitate challenges in which the child is successful in areas of sensory modulation; discrimination; postural, ocular, or oral control; and praxis, then the child will be more likely to develop skills in the challenged area.

Note. SI = sensory integration.

Figure 7.4 breaks down the types of intervention that have evolved from Ayres's theory that are evidence-informed practices. Few rigorous data support these approaches, but because they include other recognized interventions such as coaching, parent education, task-specific practice, and environmental modifications, they draw additional support for their use. It is especially important with these categories of intervention that there be clearly identified functional outcome measures that are understood by the caregivers involved.

SENSORY PROCESSING APPROACHES

Sensory Diet

The most widely used sensory processing approaches are environmental supports, and the most common of these

is the sensory diet. The term *sensory diet* was coined to explain how certain sensory experiences can be used to enhance occupational performance and support self-regulation (Foss, Swinth, McGruder, & Tomlin, 2003; Wilbarger & Wilbarger, 1991). A **sensory diet** is a caregiver-focused intervention designed to address the functional problems associated with challenges in sensory processing and integration.

Stimulation

Using information from psychology and neuroscience about sensory receptors and how they affect the nervous system, occupational therapy practitioners. Patricia Wilbarger and Julia Wilbarger (1991) noted that proprioceptive (i.e., deep pressure) stimulation had the longest effect period and might serve to help regulate (or modulate) maladaptive sensory responses. A sensory diet does

FIGURE 7.4.   Framework for conceptualizing intervention approaches.

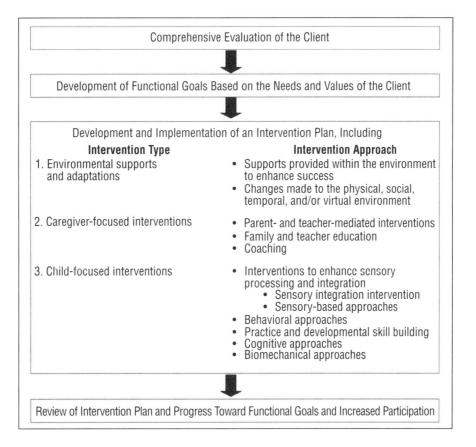

not follow a prescriptive technique or recipe but instead uses daily sensory experiences that are individualized to promote adaptive responses. Occupational therapists Mary Sue Williams and Sherry Shellenberger (1996) focused on this as part of their creative Alert Program. This program uses the analogy of a car to suggest that sometimes a person's system runs too fast, like a car revving its engine, and other times it can run too slow, such as when a car's engine is running out of gas. Optimally, a car should run "just right" depending on the needs of the driver.

Dosage

A sensory diet is an adult-mediated prescription of sensory input of varying type and qualities throughout the day, much as someone might strategically create a nutritionally based diet of protein, fruit, vegetables, and so on. Think of sensation as a dose of input to the nervous system, strategically selected for a purposeful outcome. Sensory input, then, might be facilitating (alerting), inhibiting (calming), or modulating. Doses will have varying power

and intensity, and the timing (e.g., frequency and duration, when the dose is best administered) will matter.

Sometimes the dose of sensation will be self-initiated and self-administered, and other times a caregiver may apply the sensation (e.g., massaging a child's hands before a fine motor task). The outcome of a sensory diet focuses on supporting daily routines (play, social engagement, ADLs). Sensory diets were originally introduced consistent with Ayres's theory and the ideas of Wilbarger and Wilbarger (1991) and were initially only designed for children. More recently, the idea of the sensory diet has expanded to include adults (Williams, 2017).

This expansion of a pediatric intervention grounded in a theory focused on children is an example of an emerging practice rather than an evidence-informed practice. There is little to no clinical or empirical evidence or theoretical basis indicating that the practice constitutes a substantial risk of harm to those receiving it. If any harm occurs, it is in the time invested in the approach. The use of a sensory diet with adults reflects new and untested ideas, and the decision to use one should be the end result of careful clinical reasoning.

Goals

Sensory diets are specifically aimed at the goals of self-regulation and modulation of sensation to promote adaptive responses. Goals might also include decreasing sensory defensiveness to allow participation in daily routines and support the social engagement, optimal arousal, and behavioral organization needed for classroom tasks and learning or enhancing body awareness to promote movement competence, self-esteem, and self-confidence. There is little evidence specifically supporting the sensory diet as an intervention, for many of the reasons cited earlier as difficulties in studying SI.

A sensory diet intervention should include a clear time frame for the evaluation of progress and identification of a change in the targeted behavior. Outcomes such as "reduce fight-or-flight reaction" are neither functional nor objectively measurable and should not be used. Caregivers should know what outcomes are expected and when the intervention should be altered or discontinued on the basis of actual performance data.

Science and Theory Development

Ayres's early work forms the foundation of both the SI and the sensory processing frames of reference. As noted in Chapter 5, "Behavioral Science Frames of Reference," in the discussion of the behavioral frames of reference, research supports expansion and revision of theory, often leading to distinct frames of references that share core beliefs. Two distinct frames of reference, SI and sensory processing, evolved from the original theory proposed by Ayres.

The sensory diet is an example of an intervention that uses the sensory processing frame of reference. Exhibit 7.3 outlines which aspects are common to the SI frame of reference or unique to sensory processing. Case Example 7.1 describes the use of a sensory diet as an occupational therapy intervention.

CONTROVERSY AND ARGUMENT

A prevalent misconception about EBP is that the practitioner of this standard can only use interventions that are highly empirically validated. The ongoing call for continued research supporting occupational therapy interventions in general is to help increase the scholarship supporting practices. Although strong research evidence is ideal, EBP allows consideration of less validated interventions, such as ASI or a sensory diet, when they are the best fit for the client in the real-world situation. The SI and sensory processing frames of reference offer good examples of both the challenges of generating relevant research and the use of deliberation in arguing for an intervention that is recognized but lacks strong confirmation of efficacy. Although these practices are described in this text as *evidence informed*, this distinction brings with it the need for clinicians to be able to defend their choice of these interventions.

Controversy occurs in all clinical settings and is not unique to SI and sensory processing. Occupational therapy practitioners need to understand that questioning a treatment decision, especially one that has been targeted as controversial, is integral to professional collegiality and interprofessional practice. This type of questioning should be taken not as a personal affront but rather as a request for information. Understanding a position with which one does not necessarily agree and being open to viewpoints different from one's own allow clinicians to test their own arguments.

As you deliberate and build an argument for the intervention you have selected through strong clinical reasoning, you should first strive for clarity. Educate your listeners. Listeners who cannot understand the argument are unlikely to be persuaded. Similarly, listeners who have preconceived ideas about an intervention or approach may not truly understand what you are proposing (as opposed to their idea of it).

You will want to share as much as you can about the existing data and inferences or assumptions that support your idea. If you have explored all sides of the argument, then you are most able to address the conflicting information available in the literature in a level-headed way. Overstating your case can diminish credibility, whereas realistically assessing propensity can enhance reflective consideration. Consider opposing arguments fairly, not as personal attacks. Respect is a central part of effective interprofessional and collegial communication. To create an atmosphere of mutual respect, it is important that you respect others' viewpoints as well as expect others to respect your viewpoint. Even when there is not full agreement, effective argument can move the conversation toward common ground and acceptable solutions.

SUMMARY

Perhaps the SI and sensory processing frames of reference have been victims, in part, of hasty generalization. The term *hasty generalization* was introduced in Chapter 4 to describe an error in logic when the contents of an argument's stated premises fail to adequately support its proposed conclusion. Hasty generalization among occupational therapy practitioners who found that the ideas in SI theory resonated with their own beliefs may have been why interventions attributed to SI expanded clinically so far beyond the science. While researchers continue to identify and develop fidelity measures, outcome measures, and ways to assess the neurological system, occupational therapy practitioners need to use clinical reasoning to guide intervention decisions that lead to outcomes that are observable, measurable, and occupationally focused.

(Text continued on page 140)

EXHIBIT 7.3.	SI Frame of Reference: Distinct Elements of Sensory Processing
Focus	The focus of sensory processing is on the client's ability to discriminate, modulate, and integrate sensory information needed for developmentally appropriate tasks to fully participate in daily life (Schaaf & Davies, 2010).

Basic assumptions	**Common to all approaches within the SI frame of reference:**
	▪ SI is a developmental process that mirrors human development.
	▪ The brain serves as an information processor that transforms sensory data into meaningful information that supports function and participation.
	▪ Errors in sensory information processing can occur as errors of input, errors of encoding for memory, and errors of output.
	  • Problems with the ability to process and modulate sensory input contribute to deficits in the ability to organize the behavior needed to perform developmentally appropriate tasks.
	  • Problems with the ability to store information for later use in the form of mental schema make it hard to retrieve and use this information for function.
	  • Problems in how the brain decides what to do with information and how it reacts to a stimulus can lead to inappropriate or dysfunctional behavior.
	Unique to sensory processing:
	▪ Active engagement is ideal, but passively applied sensory information (such as drinking a thick drink through a straw) may also support sensory modulation.
	▪ Providing organized sensory information tailored to the client's needs through environmental modification and the introduction of sensory experiences can lead to improved sensory processing and adaptive behaviors.

Function–disability continuum	**Common to all approaches within the SI frame of reference:** ▪ Function occurs through adaptive responses that result from effective sensory modulation, discrimination, and integration. Dysfunction, in the form of sensory defensiveness, avoidance, underregistration of sensation, or poor modulation, manifests as maladaptive behaviors such as poor postural control, praxis or bilateral integration, and participation. **Unique to sensory processing:** ▪ Function–dysfunction continuums are relevant within each sensory system.
Postulates of change	**Unique to sensory processing:** ▪ Participation in environments designed to control, support, or enhance sensory processing can support engagement and motivate adaptive responses. ▪ Occupational therapy practitioners work to develop the caregiver's ability to facilitate learning opportunities for the child and scaffold the child's participation in meaningful tasks while responding to the child's sensory needs. ▪ If occupational therapy practitioners present or facilitate challenges in which the child is successful in areas of sensory modulation; discrimination; postural, ocular, and oral control; or praxis, then the child will be more likely to develop skills in challenged area.

Note. SI = sensory integration.

CASE EXAMPLE 7.1. JESS: SENSORY PROCESSING AFFECTING PARTICIPATION IN SOCIAL OPPORTUNITIES

Jess is a 9-year-old girl with challenges in sensory processing and SI that affect her participation in daily occupations and limit her social opportunities. Exhibit 7.4 provides her occupational profile.

Jess appears to be attempting to modulate her sensory system by seeking out sensations in the environment or avoiding other sensations. The touch processing system is alerted by changes in temperature and itchy or tickly touch, all of which occur, for example, when people remove clothing in preparation for a bath, eat food of certain textures, feel a comb across the head, or even have their face washed. Jess's behaviors may be masking underlying slow processing, low energy, and heightened sensitivity to looking stupid when struggling to maintain adequate attention and modulate sensory input.

(Continued)

CASE EXAMPLE 7.1. JESS: SENSORY PROCESSING AFFECTING PARTICIPATION IN SOCIAL OPPORTUNITIES *(Cont.)*

EXHIBIT 7.4. Jess's Occupational Profile

Client	**Reason the client is seeking service and concerns related to engagement in occupations**	Jess was referred for an occupational therapy evaluation to determine appropriateness for social skills group placement and overall occupational performance needs. *Impact on occupation:* Jess's mother describes her as "high strung" and says that she can be snobbish. She has only 1 friend.	
	Occupations in which the client is successful	Jess is independent in eating, dressing, and toileting. She is good at communicating using digital technology.	
	Personal interests and values	Jess loves watching TV and YouTube. She enjoys listening to music and watching music videos.	
	Occupational history (i.e., life experiences)	Jess's mother and father are very concerned about Jess's behavior (e.g., avoidance, tantrums) and lack of interest in activities outside the house.	
	Performance patterns (routines, roles, habits, & rituals)	*Occupational roles:* Daughter, student, friend, sister. Jess's mother states that Jess grows extremely anxious when her school day is interrupted for various appointments and, if she is surprised, has difficulty recovering.	
Environment		***Supports to occupational engagement***	***Barriers to occupational engagement***
	Physical (e.g., buildings, furniture, pets)	Jess has no difficulty with physical accessibility.	Jess avoids all outdoor activities.
	Social (e.g., spouse, friends, caregivers)	Jess has a supportive family and school setting.	Jess uses immature strategies to get her needs met. For example, she would lie on the floor and kick her legs in the air with no apparent regard for the social inappropriateness of exposing her underwear to the examiner, or grab her father's hand and tightly squeeze and twist it in a clear effort to hurt him.
Context	**Cultural (e.g., customs, beliefs)**	No cultural concerns were identified in this assessment.	
	Personal (e.g., age, gender, SES, education)	9-year-old girl in elementary school.	
	Temporal (e.g., stage of life, time, year)	Jess is in middle childhood.	
	Virtual (e.g., chat, email, remote monitoring)	Jess has strong skills in these areas.	Jess has few social connections through which she can use her skills.
Client goals	**Client's priorities and desired targeted outcomes**	Parents express concerns with Jess's academic work and wonder what they can do to help Jess be more organized and more successful. Jess wants to have friends and to be able to do more outside of the family context.	

(Continued)

CASE EXAMPLE 7.1. JESS: SENSORY PROCESSING AFFECTING PARTICIPATION IN SOCIAL OPPORTUNITIES *(Cont.)*

EXHIBIT 7.4.	Jess's Occupational Profile *(Cont.)*
ANALYSIS OF PARTICIPATION	
Basic ADLs	
Eating/oral–motor	Jess is said to be a picky eater. She eats primarily carbohydrates and craves sour pickles.
Grooming	Jess is quite intolerant of having her hair combed and her face washed or touched, which creates difficulty for the family.
Bathing/transfer	Jess exhibits avoidant behaviors to bathing that are significant enough that the school has spoken to the family about their concerns regarding Jess's hygiene.
Dressing upper body	Independent (will only wear cotton or soft clothing from which tags have been removed).
Dressing lower body	Independent (will only wear elasticized sports pants such as yoga pants or leggings).
Toileting	Independent.
Problem-solving/memory	Jess showed poor ability to persist against a challenge during testing and needed many opportunities during the testing session to take breaks.
Comments:	When upset, Jess lies on the floor and kicks her legs in the air or will grab her father's hand and tightly squeeze and twist until he stops her from hurting him. Jess has difficulty with sleep routines; she is restless, has a hard time falling asleep, and wakes often. She often wakes at night and gets up to watch TV.
IADLs	
Community mobility	WNL.
Health management/ prevention	WNL.
Home management	WNL.
Financial management	WNL.
Leisure/play	Jess hates to go outside for activities, and her primary leisure pursuits are solely organized around television viewing and computer use.
Safety	Jess frequently hurts family members by running into them, pushing too hard, or squeezing too tightly. She frequently has cuts or bruises that she cannot explain.
Comments:	None.
Motor and Praxis Skills	
Sitting—static/dynamic	Jess is able to maintain dynamic sitting, although she fatigues easily and prefers to move and fidget.
Standing—static/dynamic	Jess has adequate ability in both static and dynamic standing. She has poor endurance to stand on 1 foot when asked (less than 20 seconds).
Place can on shelf	Jess is able to do this.
Retrieve item from floor	Jess is able to do this.
Screw lid on jar	Jess is able to do this.
Comb back of head	Jess is able to do this imperfectly and needs adult supervision.
Joint stability and skeletal mobility	Jess has good joint stability and ROM. Jess is unable to demonstrate supine or prone extension; when asked, she said it was too hard.

(Continued)

CASE EXAMPLE 7.1. JESS: SENSORY PROCESSING AFFECTING PARTICIPATION IN SOCIAL OPPORTUNITIES *(Cont.)*

EXHIBIT 7.4.	Jess's Occupational Profile *(Cont.)*
Writing	When grasping a writing implement, Jess uses her right hand and uses a whole-arm movement pattern. She uses an immature, 4-finger grasp pattern. The web space is closed, and her thumb is wrapped over the pencil and fingers. Jess applies heavy pencil pressure when writing, exerting a heavy force on the pencil and producing dark markings on the paper. Jess's performance deteriorated as the tasks proceeded. Jess's handwriting (i.e., letters) were large and the spacing was inconsistent, making the writing barely legible.
Lift grocery bag	Jess is able to do this imperfectly and needs adult supervision.
Coordination	Both verbal and visual praxis were measured. Jess demonstrates strong skills in imitating simple postures when given a visual demonstration (i.e., make a mirror image of a position) and significant difficulty when given a verbal direction only (i.e., follow a "Simon Says" command).
Manipulation	Jess relies on immature manipulation patterns and shifts to the ulnar side of the hand controlling the pencil. Jess is able to manage clothing fasteners and scissors.
Comments:	Jess has low postural muscle tone. Prone extension and supine flexion are each below normal limits (unable to assume positions). She fatigued easily with motor tasks and used avoidance strategies when challenged, particularly with fine motor tasks. Jess's righting and equilibrium reactions are intact in seated and standing positions. Jess had difficulty controlling her force direction during play using a ball and grew noticeably frustrated. She frequently stated, "I'm not stupid, this is stupid!"
Process Skills	
Energy for task	Jess works with her head lying on the table for most paper-and-pencil tasks. Jess has low endurance and fatigue with motor tasks.
Adaptation/praxis	Jess has difficulty learning novel tasks.
Knowledge/organization of task	Jess has general understanding but needs adult supervision.
Comments:	Jess is overly avoidant of novel experiences and shows poor persistence in challenging academic tasks. She has poor frustration tolerance, which limits her willingness to engage in new activities or complete homework assignments.
Behavioral and Cognitive Skills	
Communication and following social conventions	Jess's interactions were socially awkward, overly direct, and often inappropriately blunt and frequently improperly authoritative and directive. She was at times overly talkative (when complaining) and overly detailed about information not relevant to the social exchange.
Cognitive and emotional regulation skills	Jess hates to be interrupted or unable to get her thoughts out verbally; she clenches her fists and shakes her head. Poor eye contact was noted throughout the testing session.
Level of arousal/attention	On the SP (Dunn, 2014), Jess scored in the definite difference range on "low energy/weak" and "underresponsive/seeks sensation," which indicates a child who tires easily and has poor endurance for physical activity and difficulty modulating sensation.
Orientation	When Jess's attention was on the task at hand, she was more motivated and compliance improved.
Energy and drive	Jess presents with poor ability to control impulses, difficulty persisting against presented challenges, and difficulty resisting inappropriate behaviors during testing. She needed many opportunities during the testing session to take breaks and have a turn to direct social exchanges and multiple reminders from her father that he expected her compliance.

(Continued)

CASE EXAMPLE 7.1. JESS: SENSORY PROCESSING AFFECTING PARTICIPATION IN SOCIAL OPPORTUNITIES *(Cont.)*

EXHIBIT 7.4.	Jess's Occupational Profile *(Cont.)*
Memory and understanding	Jess needs constant reminders to complete tasks related to academic, grooming and hygiene, and household chores.
Higher level cognition	Jess has immature EF skills. In particular she has difficulty with mental flexibility and self-control.
Sensory–Perceptual Skills	
Sensory (information regarding Jess's ability to process sensory information was obtained through her mother's completion of the Short SP).	SP results indicate that Jess demonstrates difficulties with sensory processing and sensory modulation. Sensations of definite difference for Jess fall into the areas of auditory, vestibular, touch, and oral sensory processing. Modulation affecting activity levels and behavioral and emotional outcomes of sensory processing are reported to be in the definite difference range. The factor summary shows Jess has oral sensory sensitivity and inattention/distractibility, is emotionally reactive, and has fine motor/perceptual skill deficits as a result of sensory processing differences.
Self-perception	Jess is aware of her limitations and restricts her activities to hide these from her classmates.
Hearing and vision	Jess's hearing and vision are intact.
Pain	Jess gets frequents bruises and cuts but seems unaware of them. She is otherwise overly watchful and avoidant (e.g., nail clipping, doctor visits).
Skin integrity	Jess has a noticeable bruise on her left shin.
Comments:	None.

Note. Occupational profile template from American Occupational Therapy Association (2017). Analysis of participation format adapted from Skubik-Peplaski, Paris, Boyle, & Culpert (2009). ADLs = activities of daily living; EF = executive function; IADLs = instrumental activities of daily living; ROM = range of motion; SES = socioeconomic status; SP = Sensory Profile; WNL = within normal limits.

Heavy work by the muscle system (e.g., lifting, moving, carrying, running) and deep pressure (e.g., massage) or warmth can help the nervous system to achieve or maintain optimal arousal that, in turn, supports occupational engagement and self-regulation. It will be important to provide Jess with opportunities to develop her sensory–motor system as well as to establish organizing and adaptive routines with which she can feel empowered to better modulate her sensory thresholds. A sensory diet is recommended. Suggestions for a sensory diet for Jess might include

- Listening to music, especially music with strong lower notes such as from a bass, tribal drums, and so forth (e.g., *Star Wars* main theme).
- Using a vibrating toothbrush or vibrating hairbrush.
- Making sure to get heavy-work exercise each day, ideally before needing to complete challenging academic work or participate in social events.
- Performing heavy work with the oral muscles, such as sucking thick liquids through a straw, eating crunchy or chewy snacks, or chewing gum before or during tabletop activities.

- Making meals and snacks a sensory strategy to optimize performance, such as eating crunchy or chewy foods such as pickles, cereal, bagels, fruit leather, beef jerky, or other foods that require strong chewing and grinding of the teeth; sour foods (e.g., the pickles Jess craves) are encouraged.
- Using a large therapy ball to sit and bounce on when doing homework.
- Helping with cooking, mixing, and chopping; carrying dishes; and putting away heavy pans.
- Helping to set the table, using 2 hands to carry and balance a tray, or pushing chairs into and pulling them out from the table.
- Thinking about chores as a way to get Jess to do heavy work (e.g., raking leaves, carrying groceries, moving heavy items from lower to higher surfaces, mowing the lawn with a push mower, washing the car, carrying a watering can and watering plants, carrying the laundry basket).
- Setting a timer when Jess is performing written work so that she can take frequent movement breaks to prevent frustration.

Occupational therapy practitioners should be deliberative in exploring new or minimally validated interventions. When all factors, including client preferences, cost, and contextual evidence, support the intervention decision, occupational therapy practitioners should accept the challenge and advocate for their clinical judgment to best serve the needs of their clients.

LEARNING ACTIVITIES

1. As a learning tool, quiz yourself on the terms listed at the beginning of the chapter. These terms are foundational to occupational therapy practice using ASI and are widely used throughout the occupational therapy literature.
2. Challenge yourself to describe a child who would fit the types of SPD outlined in this chapter (i.e., Type 1, sensory modulation; Type 2, sensory–motor; Type 3, sensory discrimination; see Figure 7.3).
3. Read the article "An Intervention for Sensory Difficulties in Children with Autism: A Randomized Trial" (Schaaf et al., 2014). Summarize the findings presented in this article.
4. Interview an occupational therapy practitioner who uses an SI frame of reference in his or her practice. Focus your interview on how the practitioner uses clinical reasoning to measure the outcomes of the intervention. How does the practitioner explain the theory and practice of the SI frame of reference to others, especially those who ask whether their approach uses EBP?
5. Looking back on how to frame an argument, how might you create a presentation to explain and discuss SI as a reasonable approach for occupational therapy intervention? Write a short opinion paper, create a PowerPoint presentation, or develop a short TED Talk that documents your argument. (Multiple resouces are available on YouTube that discuss how to create persuasive talk, i.e., talk like TED).
6. Read the article "The Issue Is—Using a Multifaceted Approach to Working With Children Who Have Differences in Sensory Processing and Integration" (Reynolds et al., 2017). See whether you can identify the steps to making an argument the authors took in this article that follow those outlined in this chapter.

REFERENCES

American Occupational Therapy Association. (2017). AOTA occupational profile template. *American Journal of Occupational Therapy, 71*(Suppl. 2), 7112420030. https://doi.org/10.5014/ajot.2017.716S12

Argument. (2017). In *Merriam-Webster's dictionary.* Retrieved from https://www.merriam-webster.com/dictionary/argument

Autism Speaks. (2012). *Top 8 autism therapies: Reported by parents.* Retrieved from https://www.autismspeaks.org/blog/2012/09/25/top-8-autism-therapies-%E2%80%93-reported-parents

Ayres, A. J. (1972). *Sensory integration and learning disorders.* Los Angeles: Western Psychological Services.

Bear, M., Connors, B., & Paradiso, M. (2015). *Neuroscience: Exploring the Brain* (4th ed.). Philadelphia: Wolters Kluwer Health.

Berlucchi, G. (2011). Brain plasticity and cognitive neurorehabilitation. *Neuropsychological Rehabilitation, 21,* 560–578.

Boudreau, J.-P. (2009). Embodied mind and learning in infancy: A tribute to Esther Thelen. *Journal of Sport and Exercise Psychology, 31*(Suppl.), S8.

California Evidence-Based Clearinghouse. (2018). *Scientific Rating Scale.* Retrieved from http://bit.ly/1WhAxP5

Case-Smith, J., Weaver, L. L., & Fristad, M. A. (2014). A systematic review of sensory processing interventions for children with autism spectrum disorders. *Autism, 19,* 133–148. https://doi.org/10.1177/1362361313517762.

Cohn, E. S., Kramer, J., Schub, J. A., & May-Benson, T. (2014). Parents' explanatory models and hopes for outcomes of occupational therapy using a sensory integration approach. *American Journal of Occupational Therapy, 68,* 454–462. https://doi.org/10.5014/ajot.2014.010843

Dunn, W. (2014). *Sensory Profile 2: User's manual.* San Antonio, TX: Pearson.

Dunn, W., Little, L., Dean, E., Robertson, S., & Evans, B. (2016). The state of the science on sensory factors and their impact on daily life for children: A scoping review. *OTJR: Occupation, Participation and Health, 36*(Suppl. 2), S3–S26. https://doi.org/10.1177/1539449215617923

Foss, A., Swinth, Y., McGruder, J., & Tomlin, G. (2003). Sensory modulation dysfunction and the Wilbarger Protocol: An evidence review. *OT Practice, 8*(12), CE1–CE8.

Kinnealey, M., Koenig, K. P., & Smith, S. (2011). Relationships between sensory modulation and social supports and health-related quality of life. *American Journal of Occupational Therapy, 65,* 320–327. https://doi.org/10.5014/ajot.2011.001370

Kramer, P., & Hinojosa, J. (2015). *Frames of reference for pediatric occupational therapy* (3rd ed.). Philadelphia: Lippincott Williams & Wilkins.

Leong, H. M., Carter, M., & Stephenson, J. R. (2015). Meta-analysis of research on sensory integration therapy for individuals with developmental and learning disabilities. *Journal of Developmental and Physical Disabilities, 27,* 183–206. https://doi.org/10.1007/s10882-014-9408-y

Miller, L. J., Anzalone, M. E., Lane, S. J., Cermak, S. A., & Osten, E. T. (2007). Concept evolution in sensory integration: A proposed nosology for diagnosis. *American Journal of Occupational Therapy, 61,* 135–140. https://doi.org/10.5014/ajot.61.2.135

Parham, L. D., Roley, S. S., May-Benson, T. A., Koomar, J., Brett-Green, B., Burke, J. P., . . . Schaaf, R. C. (2011). Development of a fidelity measure for research on the effectiveness of the Ayres Sensory Integration® intervention. *American Journal of Occupational Therapy, 65,* 133–142. https://doi.org/10.5014/ajot.2011.000745

Pfeiffer, B., May-Benson, T. A., & Bodison, S. C. (2018). State of the science of sensory integration research with children and youth. *American Journal of Occupational Therapy, 72,* 1–4. https://doi.org/10.5014/ajot.2018.721003

Puddy, R. W., & Wilkins, N. (2011). *Understanding evidence— Part 1: Best available research evidence—A guide to the continuum of evidence of effectiveness.* Atlanta: Centers for Disease Control and Prevention. Retrieved from https://www.cdc .gov/violenceprevention/pdf/understanding_evidence-a.pdf

Reynolds, S., Glennon, T. J., Ausderau, K., Bendixen, R. M., Miller Kuhaneck, H., Pfeiffer, B., . . . Bodison, S. C. (2017). Using a multifaceted approach to working with children who have differences in sensory processing and integration. *American Journal of Occupational Therapy, 71,* 1–10. https:// doi.org/10.5014/ajot.2017.019281

Schaaf, R. C. (2015). Creating evidence for practice using data-driven decision making. *American Journal of Occupational Therapy, 69,* 690236001. https://doi.org/10.5014/ajot .2015.010561

Schaaf, R. C., Benevides, T., Mailloux, Z., Faller, P., Hunt, J., vanHooydonk, E., . . . Kelly, D. (2014). An intervention for sensory difficulties in children with autism: A randomized trial. *Journal of Autism and Developmental Disorders, 44,* 1493–1506. https://doi.org/10.1007/s10803-013-1983-8.

Schaaf, R. C., & Davies, P. L. (2010). Evolution of the sensory integration frame of references. *American Journal of Occupational Therapy, 64,* 363–367. https://doi.org/10.5014/ajot .2010.090000

Schaaf, R. C., Dumont, R. L., Arbesman, M., & May-Benson, T. A. (2018). Efficacy of occupational therapy using Ayres Sensory Integration®: A systematic review. *American Journal of Occupational Therapy, 72,* 7201119010. https://doi .org/10.5014/ajot.2018.028431

Schaaf, R. C., & Mailloux, Z. (2015). *Clinician's guide for implementing Ayres Sensory Integration®: Promoting participation for children with autism.* Bethesda, MD: AOTA Press.

Skubik-Peplaski, C., Paris, C., Boyle, D., & Culpert, A. (Eds.). (2009). *Applying the* Occupational Therapy Practice Framework: *Using the Cardinal Hill Occupational Participation*

Process in client-centered care (2nd ed.). Bethesda, MD: AOTA Press.

Smith-Roley, S., Mailloux, Z., Miller-Kuhaneck, H., & Glennon, T. (2007). Understanding Ayres Sensory Integration®. *OT Practice, 12*(17), CE1–CE8.

Theory. (2017). In *Merriam-Webster's dictionary.* Retrieved from https://www.merriam-webster.com/dictionary/theory

Tomchek, S. D., Little, L. M., & Dunn, W. (2015). Sensory pattern contributions to developmental performance in children with autism spectrum disorder. *American Journal of Occupational Therapy, 69,* 6905185040. https://doi.org/10.5014/ajot .2015.018044

Watling, R., & Hauer, S. (2015). Effectiveness of Ayres Sensory Integration® and sensory-based interventions for people with autism spectrum disorder: A systematic review. *American Journal of Occupational Therapy, 69,* 6905180030. https://doi.org/10.5014/ajot.2015.018051

Whitney, R., & Pickren, W. (2014). *Self-regulation: A family systems approach for children with autism, learning disabilities, ADHD, and sensory disorders.* Eau Claire, WI: PESI.

Wilbarger, J., & Wilbarger, P. (1991). *Sensory defensiveness in children aged 2–12: An intervention guide for parents and other caretakers.* Santa Barbara, CA: Avanti Educational Programs.

Williams, K. L. (2017). Understanding the role of sensory processing in occupation: An updated discourse with cognitive neuroscience. *Journal of Occupational Science, 24*(3), 302–313. https://doi.org/10.1080/14427591.2016.1209425

Williams, M. S., & Shellenberger, S. (1996). *How does your engine run? A leader's guide to the Alert Program for Self-Regulation.* Albuquerque, NM: TherapyWorks.

Zimmer, M., & Desch, L. (2012). Sensory integration therapies for children with developmental and behavioral disorders. *Pediatrics, 129,* 1186–1189. https://doi.org/10.1542/ peds.2012-0876

PART III.

Intervention

Occupation-Focused Practice Models

8

Anne Cronin, PhD, OTR/L, ATP, FAOTA, and Garth Graebe, MOT, OTR/L

CHAPTER HIGHLIGHTS

- Distinguishes between frames of reference and models.
- Provides an overview of occupation-based practice.
- Considers reductionism vs. holism in clinical reasoning.
- Introduces readers to the Model of Human Occupation (MOHO) and includes a case example using the MOHO to guide clinical reasoning.
- Describes the Person–Environment–Occupation–Performance (PEOP) Model and includes a case example using the PEOP Model to guide clinical reasoning.
- Describes the Canadian Model of Occupational Performance and Engagement.
- Presents strategies for considering and comparing occupation-focused models and frames of reference.
- Delineates innovations in occupation-based practice.

KEY TERMS AND CONCEPTS

Canadian Model of Occupational Performance and Engagement
Frame of reference
Habituation
Holism
Kawa Model
Model

Model of Human Occupation
Occupation-based practice
Occupation-focused models
Organizational narrative
Performance
Personal causation
Personal narrative

Person–Environment–Occupation–Performance Model
Population narrative
Reductionism
Volition

In this chapter, readers will gain an understanding of occupation-focused practice models, both as they serve as models for clinical decision making and also how they might be applied as frames of reference for intervention decisions. This chapter argues for the inclusion of occupation-based reasoning in both the formulation and the refinement of the clinical hypothesis. This is important because much of the science and theory that guide intervention are drawn from outside the occupational therapy profession and do not consider occupation in its original form. With the exception of the sensory integration frame of reference, all of the frames of reference discussed in the earlier chapters originated from outside the discipline of occupational therapy and were adopted by the profession as effective tools to guide clinical reasoning.

This chapter begins by distinguishing between models and frames of reference, followed by an overview of occupation-based practice. It then describes the Model of Human Occupation (MOHO), Person–Environment–Occupation–Performance (PEOP) Model, and Canadian Model of Occupational Performance and Engagement (CMOP-E), followed by a discussion of strategies to compare occupation-focused practice models and innovations in occupation-based practice.

MODELS VS. FRAMES OF REFERENCE

Earlier in this text, a distinction was made between frames of reference and models. A *frame of reference* is defined as a set of assumptions or concepts, often drawn from theory, that explains how occupational therapy works in routine practice. A frame of reference organizes aspects of theories, models, and science into a functional perspective that will guide clinical evaluation, intervention, and outcome identification. Frames of reference serve as guidelines for clinical decisions about how to assess a client's functional capacities, what functional capacities should be the focus of the assessment, how to implement an intervention, and how to formulate purposeful interventions to support performance and participation.

In contrast, a *model* is an abstract way of schematizing a process. A model typically defines concepts and phenomena under the umbrella of the perspective it proposes. Models are more general than frames of reference. The intent of a model is to guide clinical reasoning and the process without being directive about the specifics of implementing the concepts in clinical practice.

145

These 2 definitions distinguish between frames of reference and models, but in practice the distinction is not so clear. As noted earlier, several assessment tools have been developed to be used with MOHO in clinical interventions, adding to this model aspects of a frame of reference. Other frames of reference, such as the sensory integration frame of reference, include a broad theoretical viewpoint with unique definitions of concepts and phenomena, which give them aspects of a model.

OVERVIEW OF OCCUPATION-BASED PRACTICE

Domain and Hypothesis

Wong and Fisher (2015) noted that occupational therapy practitioners' ability to synthesize and apply occupational concepts is what uniquely distinguishes occupational therapy from other health professions. Earlier chapters in this text introduced the clinical hypothesis as an entry into the clinical reasoning process. The occupational therapy practice domain itself is not prescriptive as to the type of assessment that should be done or of intervention approaches that best respond to the needs identified through assessment. The clinical hypothesis emerges from the occupational therapy domain of practice as it is informed by science, and it is an excellent tool to guide the occupational therapy process from evaluation through outcomes. Although clinical reasoning was first presented in this text as a structured clinical question leading to a hypothesis, the occupational therapy practitioner' paradigm influences the formulation of the hypothesis.

Reductionism

Most of the frames of reference presented in earlier chapters are reductionistic. *Reductionism* is an approach to reasoning that assumes that all complex systems can be completely understood in terms of their components. Reductionism is not inherently either good or bad. It is an essential tool in science and clinical reasoning. The classic medical diagnostic hypothesis is usually based on body structure and function-level reductionistic reasoning. The pitfall of this type of reasoning is that it reduces the complexity of the individual to a disease or injury label, and the essential intrinsic and extrinsic factors that support change may be lost. The idiom "can't see the forest for the trees" characterizes reductionism.

Holism

The opposite of reductionism is *holism,* an approach that assumes that a system can be understood only as a whole. Another idiom, "the whole is greater than the sum of its parts," characterizes this approach to reasoning. Holism, like reductionism, is not inherently either good or bad.

At times, the reductionistic approach offers the fastest and most complete return to daily occupations and participation for the individual. Concerns arise in that traditional medical models are highly reductive, and the holistic viewpooint may be lost. The ability to assimilate the reductionistic details of the clinical environment while retaining a holistic view is the ideal sought in occupational therapy practice.

When discussing frames of reference in this text, we have been careful to identify them "as used in occupational therapy." The intent here was to assure readers that occupational therapy pratitioners can authentically use these approaches because they are consistent with the occupational therapy domain of practice and can be applied while holistically integrating occupational concepts.

Occupation-Based Practice

Occupation-based practice is a term describing the use of a client's engagement in occupations as "the therapeutic agent of change" (Fisher, 2013, p. 164). The *Occupational Therapy Practice Framework: Domain and Process* (*OTPF–3*; American Occupational Therapy Association [AOTA], 2014) defines *occupational therapy* as "the therapeutic use of everyday life activities (occupations) with individual people or groups for the purpose of enhancing or enabling participation in roles, habits, and routines in home, school, workplace, community, and other settings" (p. S1). The *OTPF–3* also affirms that occupational therapy practitioners "are concerned with the end result of participation" (p. S1). Occupation-based practice is the end result of clinical reasoning grounded in the paradigm of occupation.

Both occupation-based practice and occupation-focused models are inherently holistic and offer a balance to reductionistic reasoning. This chapter presents holistic approaches based on organized theories that offer a framework for considering occupation while delineating rules, patterns, and generalizations about occupation that can be explored through research and measured in functional client outcomes.

Occupation-Focused Models

In clinical reasoning, a *model* is an abstract way of schematizing a process so that the foundational theory can be generalized. In this chapter, we introduce models that are designed to embed core concepts of occupation throughout the occupational therapy process. *Occupation-focused models* incorporate a systematic description of human participation and engagement while also considering skills, roles, habits, routines, and contexts of a client's lifestyle. Occupation-focused models consider the effects of engagement in daily occupations and the potential performance-enhancing effects of occupational engagement as tools to support health, development, recovery of function, and satisfaction with participation in daily life activities. These models are essential to understanding occupational therapy clinical reasoning because they both support and challenge occupational therapy practitioners and scientists to clearly articulate their distinct contribution both to science and to the health care team.

Any frame of reference can be applied in the context of occupation-based practice, but this application requires creativity and ingenuity on the part of occupational therapy practitioners. Prodinger, Shaw, Stamm, and Rudman (2014) noted that although occupation-based practice is presented as an ideal, there are many obstacles to enacting this approach. One obstacle cited by these authors is practice in a medical institutional setting that is focused on disease and disease-related issues. Another obstacle is the profession's borrowing of frames of reference that emerged outside the profession of occupational therapy.

The first known effort to describe a general theory of occupational therapy was the work of Mary Reilly (1977). Since then, many theorists have built on her work. Today, there are several published occupation-focused models, all of which are consistent with the paradigm of occupational therapy (see below). Occupation-focused models consistently reflect that occupation is essential to humans and that occupation organizes human behavior. In this broad sense, occupation gives meaning to life. Occupation-focused models are built on the assumption that healthy patterns of occupation enable a healthy lifestyle and a sense of life satisfaction. All occupation-focused approaches put occupation at the core of the profession. Frames of reference, such as those presented earlier in this text, fall in the occupational therapy domain only when they are assimilated through the use of an occupational lens.

There is nothing inherently wrong with using knowledge from a broad variety of sources to provide the best possible care for clients. The caveat is that practitioners must actively and thoughtfully consider how to integrate frames of reference within the occupational therapy domain of practice. Occupational therapy practitioners using the biomechanical or the motor learning frame of reference should apply these frames of reference in the context of enhancing or enabling participation in roles, habits, and routines in the home, school, workplace, community, and other settings. The functional outcomes that result from occupational therapy interventions should be grounded in occupation and occupational performance to reflect the distinctive contribution of occupationl therapy to clients and the health care teams.

A major reason for the development of occupation-focused practice models for occupational therapy was the difficulty of retaining an occupational focus in practice when working in a medical, disease-focused environment using frames of reference that are not occupation oriented. MOHO, introduced by Kielhofner and Burke (1980), was the first conceptual practice model to emerge from occupational therapy. Kielhofner and Burke built on Reilly's (1977) theoretical work in occupational behavior, knowledge from the social sciences, and von Bertalanffy's (1974) general systems theory. Since the early work on MOHO, several other occupational-focused practice models have been developed. This chapter's discussion is limited to the MOHO and PEOP Model, the most researched and most widely used occupation-focused models.

MOHO

MOHO describes a dynamic process in which the occupational therapy process, from assessment to outcome measures, focuses on the occupations of interest to clients (Kielhofner, 2008). Unlike the frames of reference presented in Parts 1 and 2 of this text, MOHO offers both a theoretical focus and a language specific to occupation that supports occupational therapy practitioners in understanding how their clients' occupations "are motivated, transformed into routines and habits, and performed capably within given social and physical environments" (Lee et al., 2012, p. 450).

Theoretical Focus

MOHO draws from general systems theory, from the work in occupational behavior begun by Reilly (1977) and from the social sciences. It describes a human being as a self-organizing open system in interaction with the environment. The model emphasizes the dynamic adaptation of the individual that results from occupational participation. Individuals, as open systems, have the ability to both take in information from the environment and affect the environment through output, making them dynamic agents of change within the environment.

MOHO postulates that it is through the self-organizing aspects of systems that occupational behavior is organized and structured. It explains occupation in terms of 3 main aspects:
1. Volition (how occupation is motivated),
2. Habituation (how occupation is organized), and
3. Performance (how occupation occurs; Kielhofner, 2008). These aspects of occupation are part of a dynamic open system that is self-organizing and self-regulating through the assimilation of feedback.

Volition

Volition is the use of one's will to choose what to do. Volition is a process that begins with a drive for action and results in a lived experience that the person learns from and interprets to inform future action choices. When the occupational therapy practitioner supports a client's volition, the client is motivated to choose. When the client feels confident of his or her abilities, a sense of personal capacity and self-efficacy results. Within MOHO, this result is called ***personal causation.*** Supporting client volition also involves encouraging choices that the client believes are meaningful and reflective of his or her values. A final aspect of volition addresses a focus on interests, those things the client likes or wants to do.

Habituation

Habituation, in the context of MOHO, reflects the individual's intrinsic readiness to demonstrate a consistent pattern of behavior in the form of a habit or a role. Habits and roles organize daily occupation. They may be affected by intrinsic factors such as disability or extrinsic factors such as social expectations. The *OTPF–3* has assimilated aspects of MOHO in its definition of *performance patterns* as "the habits, routines, roles, and rituals used in the process of engaging in occupations or activities that can support or hinder occupational performance" (AOTA, 2014, p. S8).

Performance

Finally, ***performance,*** as defined in MOHO, is what enables clients to actually "do" their valued occupations. Performance relies on the ability to recruit body structures and body functions to support action. The performance described in MOHO relates to the performance skills described in the *OTPF–3*. "*Performance skills* are goal-directed actions that are observable as small units of engagement in daily life occupations" (AOTA, 2014, p. S7). Performance skills are learned and developed over time and are situated in specific contexts and environments (Fisher & Griswold, 2014).

MOHO considers the environment of the open system as a facilitator of or a constraint to the person's performance of occupations. Environments can be physical, including natural and built nonhuman surroundings and objects. The *OTPF–3* elaborates on physical environments as inclusive of geographic terrain, plants, and animals as well as the sensory qualities of the surroundings (AOTA, 2014).

Environments can also be social, including the presence of others in the physical environment as well as the expectations of persons, groups, or populations whom the client values or has contact with. The *OTPF–3* elaborates on social environments as including the availability and expectations of significant people; relationships with individual people, groups, or populations; and even relationships with systems (e.g., political, legal, economic, institutional) that influence norms, role expectations, and social routines (AOTA, 2014). Wong and Fisher (2015) stated that "the focus in MOHO is on understanding and developing the person's motivation for occupation, with the assumption that skills, performance, and, ultimately adaptation, will follow" (p. 303). Case Example 8.1 applies MOHO, emphasizing the importance of developing the client's motivation for occupation.

State of Science and Evidence-Based Considerations

MOHO has the most substantial research support of all of the occupation-focused models. Lee (2010) reported on 433 peer-reviewed journal articles that focused on MOHO. The scope of the journal articles was broad and related to many aspects of occupational therapy practice. The greatest clinical use of MOHO has been in support of emotional and behavioral challenges that result in disruptions to desired daily activities.

An example of this is offered in Gindi, Galili, Volovic-Shushan, and Adir-Pavis (2016), who studied the impact of combat stress on occupation and, through the application of MOHO, developed an intervention aimed at promoting adaptive and efficient functioning by engaging soldiers in occupation-centered tasks. The intent of this treatment approach was to restore the soldiers' sense of control, to renew and strengthen interpersonal relations, and to build motivation and self-efficacy to support motivation for future activity. The authors noted that "this proposed model has 2 main therapeutic goals: preventing soldiers' fixation on their role as patients, and promoting their rapid return to efficient and adaptive functioning" (p. 739). Their article presents a therapeutic model that uses MOHO and MOHO-based assessments to guide occupational therapy intervention for people with mental health challenges. It clearly reflects the MOHO's top-down perspective, emphasizing volition and habituation to drive change at the performance level.

PEOP MODEL

The ***PEOP Model*** was first published in 1991 and, like the MOHO, was developed in response to a need for more occupation-focused models (Christiansen & Baum, 1991). As with MOHO, the PEOP Model emphasizes occupation and the specific contributions of occupational performance and participation. It holds that the individual has many intrinsic influences that are the building blocks of his or her set of skills and abilities. In this model, occupations are grouped in a meaningful way so that the person can perform life roles. Extrinsic environmental influences play a major role in the performance of occupations, and participation is always affected by the extrinsic characteristics of the environment in which it occurs.

Theoretical Focus

The primary assumption guiding the PEOP Model is that occupational performance is influenced by the relationship between a person and his or her environment. As with the MOHO, the PEOP Model draws from general systems theory and from the social sciences. In addition, it incorporates aspects of environmental theory, neurobehavioral theories,

CASE EXAMPLE 8.1. COLLIN: MOHO APPLICATION

Collin, age 10 years, is struggling in his occupational roles and in his performance due to cognitive and self-regulation challenges. His occupational profile is shown in Exhibit 8.1.

The occupational therapy practitioner's intervention involved working on 2 basic assumptions:

1. By teaching Collin to work more slowly and deliberately, he would soon discover that he would get his homework done more quickly than in the past, thus allowing him more time to do other things, and
2. Using a brightly colored folder for Collin's homework and a timer to indicate work periods and break periods would help him to increase his organizational skills.

With the help of his occupational therapy practitioner, Collin began to use a red folder to bring his homework assignments home and to return the completed assignments to school. With his parents' support, he would check to make sure he had the red folder in his backpack before leaving both school and his home. Collin and his occupational therapy practitioner also worked together to complete his homework in a quiet environment, focusing on working slowly and methodically.

After determining Collin's homework time, the occupational therapy practitioner set up a schedule of 15 minutes of work followed by a 3-minute break.

Because his usual homework time was 60 minutes, the practitioner broke it into 4 work periods. Collin was encouraged to be deliberate and focused during these 15-minute periods. Soon Collin was doing his homework more efficiently and was consistently finishing it in 45 minutes. His parents reported that homework time was less stressful and that there were no longer fights because he was more willing to do his work. His grades began to improve considerably. As Collin's grades began to improve, his self-efficacy improved which, in turn, helped him to choose to do his homework (volition) and increased his occupational competence.

Using MOHO as a guide to clinical reasoning, the occupational therapy practitioner chose intervention strategies that were designed to support Collin in understanding how he was using his time and provided strategies that offered clear data so that Collin could measure and recognize his own progress. This helped motivate him and supported positive changes in his behavior. MOHO does not specifically direct the occupational therapy practitioner to intervention strategies. This distinguishes it from many of the frames of reference discussed earlier in this text. MOHO assumes that the occupational therapy practitioner can effectively draw from a variety of strategies when the desired clinical outcome, in this case improved motivation and self-efficacy, is clear.

EXHIBIT 8.1.	Collin's Occupational Profile	
Client	**Reason the client is seeking service and concerns related to engagement in occupations**	Referred to occupational therapy because of behavioral problems at school and at home. Collin is failing in school because he does not complete or turn in his homework. *Impact on occupation:* Collin's parents value school-based achievement. Although Collin wants to please his parents, he feels that he is incapable of getting good grades, so he has given up trying.
	Occupations in which the client is successful	Collin has a group of friends who hang out together.
	Personal interests and values	Collin loves dirt bikes and trail bicycle racing. Collin also enjoys videogames.
	Occupational history (i.e., life experiences)	Collin has a diagnosis of ADHD and has been on medication for several years. His parents report that the medication helps him control his impulsiveness and improves his focus, but homework time is fraught with arguments.
	Performance patterns (routines, roles, habits, & rituals)	When he was interviewed by the occupational therapist, Collin stated that he wants to be a good student, but on the basis of past failures, he does not think he has the ability. He feels that even if he does his homework, it will "probably be wrong anyway." He indicated that he does not like the fighting over homework at home, but he gets frustrated because it takes too long and he has to keep redoing it until it is acceptable to his parents. In short, when it comes to doing his homework, Collin has given up. Collin often forgets to bring work home and sometimes forgets to turn it in when it has been completed.

(Continued)

CASE EXAMPLE 8.1. COLLIN: MOHO APPLICATION *(Cont.)*

EXHIBIT 8.1.	Collin's Occupational Profile *(Cont.)*		
Environment		**Supports to occupational engagement**	**Barriers to occupational engagement**
	Physical (e.g., buildings, furniture, pets)	Collin easily accesses his physical environment.	
	Social (e.g., spouse, friends, caregivers)	Collin has a group of close friends.	Collin's difficulty with school performance leads to restriction in his social time.
Context	**Cultural** (e.g., customs, beliefs)	No issues related to culture, customs, or beliefs were identified in during assessment.	
	Personal (e.g., age, gender, SES, education)	10 year old male.	
	Temporal (e.g., stage of life, time, year)	Middle childhood.	
	Virtual (e.g., chat, email, remote monitoring)	Collin is able to effectively use his smartphone, tablet, and computer to access virtual contexts.	
Client goals	**Client's priorities and desired targeted outcomes**	Collin and his parents want homework to be less stressful and more successful. They are hoping that the OT can help Collin become more organized.	

ANALYSIS OF PARTICIPATION

Basic ADLs

Eating/oral motor	Collin has no difficulty in this area.
Grooming	Collin has no difficulty in this area.
Bathing/transfer	Collin has no difficulty in this area.
Dressing upper body	Collin has no difficulty in this area.
Dressing lower body	Collin has no difficulty in this area.
Toileting	Collin has no difficulty in this area.
Problem-solving/memory	Collin seems to be having a lot of difficulty remembering to do (and turn in) his homework. He finds it very difficult and time consuming. He has difficulty organizing other routine tasks such as assigned housework.
Comments:	Collin's behavior seems to be based on past choices and experiences. In other words, his difficulties are based in volition.

IADLs

Community mobility	N/A
Health management/prevention	N/A
Home management	Collin has limited home management responsibilities, but he does not initiate or persist at chores in the home.
Financial management	N/A

(Continued)

CASE EXAMPLE 8.1. COLLIN: MOHO APPLICATION *(Cont.)*

EXHIBIT 8.1.	**Collin's Occupational Profile** *(Cont.)*
Leisure/play	Collin enjoys all sports and is very active. He does not have a high level of achievement in any single sport.
Safety	Collin has poor safety awareness as a result of his impulsiveness.
Comments:	Collin relies on his parents for many IADLs. He is not involved in child care or the care of pets.
Motor and Praxis Skills	
Sitting—static/dynamic	Collin has no difficulty in this area.
Standing—static/dynamic	Collin has no difficulty in this area.
Joint stability and skeletal mobility	Collin has no difficulty in this area.
Place can on shelf	Collin has no difficulty in this area.
Retrieve item from floor	Collin has no difficulty in this area.
Screw lid on jar	Collin has no difficulty in this area.
Comb back of head	Collin has no difficulty in this area.
Writing	Collin has no difficulty in this area.
Lift grocery bag	Collin has no difficulty in this area.
Coordination	Collin has no difficulty in this area.
Manipulation	Collin has no difficulty in this area.
Comments:	None.
Process Skills	
Energy for task	Collin has no difficulty in this area.
Knowledge/organization of task	Collin is very disorganized with respect to his schoolwork. When playing sports, he is much more focused; he is able to follow the directions of his coaches and is considered a good team player.
Adaptation/praxis	Collin has no difficulty in this area.
Comments:	The organizational differences among academics, housework, and sports suggest that Collin's difficulties are related to volition.
Behavioral and Cognitive Skills	
Communication and following social conventions	Collin does not seem to care whether he gets poor grades or disappoints his parents, although he says that both of these things bother him very much.
Cognitive and emotional regulation skills	Collin demonstrates poor self-regulation during quiet occupations because of his ADHD.
Level of arousal/attention	Collin's attention is moderately to severely impaired.
Orientation	Collin is alert and oriented to person, place, time, and event.
Energy and drive	Collin stated that he would like to change the way things are but does not think he has the ability to do any better.
Memory and understanding	Collin does not have a strategy to help him remember his assignments.
Higher level cognition	Educational testing has revealed that Collin is of average to slightly above average in intelligence.

(Continued)

CASE EXAMPLE 8.1. COLLIN: MOHO APPLICATION *(Cont.)*

EXHIBIT 8.1.	Collin's Occupational Profile *(Cont.)*
	Sensory–Perceptual Skills
Sensory	Collin has no difficulty in this area.
Self-perception	Collin has poor self-awareness and very low self-efficacy. He uses an avoidance strategy when it comes to homework, which causes more failure and reduces his self-efficacy even more.
Pain	Collin has no difficulty in this area.
Skin integrity	Collin has no difficulty in this area.
Comments:	The OT theorizes that Collin's self-efficacy will begin to increase as he becomes more successful with his organizational skills. This increase in self-efficacy with enhance his volition, leading to his choosing to do his homework well.

Note. Occupational profile template from American Occupational Therapy Association (2017). Analysis of participation format adapted from Skubik-Peplaski, Paris, Boyle, & Culpert (2009). ADHD = attention deficit hyperactivity disorder; ADLs = activities of daily living; IADLs = instrumental activities of daily living; N/A = not applicable; OT = occupational therapist; SES = socioeconomic status.

and behavioral psychology (Cole & Tufano, 2008). In this approach, the client's view of the problem is of primary concern during intervention. This model also includes extensive consideration of adaptation as a process of using resources to master challenges of daily living. The authors of this model note that "for a given situation, the applicability of importance of the person and environmental factors will vary" (Christiansen, Baum, & Bass, 2014, p. 5).

Narrative

The PEOP *personal narrative* is the personal story from the client's point of view. The focus of the narrative is the client's perceptions of his or her problems and their meaning within the broader context of the client's life. Other aspects of the narrative are the exploration of client choices, responsibilities, attitudes, motivations, needs, and goals. In the PEOP Model, the consideration goes beyond the personal. The model may include organizational or population influences as an aspect of the environmental influences affecting an individual client. It is also possible with this model for the focus of analysis and intervention to be organization- or population-level interactions.

The *organizational narrative* is the story presented in the mission and history of the organization, together with the organization's focus and priorities. This narrative tells the organizational story and incorporates influences of key stakeholders and the perceived needs and goals of the organization. The final narrative included in the PEOP Model is the population narrative.

The *population narrative* describes the perceived impacts of environments and behaviors within the population. Features of the population narrative include

population demographics, disparities, and epidemiology, as well as perceived needs and goals. The gathering and analysis of these narratives is the beginning of the PEOP occupational therapy process. This stage in the process is followed by assessment to identify specific constraints or barriers to achieving the identified goals and specific capabilities or enablers to support achievement of goals. The next stage in the process is targeted intervention, and the final stage includes the outcomes, which may be in the areas of performance, participation, and well-being. Figure 8.1 characterizes the PEOP Model. Case Example 8.2 shows use of the PEOP Model in intervention with Maria.

Although both the PEOP Model and MOHO approaches focus on occupation, using the MOHO approach allowed the occupational therapy practitioner to find support for clinical reasoning and problem-solve the client's needs. The focus was on using intervention strategies to support volition. The PEOP Model differs from MOHO in that it led the occupational therapy practitioner to consider Maria's perceptions and values and to build strategies to specifically change her self-appraisal in terms of her role performance. In Collin's and Maria's cases, the end result was improved self-efficacy and improved role performance, although the path to these goals was slightly different, reflecting the different frames of reference guiding clinical reasoning.

State of Science and Evidence-Based Considerations

The narrative assessment used in Maria's case is also used in the following discussion of Boyle (2014). In this article, the use of narrative in assessment; the consideration

FIGURE 8.1. PEOP Model.

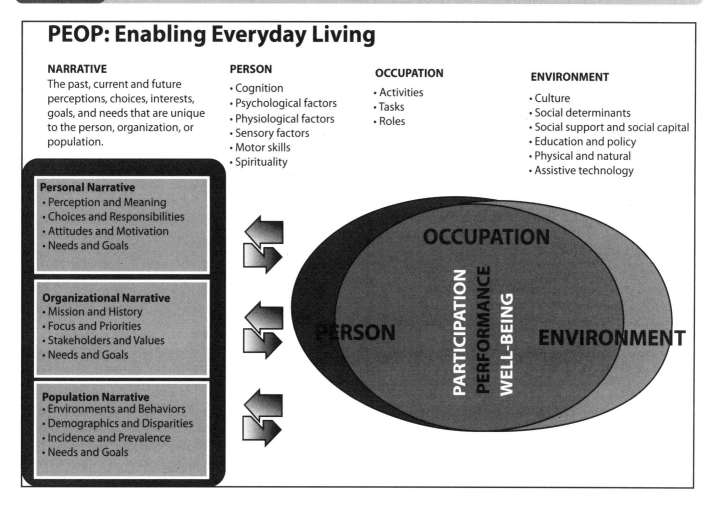

PEOP: Enabling Everyday Living

NARRATIVE
The past, current and future perceptions, choices, interests, goals, and needs that are unique to the person, organization, or population.

PERSON
- Cognition
- Psychological factors
- Physiological factors
- Sensory factors
- Motor skills
- Spirituality

OCCUPATION
- Activities
- Tasks
- Roles

ENVIRONMENT
- Culture
- Social determinants
- Social support and social capital
- Education and policy
- Physical and natural
- Assistive technology

Personal Narrative
- Perception and Meaning
- Choices and Responsibilities
- Attitudes and Motivation
- Needs and Goals

Organizational Narrative
- Mission and History
- Focus and Priorities
- Stakeholders and Values
- Needs and Goals

Population Narrative
- Environments and Behaviors
- Demographics and Disparities
- Incidence and Prevalence
- Needs and Goals

OCCUPATION

PERSON

PARTICIPATION
PERFORMANCE
WELL-BEING

ENVIRONMENT

Source. From "Theory, Models, Frameworks, and Classifications," by C. M. Baum, J. D. Bass, & C. H. Christiansen, p. 39. In C. H. Christiansen, C. M. Baum, and J. D. Bass (Eds.), *Occupational Therapy: Performance, Participation, and Well-Being* (4th ed.), 2014, Thorofare, NJ: Slack. Copyright © 2014 by Slack. Reprinted with permission.

CASE EXAMPLE 8.2. MARIA: USING THE PEOP MODEL

Maria, age 32, has been hospitalized for mental health problems and is facing challenges to the occupational role performance as she tries to return to living on her own. Maria's occupational profile is shown in Exhibit 8.2.

Maria's occupational therapy practitioner decided to use the PEOP Model to help Maria begin to achieve some success in an effort to change her personal narrative. Maria and her occupational therapy practitioner decided to concentrate on daily meal preparation as a starting point in her treatment because it is an important aspect of her maternal role. Because Maria is easily overwhelmed and has great difficulty making choices, her occupational therapy practitioner suggested they change Maria's meal planning occupation by

eliminating choices. Instead of deciding what to make on a daily basis, Maria chose specific meals for specific days, creating a weekly menu. For example, she chose Monday as spaghetti day, Tuesday as taco day, and so on for every day of the week. This eliminated the necessity of choosing a meal every day.

To help her with grocery shopping, Maria and her occupational therapy practitioner used the weekly menu to prepare a grocery list so that Maria did not have to rely on her memory, which offers a compensatory strategy to support the performance aspect of the model. They further refined the list by grouping the items on the basis of their location in the store so that Maria could shop more efficiently, which addressed

(Continued)

CASE EXAMPLE 8.2. MARIA: USING THE PEOP MODEL *(Cont.)*

EXHIBIT 8.2.	Maria's Occupational Profile	
Client	**Reason the client is seeking service and concerns related to engagement in occupations**	Referred to occupational therapy for impairments in basic organizational skills, homemaking skills, and behavioral issues after an inpatient psychiatric hospital stay for major depression with psychotic features. *Impact on occupation:* Maria is a divorced mother of 2 children, David, age 10 years, and Elena, age 7 years. She does not currently work and relies on child support and disability income.
	Occupations in which the client is successful	Maria is able to get her children fed, dressed, and to school regularly.
	Personal interests and values	Maria values her role as mother. She wants to be a good mother, but she feels that she is failing in this role. Maria likes to watch daytime TV.
	Occupational history (i.e., life experiences)	Maria has a long history of major depressive disorder, recurring. She divorced her ex-husband because he was physically abusive toward her. She has been trying to raise her children by herself, but she has been having great difficulty as a result of bouts of depression, very low self-esteem, and poor coping and organizational skills.
	Performance patterns (routines, roles, habits, & rituals)	Maria relies on her elderly parents when there are problems, which increases her self-perception of not being a good mom.

Environment		*Supports to occupational engagement*	*Barriers to occupational engagement*
	Physical (e.g., buildings, furniture, pets)	Maria easily accesses her physical environment.	
	Social (e.g., spouse, friends, caregivers)		Maria feels very isolated as a single parent.
Context	**Cultural** (e.g., customs, beliefs)	Maria is of Puerto Rican heritage.	
	Personal (e.g., age, gender, SES, education)	32-year-old female.	
	Temporal (e.g., stage of life, time, year)	Middle adulthood.	
	Virtual (e.g., chat, email, remote monitoring)	Maria uses her cell phone but does not use other virtual contexts.	
Client goals	**Client's priorities and desired targeted outcomes**	Maria claims her home is a mess, and she is only able to feed her children takeout fast food because she is too overwhelmed by the grocery store.	

ANALYSIS OF PARTICIPATION	
Basic ADLs	
Eating/oral–motor	Maria has no difficulty in this area.
Grooming	Maria has no difficulty in this area.
Bathing/transfer	Maria has no difficulty in this area.
Dressing upper body	Maria has no difficulty in this area.
Dressing lower body	Maria has no difficulty in this area.

(Continued)

CASE EXAMPLE 8.2. MARIA: USING THE PEOP MODEL *(Cont.)*

EXHIBIT 8.2. **Maria's Occupational Profile** *(Cont.)*

Toileting	Maria has no difficulty in this area.
Problem-solving/memory	Maria has significant difficulty with problem solving. She becomes very anxious and is easily overwhelmed. She tends to give up when faced with even simple problems.
Comments:	Maria arrived at the clinic dressed neatly and well groomed. She is able to fix her children cereal for breakfast and then takes them to school. She watches TV until it is time to pick them up.
	IADLs
Community mobility	Maria drives and owns a car. She has no difficulty in this area.
Health management/prevention	Maria tends to ignore health problems. Although she recognizes her depression symptoms, she will not contact her health care provider. Her son called Maria's parents during the last episode to tell them that she was hearing voices and the children were afraid, which prompted her parents to have her admitted to a psychiatric hospital.
Home management	Maria is unable to accomplish most household management tasks. She is so far behind in routine cleaning and maintenance that even beginning to work on these things causes an increase in her anxiety, leading to an avoidance strategy.
Financial management	Maria has sufficient financial resources, but she is often behind in her bills because she forgets to pay them.
Leisure/play	Maria's only leisure activities are watching television and occasionally playing games with her children.
Safety	Maria demonstrates good safety awareness.
Comments:	Maria relies on her elderly parents when there are problems, which increases her self-perception of not being a good mom.
	Motor and Praxis Skills
Sitting—static/dynamic	Maria has no difficulty in this area.
Standing—static/dynamic	Maria has no difficulty in this area.
Joint stability and skeletal mobility	Maria has no difficulty in this area.
Place can on shelf	Maria has no difficulty in this area.
Retrieve item from floor	Maria has no difficulty in this area.
Screw lid on jar	Maria has no difficulty in this area.
Comb back of head	Maria has no difficulty in this area.
Writing	Maria has no difficulty in this area.
Lift grocery bag	Maria has no difficulty in this area.
Coordination	Maria has no difficulty in this area.
Manipulation	Maria has no difficulty in this area.
Comments:	None.
	Process Skills
Energy for task	Maria has no difficulty in this area.
Knowledge/organization of task	Maria has no difficulty in this area.
Adaptation/praxis	Maria has no difficulty in this area.

(Continued)

CASE EXAMPLE 8.2. MARIA: USING THE PEOP MODEL (Cont.)

EXHIBIT 8.2.   Maria's Occupational Profile (Cont.)

Comments:	Although Maria is able to perform most if not all tasks, she lacks volition and motivation because of her excessive fear of failure.
Behavioral and Cognitive Skills	
Communication and following social conventions	Maria has no difficulty in this area.
Cognitive and emotional regulation skills	Maria demonstrates very poor coping skills. Her mental-processing speed is extremely slow.
Level of arousal/attention	Maria's attention is moderately to severely impaired.
Orientation	Maria is alert and oriented to person, place, time, and event.
Energy and drive	Maria is motivated to change her behavior, but she does not know where to begin.
Memory and understanding	Maria is very forgetful and uses no compensatory strategies to assist her memory.
Higher level cognition	Maria's higher level executive function was hard to assess because of her tendency to give up easily when tested.
Sensory–Perceptual Skills	
Sensory	Maria has no difficulty in this area.
Self-perception	Maria has poor self-awareness and very low self-efficacy. She uses an avoidance strategy with most tasks to avoid failing, although she causes herself more problems in the process.
Pain	Maria has no difficulty in this area.
Skin integrity	Maria has no difficulty in this area.
Comments:	Maria demonstrates a high degree of dysfunction in her daily life. She reports that she has been trying every day to fix a nourishing meal for her children. Her typical afternoon consists of picking her children up from school and then going to the grocery store to purchase food to cook for dinner. At the store, she has difficulty deciding what type of meal to make and wanders the aisles until she becomes frustrated and overwhelmed. At this point, she leaves the store and takes her children to a local fast-food restaurant for takeout. She reports that feeding her children fast food every day makes her feel like a bad mother and is just another way in which she fails.

Note. Occupational profile template from American Occupational Therapy Association (2017). Analysis of participation format adapted from Skubik-Peplaski, Paris, Boyle, & Culpert (2009). ADLs = activities of daily living; IADLs = instrumental activities of daily living; SES = socioeconomic status.

the environmental aspect. Maria was instructed to buy only those items that appeared on the list. This approach refined the grocery shopping task to help her avoid becoming anxious and overwhelmed and reduced the number of shopping trips to 1 per week.

This approach helped Maria feel more confident and that she is living up to her role expectations. In addition, because shopping and meal planning were simplified,

she had more time to spend with her children and help them with their homework, which served to increase her task performance and her expanded role as parent. Although Maria and her therapist continued to work on other areas of dysfunction, because preparing meals for her children was an essential part of Maria's personal narrative, use of the PEOP Model was clearly a good starting point for Maria's rehabilitation.

of broad physical, social, and political influences; and the conclusion that

an occupational therapist's ability to assess the interaction between a person's or organization's skills, the environment in which that person or organization is

functioning, and the desired occupational outcomes of that person or organization, enables a unique and valuable contribution as a volunteer. (p. 6)

clearly mirrors the factors we have described in the PEOP Model. Boyle did not cite the PEOP Model as an influence in her reasoning, but in her description of the Sudanese refugee community in Toowoomba, Queensland, Australia, and her experience as a volunteer in Bhutan, she expressed a rich narrative that includes personal, organizational, and population perspectives and resulted in an identification of needs and goals. Boyle then identified specific constraints and barriers to achieving the identified goals and specific capabilities and enablers to support goal achievement. Boyle only briefly mentioned targeted intervention, but she did discuss positive outcomes in the areas of performance, participation, and well-being.

The Boyle (2014) article was selected for review because, even though it does not explicitly cite the PEOP Model, it is constructed and presented in a manner highly consistent with this model. In addition, it provides a perspective that focuses on volunteerism and social justice rather than specific clinical practice. Because the PEOP Model explicitly considers clients at the individual, organizational, and population levels, this article shows that the PEOP Model has the potential to be applied at other levels.

Although the literature review by Lee (2010) cited earlier included 433 peer-reviewed journal articles focused on MOHO, it included only 27 related to the PEOP Model. One difference between these models is that since its inception, assessment tools have been developed and published for clinical use with MOHO that support occupation-based clinical practice. These assessments have been developed over time, have authors from diverse areas of practice and, in many cases, are reviewed and revised as aspects of the model are expanded based on research. The value of these assessment tools is immense. Not only have they guided the development of the occupational profile to focus on occupation, they are effective tools to use in developing research on the model. One of the reasons for the wider research presence of MOHO is the high utility of MOHO-based assessment tools for measuring the constructs of occupation in a scientific manner.

COMPARISION OF MODELS AND FRAMES OF REFERENCE

Both of the occupation-focused models introduced in this chapter are client centered, consider the environment as a significant influence on occupation, and emphasize the need to identify valued outcomes through a collaborative process between the occupational therapy practitioner and the client. The environment, which consists of physical, cultural, and social components, is where occupational performance takes place, but the PEOP model has a greater focus on environment.

Both MOHO and the PEOP Model direct the occupational therapy practitioner to look at the fit between the individual client and the environment. The PEOP Model charges the occupational therapy practitioner to "not only address the immediate social and physical context of the individual but also actively incorporate the interplay of concurrent institutional and cultural factors" (Wong & Fisher, 2015, p. 304). With a significantly different focus than MOHO, the PEOP Model challenges the practitioner to specifically assess the environment in terms of whether it enables performance or acts as a barrier to performance (Christiansen et al., 2014).

The PEOP Model focuses more on the therapeutic process between the therapist and client than MOHO, providing a strong clinical reasoning tool without the emphasis on process. A final distinction between MOHO and the PEOP Model is that the PEOP Model can be applied with consideration of group and institutional needs and can be used as a tool to support clinical reasoning with an individual client. Table 8.1 reflects the distinctions between these occupation-focused models.

CMOP–E

In this chapter, we chose to present the topic of occupation-focused models using 2 models as examples. They were chosen because they are widely used, are well documented, and had clear differences in their approaches to the clinical reasoning process.

Another occupation-focused model, and one of the most globally used, is **CMOP–E** (Canadian Association of Occupational Therapists [CAOT], 2002). The CMOP–E is the end result of a series of 5 consensus guidelines developed by CAOT (Wong & Fisher, 2015).

TABLE 8.1.	**Distinctions Between MOHO and PEOP**		
MODEL	**FOCUS**	**PERFORMANCE OUTCOMES**	**PARTICIPATION OUTCOMES**
MOHO	Volition and habituation	Occupational competence and occupational identity	Occupational adaptation
PEOP	Personal narrative Organizational narrative Population narrative	Occupational performance	Occupational participation

Source. From "Comparing and Using Occupation-Focused Models," by S. R. Wong and G. Fisher, 2015, *Occupational Therapy in Health Care, 29,* p. 315. Copyright © 2015 by Haworth Press. Adapted with permission.
Note. MOHO = Model of Human Occupation; PEOP = Person–Environment–Occupation–Performance Model.

Like MOHO and the PEOP Model, the CMOP–E has evolved with the growth of knowledge and science for more than 25 years, and advances in each model inform those in the others. From its introduction in 1991, CMOP–E has incorporated the core concepts of the environment (Law, 1991), of enablement (Polatajko, 1992), and of social justice (Townsend, 1993). Like the PEOP Model, the CMOP–E includes an emphasis on the therapeutic process. A focus on engagement was incorporated into the original Canadian Model of Occupational Performance, resulting in the addition of "and Engagement" to its name (Townsend & Polatajko, 2007). Although it shares many commonalities with the other 2 models presented in this chapter, the CMOP–E emphasizes occupational engagement and experience (Townsend & Polatajko, 2007; Turpin & Iwama, 2011).

Like MOHO, CMOP–E is associated with a model-informed assessment tool, the Canadian Occupational Performance Measure (COPM; Law et al., 2014). Most of the research relevant to CMOP–E is focused on the COPM rather than on the model as a whole. This underscores the importance of occupation-focused models in guiding occupational therapy practice. The COPM is one of the mostly widely used and widely respected assessment tools in occupational therapy. It has been adopted by occupational therapy practitioners but also by multidisciplinary health care teams, widely extending the application of client-centered and occupation-based assessment.

INNOVATIONS IN OCCUPATION-BASED CLINICAL REASONING

As the field of occupational science grows, we can expect to see new and innovative occupationally focused approaches. An example of this is Iwama's (2006) Kawa Model. The 3 occupation-focused models presented so far in this chapter emerged from North America. Although these models have been widely adopted globally, there has been some concern that they are grounded in Western philosophy, which is more reductionistic and integrates aspects such as a Protestant work ethic that are not applicable to non-Western populations. The **Kawa Model** is described as broad in its application as a model, a frame of reference, an assessment tool, and a modality for occupation-based intervention (Kawamodel.com, 2016).

The Kawa Model is unique in that it is decribed in metaphor rather than as a process schematic, such as those for MOHO and the PEOP Model. This approach has drawn much interest from occupational therapy practitioners worldwide and has led to the growing use of metaphor in the occupational therapy process. Support for and the research foundation of this newer occupation-focused model has been growing in recent years. Unlike the other models presented, the Kawa Model allows for nonlinear thinking.

Leadley (2015) described this model's use in forensic occupational therapy practice as a means of supporting the goal of culturally sensitive practice. In many instances, occupational therapy practitioners work with people who are disenfranchised or alienated from the social mainstream. These people may have difficulty relating to science-driven clinical processes and may not fully express their own perspectives in the evaluation and goal identification processes in occupational therapy. In the Leadley case report, the narrative-based, open-ended nature of the Kawa Model's tools supported a recovery focus rather than an illness focus.

There is a lot of focus in occupational therapy on keeping practice "authentic" and supporting the use of occupation-based practice. An essential part of occupational therapy practice is being reflective and understanding humans as occupational beings throughout the occupational therapy process, from evaluation through outcomes. Occupation-based practice is not an activity choice; it is a mindset. As suggested in Practice Wisdom 8.1, occupation-based practice is something practitioners must work for, something that requires a deliberate change in thinking and an openness to new ideas and new approaches. Building a new approach requires more than a good idea; it requires deliberate, committed action that includes research and data collection.

Earlier in the text, the concept of the *half-life of knowledge* was introduced. Occupational science is in its infancy as far as sciences go, and readers can expect to see many revisions of existing occupation-based practice models and many new models as knowledge specific to occupation grows. Good clinical reasoning includes the ability to critically consider emerging ideas and practices. It is natural to be drawn to new things and new practices. New ideas seldom have strong supporting evidence, so occupational therapy practitioners must be able to consider the consistency of emergent information or practice with existing, more tested practices to determine whether the innovation is based on sound foundational knowledge. With solid client-specific data, practitioners can effectively and ethically consider intervention approaches that are less scientifically grounded than motor learning theory. Data that reflect the goals and context of the client should be at the core of occupational therapy clinical reasoning and are central to occupation-based practice.

PRACTICE WISDOM 8.1.   Embracing Change

"We are addicted to our thoughts. We cannot change anything if we cannot change our thinking." —*Santosh Kalwar (2010)*

SUMMARY

Using occupation-focused models serves as a heuristic shortcut to holistic occupation-based diagnostic hypothesis generation. These models support a holistic view of the client while supporting the attention to reductionistic features of disease, disability, and injury. Although occupational therapy practitioners can be very effective and occupation based while using any frame of reference, occupation-focused models serve as heuristic tools to support and build the holistic focus that is considered best practice in occupational therapy.

A systematic and reflective occupational therapy process, as described in all of the occupation-focused models, results in collaborative occupation-based functional goals. Occupational therapy intervention strategies are designed to move the client toward achievement of these goals, although neither approach prescribes specific intervention approaches. It is common for occupational therapy practitioners to see the use of occupation-based models as an "either–or" phenomenon. In this conceptualization, if one is not using a specific occupation-focused model to guide clinical reasoning, one's occupational therapy goals and outcomes will not be occupation based. This is a hasty generalization—a conclusion made without considering all of the variables.

Rather, practitioners can use an occupation-focused model and still elect to use a biomechanical frame of reference to treat a hand injury. The actual intervention strategies selected should be evidence informed and support the client's outcome goals. Exercise is a valued occupation for many people. A client with a tendon injury who wants to play the piano again may prefer a set of home exercises for rebuilding strength to a more occupationally centered intervention involving the piano. The client may be disheartened by repetitive plinking at the piano as movement patterns are strengthened. The need for repetition and practice will be the same regardless of the intervention selected, so this client may prefer a traditional home exercise program to a more occupationally embedded home program.

Clients are the essential factor in what makes the process and the outcomes occupationally grounded. As suggested by Wong and Fisher (2015), the use of occupation-focused models ensures that the client is considered holistically. Within this occupation-based lens, the selection of intervention approaches is guided by the client and by scientific evidence. The pianist described earlier may have a traditional home exercise program but should also have goals and outcome measures tied to returning to the desired occupation of musician. The outcome measure should be identified collaboratively with the client; the measure should not be strength or range of motion but might instead be the ability to play the piano at a level acceptable to the client.

All of the occupation-focused models introduced in this chapter have distinctive aspects. The choice of which one to use should be based on the client and the client's needs. These models have more consistency among them than differences. This makes it possible for the reflective occupational therapy practitioner to combine aspects of each occupation-based model to address the client's holistic needs. Wong and Fisher (2015) delineated specific characteristics of the MOHO, PEOP Model, and CMOP–E for their readers, and their article is a good source for readers wanting to delve more deeply into the comparisons among and use of these models. These authors argue that

> it is imperative that therapists do not just "go with the flow" or claim "eclectic" use of models but attempt to critically analyze available models in terms of their concepts, research evidence and practical use. It may be common to find that one model may not suffice all the time and occupation-focused models can be used to supplement each other. (p. 309)

It may seem easier to use a focused frame of reference in medical environments that are inherently impairment focused. Indeed, expert occupational therapy practitioners may articulate these focused frames of reference when asked to describe their approaches. Holistic, occupationally grounded reasoning is an essential feature of the occupational therapy process, regardless of the frame of reference used. For expert clinicians, the occupational focus becomes a background that is assumed but not always articulated. Focused frames of reference can be very effective tools, but in the absence of a structured assessment of occupation throughout the process, the result may be reductionistic practice that is indistinguishable from the services provided by practitioners in other disciplines. Wong and Fisher (2015) remarked,

> A therapist who begins with an occupation-focused model as the organizing model of practice will have gathered essential information about occupational roles and priorities up front, and will be reminded to ensure that therapy sessions reflect client-centered goals and interests. Blending the impairment-focused frame of reference with models that address issues of learning and motivation in the context of occupation is recommended. (p. 310)

LEARNING ACTIVITIES

1. As a learning tool, quiz yourself on the key terms and concepts listed at the beginning of this chapter. These terms are foundational to occupational therapy practice and are widely used throughout occupational therapy literature.
2. Choose an occupation-focused practice model (other than MOHO, PEOP or CMOP–E), and describe it in terms of focus, performance outcomes, and

participation outcomes. Discover what is unique to the model you choose, and write a short paragraph to present it.

3. Read the Wong and Fisher (2015) article. These authors offer a methodology to compare occupation-focused models. In a short paper, summarize the findings presented in this article.

4. Interview an occupational therapy practitioner about what models he or she uses in practice. Delve into the respondent's answers to ascertain whether he or she uses occupationally based clinical reasoning but does not identify a model, whether he or she identifies strongly with a specific frame of reference, and whether he or she expressed a positive or a negative attitude toward the concepts of occupation-based practice.

5. One distinction between MOHO and the PEOP Model is that MOHO emphasizes the individual and the PEOP Model can be applied to both individual people and groups. Another occupation-focused model, the Kawa Model, also addresses groups. Read Lape and Scaife (2017), and write a short statement regarding whether you think the PEOP Model could be used to support a similar study.

6. Read the case of Surya presented in Chapter 3. Many aspects of Surya's case would benefit from a more occupation-based clinical reasoning focus. Choose an occupation-based model to use with this case and, applying this model, identify specific occupation-based intervention goals for Surya.

REFERENCES

American Occupational Therapy Association. (2014). Occupational therapy practice framework: Domain and process (3rd ed.). *American Journal of Occupational Therapy, 68*(Suppl.), S1–S48. https://doi.org/10.5014/ajot.2014.682006

American Occupational Therapy Association. (2017). AOTA occupational profile template. *American Journal of Occupational Therapy, 71*(Suppl. 2), 7112420030. https://doi.org/10.5014/ajot716S12

Baum, C. M., Bass, J. D., & Christiansen, C. H. (2014). Theory, models, frameworks, and classifications. In C. H. Christiansen, C. M. Baum, & J. D. Bass (Eds.), *Occupational therapy: Performance, participation, and well-being* (4th ed.). Thorofare, NJ: Slack.

Boyle, M. (2014). Occupational performance and self-determination: The role of the occupational therapist as volunteer in two mountain communities. *Australian Occupational Therapy Journal, 61*, 6–12. https://doi.org/10.1111/1440-1630.12104

Canadian Association of Occupational Therapists. (2002). *Enabling occupation: An occupational therapy perspective* (2nd ed.). Ottawa, Ontario: CAOT Publications.

Christiansen, C., & Baum, C. (1991). *Occupational therapy: Overcoming human performance deficits.* Thorofare, NJ: Slack.

Christiansen, C., Baum, C., & Bass, J. (Eds.). (2014). *Occupational therapy: Performance, participation, and well-being* (4th ed.). Thorofare, NJ: Slack.

Cole, M., & Tufano, R. (2008). *Applied theories in occupational therapy: A practical approach.* Thorofare, NJ: Slack.

Fisher, A. G. (2013). Occupation-centered, occupation-based, occupation-focused: Same, same or different? *Scandinavian Journal of Occupational Therapy, 20*, 162–173. https://doi.org/10.3109/11038128.2012.754492

Fisher, A. G., & Griswold, L. A. (2014). Performance skills: Implementing performance analyses to evaluate quality of occupational performance. In B. A. Boyt Schell, G. Gillen, & M. Scaffa (Eds.), *Willard and Spackman's occupational therapy* (12th ed., pp. 249–264). Philadelphia: Lippincott Williams & Wilkins.

Gindi, S., Galili, G., Volovic-Shushan, S., & Adir-Pavis, S. (2016). Integrating occupational therapy in treating combat stress reaction within a military unit: An intervention model. *Work, 55*, 737–745. https://doi.org/10.3233/WOR-162453

Iwama, M. K. (2006). *The Kawa model: Culturally relevant occupational therapy.* Edinburgh: Churchill Livingstone/Elsevier.

Kalwar, S. (2010). *Quote me everyday.* Morrisville, NC: LuLu Press. Retrieved from https://www.goodreads.com/quotes/tag/life-lessons

Kawamodel.com. (2016). *About.* Retrieved from http://www.kawamodel.com/v1/index.php/about/

Kielhofner, G. (2008). *Model of Human Occupation: Theory and application* (4th ed.). Baltimore: Lippincott Williams & Wilkins.

Kielhofner, G., & Burke, J. (1980). A Model of Human Occupation, Part 1. Conceptual framework and content. *American Journal of Occupational Therapy, 34*, 572–581. https://doi.org/10.5014/ajot.34.9.572

Lape, J., & Scaife, B. (2017). Use of the Kawa Model for team-building with rehabilitative professionals: An exploratory study. *Internet Journal of Allied Health Sciences and Practice, 15*(1), Article 10. Retrieved from http://nsuworks.nova.edu/ijahsp/vol15/iss1/10/

Law, M. (1991). 1991 Muriel Driver Lecture—The environment: A focus for occupational therapy. *Canadian Journal of Occupational Therapy, 58*, 171–179. https://doi.org/10.1177/000841749105800404

Law, M., Baptiste, S., Carswell, A., McColl, M. A., Polatajko, H., & Pollock, N. (2014). *Canadian Occupational Performance Measure* (5th ed.). Ottawa, ON: CAOT Publications.

Leadley, S. (2015). The Kawa Model: Informing the development of a culturally sensitive, occupational therapy assessment tool in Aotearoa/New Zealand. *New Zealand Journal of Occupational Therapy, 62*(2), 48–54.

Lee, J. (2010). Achieving best practice: A review of evidence linked to occupation-focused practice models. *Occupational Therapy in Health Care, 24*, 206–221. https://doi.org/10.3109/07380577.2010.483270

Lee, S. W., Kielhofner, G., Morley, M., Heasman, D., Garnham, M., Willis, S., . . . Taylor, R. R. (2012). Impact of using the Model of Human Occupation: A survey of occupational therapy mental health practitioners' perceptions. *Scandinavian Journal of Occupational Therapy, 19*, 450–456. https://doi.org/10.3109/11038128.2011.645553

Polatajko, H. J. (1992). Muriel Driver Lecture 1992—Naming and framing occupational therapy: A lecture dedicated to the life of Nancy B. *Canadian Journal of Occupational Therapy, 59,* 189–200. https://doi.org/10.1177/000841749205900403

Prodinger, B., Shaw, L., Stamm, T., & Rudman, D. L. (2014). Enacting occupation-based practice: Exploring the disjuncture between the daily lives of mothers with rheumatoid arthritis and institutional processes. *British Journal of Occupational Therapy, 77,* 491–498. https://doi.org/10.4276/0308 02214X14122630932359

Reilly, M. (1977). A response to: Defining occupational therapy: The meaning of therapy and the virtues of occupation. *American Journal of Occupational Therapy, 31,* 673–674.

Skubik-Peplaski, C., Paris, C., Boyle, D. & Culpert, A. (Eds.). (2009*). Applying the* Occupational Therapy Practice Framework: *Using the Cardinal Hill Occupational Participation*

Process in client-centered care (2nd ed.). Bethesda, MD: AOTA Press.

Townsend, E. (1993). Occupational therapy's social vision. *Canadian Journal of Occupational Therapy, 60,* 174–184. https://doi.org/10.1177/000841749306000403

Townsend, E., & Polatajko, H. (2007). *Enabling occupation II: Advancing an occupational therapy vision for health, well-being, and justice through occupation.* Ottawa, ON: CAOT Publications.

Turpin, M., & Iwama, M. (2011). *Using occupational therapy models in practice: A field guide.* Edinburgh: Elsevier.

von Bertalanffy, L. (1974). *Perspectives on general system theory.* New York: George Braziller.

Wong, S. R., & Fisher, G. (2015). Comparing and using occupation-focused models. *Occupational Therapy in Health Care, 29,* 297–315. https://doi.org/10.3109/07380577.2015 .1010130

Occupational Therapy Intervention Process

Anne Cronin, PhD, OTR/L, ATP, FAOTA, and Garth Graebe, MOT, OTR/L

9

CHAPTER HIGHLIGHTS

- Outlines occupational therapy intervention strategies to improve a situation or address a client concern through actions to create or promote positive change; to establish, restore, or maintain occupational performance; to modify task performance to increase function; or to prevent loss of occupational performance or valued occupations as described in the *Occupational Therapy Practice Framework*.
- Includes an explanation of strategic thinking and reasoning in client-centered occupational therapy interventions.
- Provides an overview of the process of theory-driven activity analysis in occupational therapy intervention.
- Explores reasoning in the intervention process, including education and training, advocacy, and group interventions.

KEY TERMS AND CONCEPTS

Activities	Intervention algorithm	Preparatory methods
Activity analysis	Intervention implementation	Preparatory tasks
Advocacy	Intervention plan	Reflective practice
Education	Intervention process	Strategic thinking
Evidence-informed practice	Intervention review	Systems perspective
Group intervention	Occupation	Training
Intelligent opportunism	Practical reasoning	

In this chapter, readers will further their understanding of occupation-based occupational therapy practice through the intervention process. The ***intervention process*** is an action process by occupational therapy practitioners to improve a situation or address a client concern as part of the occupational therapy process. The intervention process, as it is presented in the *Occupational Therapy Practice Framework: Domain and Process* (*OTPF–3*; American Occupational Therapy Association [AOTA], 2014) has 3 components:

1. Plan,
2. Implement, and
3. Review.

These components rely on reflective practice and theory-driven activity analysis. The occupational therapy process, as described in the *OTPF–3*, is illustrated in Exhibit 9.1.

It is in the intervention stage of the occupational therapy process that occupational therapy practitioners must reflectively weigh the relative value of reductionist approaches and holistic approaches within the context of each individual client. It is also in the intervention stage that organizational pressures to speed client discharge; to limit visits with clients; to consider standardized treatment protocols; and to fit interventions within a prescribed, predetermined time frame challenge occupational therapy practitioners' decision making.

Although the iterative nature of occupational therapy clinical reasoning is emphasized throughout this text, it is in the intervention that this becomes the most evident. In reviewing Exhibit 9.1, note that targeted outcomes are identified during the evaluation stage of the occupational therapy process. They reflect clinical reasoning that is informed by client assessment and lead to the following actions that will inform and guide the intervention process:

- Creating goals in collaboration with the client that address desired outcomes,
- Determining procedures to measure the outcomes of intervention, and
- Delineating a potential intervention on the basis of best practices and available evidence (AOTA, 2014).

REFLECTIVE PRACTICE

Reflective practice was first introduced in Chapter 2, "Clinical Reasoning and Occupational Therapy's Domain of Practice," and is the use of experiential knowledge that is considered critically to link theory and practice. Reflective practice involves critically considering the practical values and theories that inform the

EXHIBIT 9.1.	**Operationalizing the Occupational Therapy Intervention Process**

Evaluation		Intervention			Targeting of Outcomes
Occupational Profile	**Analysis of Occupational Performance**	**Intervention Plan**	**Intervention Implementation**	**Intervention Review**	**Outcomes**
Identify the following: • Why is the client seeking service, and what are the client's current concerns relative to engaging in activities and occupations? • In what occupations does the client feel successful, and what barriers are affecting his or her success? • What aspects of the contents or environments does the client see as supporting and as inhibiting engagement in desired occupations? • What is the client's occupational history? • What are the client's values and interests? • What are the client's daily life roles? • What are the client's patterns of engagement in occupations, and how have they changed over time? • What are the client's priorities and desired targeted outcomes related to occupational performance, prevention, participation, role competence, health and wellness, quality of life, well-being, and occupational justice?	• Synthesize information from the occupational profile to focus on specific occupations and contexts. • Observe the client's performance during activities relevant to desired occupations. • Select and use specific assessments to identify and measure contexts or environments, activity and occupational demands, client factors, and performance skills and patterns. • Select outcome measures. • Interpret assessment data to identify supports for and hindrances to performance. • Develop and refine hypotheses about the client's occupational performance strengths and limitations. • Create goals in collaboration with the client that address desired outcomes. • Determine procedures to measure the outcomes of intervention. • Delineate a potential intervention based on best practices and available evidence.	1. Develop the plan, which involves selecting • Objective and measurable occupation-focused goals and related time frames; • Occupational therapy intervention approach or approaches, such as create or promote establish or restore, maintain, modify, or prevent; and • Methods for service delivery, including who will provide the intervention, types of intervention, and service delivery models. 2. Consider potential discharge needs and plans. 3. Recommend or refer to other professionals as needed.	1. Determine and carry out occupational therapy intervention or interactions, which may include the following: • Therapeutic use of occupations and activities • Preparatory methods and tasks • Education and training • Advocacy • Group interventions 2. Monitor the clients response through ongoing evaluation and reevaluation.	1. Reevaluate the plan and implementation relative to achieving outcomes. 2. Modify the plan as needed. 3. Determine the need for continuation or discontinuation of occupational therapy services and for referral.	1. Early in the intervention process, select outcomes and measures that are • Valid, reliable, sensitive to change, and consistent with outcomes • Congruent with client goals • Based on their actual or purposed ability to predict future outcomes 2. Apply outcomes to measure progress and adjust goals and interventions. • Compare progress toward goal achievement to outcomes throughout the intervention process. • Assess outcome use and results to make decisions about the future direction of intervention.

←——— Continue to renegotiate intervention plans and targeted outcomes. ———→

←——— Ongoing interaction among evaluation, intervention, and outcomes occurs throughout the process. ———→

Source. From *Occupational Therapy Practice Framework: Domain and Process* (3rd ed.), by the American Occupational Therapy Association, *American Journal of Occupational Therapy, 68*(Suppl. 1), p. S17. Copyright © 2014 by the American Occupational Therapy Association. Used with permission.

intervention process. Reflective practice enables professional and personal development while reinforcing continuous learning and supporting best practice ideals.

The intervention process requires continual reflection before, during, and after action.

- *Reflection before action* involves thinking about the intervention strategies best suited to supporting progress toward client goals.
- *Reflection during action* involves considering the impact of what one is doing in real time during the provision of occupational therapy intervention.

- *Reflection after action* is the process of looking retrospectively at what happened and analyzing the information gathered. Reflection after action is involved in the hypothesis testing and refinement that goes on throughout occupational therapy intervention.

ACTIVITY ANALYSIS IN OCCUPATIONAL THERAPY

Activity analysis was described in Chapter 4, "Psychodynamic and Developmental Systems Frames of Reference," as an essential tool that can be used in all 3 stages of the occupational therapy intervention process. *Activity analysis* is defined in the *OTPF–3* as direct observation of the person performing a defined task and the specific analysis of "the demands of an activity or occupation to understand the specific body structures, body functions, performance skills, and performance patterns that are required and to determine the generic demands the activity or occupation makes on the client" (AOTA, 2014, p. S12).

In the evaluation stage, activity analysis can clarify client impairments and limitations in the performance of daily occupations. During the intervention process, activity analysis can also be invaluable as a tool to break down functional activities and identify steps toward the achievement of functional outcomes.

Activity analysis is often a theory-driven strategy that informs and supports the intervention process. What occupational therapy practitioners choose to document in relation to the skills and context needed for successful activity performance is informed by the paradigm through which they organize information. In occupational therapy, activity analysis should be grounded in the occupational therapy paradigm and be inherently occupation based. Occupation-based activity analysis can be focused on an individual person, a group of people, or a population. The human focus of activity analysis guides the identification of which occupation-based concepts need to be explored to obtain the necessary information. For example, communication and interaction skills may be an essential part of toileting for a 3-year-old child but may be omitted from the activity analysis of a young adult woman because toileting is a solitary activity in adulthood.

Both Thomas (2015) and Kielhofner and Forsyth (2009) described occupation-based activity analysis as a multistep process. Exhibit 9.2 presents the general process of activity analysis informed by both of these sources. Readers should note that the process largely mirrors the "Activity and Occupational Demands" table in the *OTPF–3* (AOTA, 2014, Table 7, p. S32). There is great emphasis on consistency in the structure of the activity analysis process across all current occupation-focused practice models.

Keeping the process of activity analysis based on occupation relies on an exploration of the relevance and importance of the occupation to be analyzed. Once client-centered goals have been identified during the analysis of occupational performance, the occupational

> **EXHIBIT 9.2.** **Theory-Driven Activity Analysis Process**
>
> - Explore the relevance and importance of the occupation to be analyzed.
> - Use theoretical reasoning to identify the appropriate practice model to guide analysis.
> - Identify the steps required.
> - Determine the objects and environmental supports that may be needed.
> - Determine the space demands.
> - Determine the social demands.
> - Determine the required body structures.
> - Determine the required performance skills.
> - Determine the required process skills.
> - Analyze the possibility of adapting or grading the activity.
>
> *Note.* Kielhofner and Forsyth (2009) and Thomas (2015).

therapy practitioner needs to translate those goals into measurable outcomes that express what the client hopes to accomplish, are attainable, and can be measured objectively. Activity analysis is inherently objective and empirical, which makes it a valuable tool for generating measurable goals for intervention. In the intervention stage, activity analysis can serve as a tool to help the occupational therapy practitioner use "an occupation to achieve some therapeutic benefit or allow a person to engage in a former or new occupational role" (Kielhofner & Forsyth, 2009, p. 91).

INTERVENTION PLAN

The intervention phase of the occupational therapy process begins with the development of an intervention plan. The *intervention plan,* which is a guide to actions taken by the occupational therapy practitioner in collaboration with the client, is a result of the evaluation stage described in the *OTPF–3* (AOTA, 2014). It is ideally occupation based and is drawn from science-driven frames of reference and evidence. It confirms the outcomes to be targeted during the intervention. Developing an intervention plan involves the selection of

- Objective and measurable occupation-focused goals and related time frames;
- Occupational therapy intervention strategies, such as those that aim to create or promote, establish or restore, maintain, modify, or prevent; and
- Methods for service delivery, including who will provide the intervention, types of intervention, and service delivery models. (AOTA, 2014, p. S17)

The occupational therapy practitioner makes every effort to be conscientious and use the current best evidence in making decisions about occupational therapy interventions. To provide high-quality services that reflect clients' interests, values, needs, and choices, occupational therapy practitioners rely on the standards of evidence-informed practice.

Evidence-informed practice is the conscientious use of the current best evidence to identify the potential benefits, harms, and costs of an intervention while acknowledging that what works in one context may not be appropriate or feasible in another. Evidence-informed practice integrates the best available research evidence; clients' needs, values, and preferences; practitioner wisdom; and theory as filtered through the lens of client and community culture into the clinical decision-making process.

INTERVENTION IMPLEMENTATION

Intervention implementation is the process of initiating the strategies to address client-centered goals identified through occupational therapy evaluation (AOTA, 2014). Occupational therapy interventions "may focus on a single aspect of the domain, such as a specific occupation, or on several aspects of the domain, such as context and environment, performance patterns, and performance skills" (AOTA, 2014, p. S15). Exhibit 9.3 describes types of occupational therapy intervention (pp. S29–S31).

Occupation and Activities

Occupation as an intervention tool involves "client-directed daily life activities that match and support or address identified participation goals" (AOTA, 2014, p. S29). In the context of occupational therapy intervention, *activities* are defined as "actions designed and selected to support the development of performance skills and performance patterns to enhance occupational

EXHIBIT 9.3.	Types of Occupational Therapy Interventions	
CATEGORY	**DESCRIPTION**	**EXAMPLES**
▪ **OCCUPATIONS AND ACTIVITIES**—Occupations and activities selected as interventions for specific clients and designed to meet therapeutic goals and address the underlying needs of the mind, body, and spirit of the client. To use occupations and activities therapeutically, the practitioner considers activity demands and client factors in relation to the client's therapeutic goals, contexts, and environments.		
Occupations	Client-directed daily life activities that match and support or address identified participation goals.	The client ▪ Completes morning dressing and hygiene using adaptive devices ▪ Purchases groceries and prepares a meal ▪ Visits a friend using public transportation independently ▪ Applies for a job in the retail industry ▪ Plays on a playground with children and adults ▪ Participates in a community festival by setting up a booth to sell baked goods ▪ Engages in a pattern of self-care and relaxation activities in preparation for sleep ▪ Engages in a statewide advocacy program to improve services to people with mental illness
Activities	Actions designed and selected to support the development of performance skills and performance patterns to enhance occupational engagement. Activities often are components of occupations and always hold meaning, relevance, and perceived utility for clients at their level of interest and motivation.	The client ▪ Selects clothing and manipulates clothing fasteners in advance of dressing ▪ Practices safe ways to get into and out of the bathtub ▪ Prepares a food list and practices using cooking appliances ▪ Reviews how to use a map and transportation schedule ▪ Writes answers on an application form ▪ Climbs on and off playground and recreation equipment ▪ Greets people and initiates conversation in a role-play situation ▪ Develops a weekly schedule to manage time and organize daily and weekly responsibilities required to live independently ▪ Uses adaptive switches to operate the home environmental control system ▪ Completes a desired expressive activity (e.g., art, craft, dance) that is not otherwise classified ▪ Plays a desired game either as a solo player or in competition with others

(Continued)

EXHIBIT 9.3.	Types of Occupational Therapy Interventions *(Cont.)*	
CATEGORY	**DESCRIPTION**	**EXAMPLES**

- **PREPARATORY METHODS AND TASKS**—Methods and tasks that prepare the client for occupational performance, used as part of a treatment session in preparation for or concurrently with occupations and activities or provided to a client as a home-based engagement to support daily occupational performance.

CATEGORY	DESCRIPTION	EXAMPLES
Preparatory methods	Modalities, devices, and techniques to prepare the client for occupational performance. Often preparatory methods are interventions that are "done to" the client without the client's active participation.	The practitioner - Fabricates and issues a splint or orthotic to support a weakened hand and decrease pain - Fabricates and issues a wrist splint to facilitate movement and enhance participation in household activities
Splints	Construction and use of devices to mobilize, immobilize, and support body structures to enhance participation in occupations.	The practitioner - Fabricates and issues a splint or orthotic to support a weakened hand and decrease pain - Fabricates and issues a wrist splint to facilitate movement and enhance participation in household activities
Assistive technology and environmental modifications	Identification and use of assistive technologies (high and low tech), application of universal design principles, and recommendations for changes to the environment or activity to support the client's ability to engage in occupations. This preparatory method includes assessment, selection, provision, and education and training in use of devices.	The practitioner - Provides a pencil grip and slant board - Provides electronic books with text-to-speech software - Recommends visual supports (e.g., a social story) to guide behavior - Recommends replacing steps with an appropriately graded ramp - Recommends universally designed curriculum materials
Wheeled mobility	Use of products and technologies that facilitate a client's ability to maneuver through space, including seating and positioning, and that improve mobility, enhance participation in desired daily occupations, and reduce risk for complications such as skin breakdown or limb contractures.	The practitioner - Recommends, in conjunction with the wheelchair team, a sip-and-puff switch to allow the client to maneuver the power wheelchair independently and interface with an environmental control unit in the home
Preparatory tasks	Actions selected and provided to the client to target specific client factors or performance skills. Tasks involve active participation of the client and sometimes comprise engagements that use various materials to simulate activities or components of occupations. Preparatory tasks themselves may not hold inherent meaning, relevance, or perceived utility as stand-alone entities.	The client - Refolds towels taken from a clean linen cart to address shoulder range of motion - Participates in fabricated sensory environment (e.g., through movement, tactile sensations, scents) to promote alertness - Uses visual imagery and rhythmic breathing to promote rest and relaxation - Performs a home-based conditioning regimen using free weights - Does hand-strengthening exercises using therapy putty, exercise bands, grippers, and clothespins - Participates in an assertiveness training program to prepare for self-advocacy

- **EDUCATION AND TRAINING**

CATEGORY	DESCRIPTION	EXAMPLES
Education	Imparting of knowledge and information about occupation, health, well-being, and participation that enable the client to acquire helpful behaviors, habits, and routines that may or may not require application at the time of the intervention session.	The practitioner - Provides education regarding home and activity modifications to the spouse or family member of a person with dementia to support maximum independence - Educates town officials about the value of and strategies for making walking and biking paths accessible for all community members - Educates providers of care for people who have experienced trauma on the use of sensory strategies

(Continued)

EXHIBIT 9.3.	Types of Occupational Therapy Interventions *(Cont.)*	
CATEGORY	**DESCRIPTION**	**EXAMPLES**
		▪ Provides education to people with mental health issues and their families on the psychological and social factors that influence engagement in occupation
Training	Facilitation of the acquisition of concrete skills for meeting specific goals in a real-life, applied situation. In this case, skills refers to measurable components of function that enable mastery. Training is differentiated from education by its goal of enhanced performance as opposed to enhanced understanding, although these goals often go hand in hand (Collins & O'Brien, 2003).	The practitioner ▪ Instructs the client in how to operate a universal control device to manage household appliances ▪ Instructs family members in the use and maintenance of the father's power wheelchair ▪ Instructs the client in the use of self range of motion as a preparatory technique to avoid joint contracture of wrist ▪ Instructs the client in the use of a handheld electronic device and applications to recall and manage weekly activities and medications ▪ Instructs the client in how to direct a personal care attendant in assisting with self-care activities ▪ Trains parents and teachers to focus on a child's strengths to foster positive behaviors
▪ **ADVOCACY**—Efforts directed toward promoting occupational justice and empowering clients to seek and obtain resources to fully participate in daily life occupations. The outcomes of advocacy and self-advocacy support health, well-being, and occupational participation at the individual or systems level.		
Advocacy	Advocacy efforts undertaken by the practitioner.	The practitioner ▪ Collaborates with a person to procure reasonable accommodations at a work site ▪ Serves on the policy board of an organization to procure supportive housing accommodations for people with disabilities ▪ Serves on the board of a local park district to encourage inclusion of children with disabilities in mainstream district sports programs when possible ▪ Collaborates with adults who have serious mental illness to raise public awareness of the impact of stigma ▪ Collaborates with and educates staff at federal funding sources for persons with disabling conditions
Self-advocacy	Advocacy efforts undertaken by the client, which the practitioner can promote and support.	▪ A student with a learning disability requests and receives reasonable accommodations such as textbooks on tape. ▪ A grassroots employee committee requests and procures ergonomically designed keyboards for their work computers. ▪ People with disabilities advocate for the use of universal design principles with all new public construction. ▪ Young adults contact their Internet service provider to request support for cyberbullying prevention.
▪ **GROUP INTERVENTIONS**—Use of distinct knowledge and leadership techniques to facilitate learning and skill acquisition across the life-span through the dynamics of group and social interaction. Groups may also be used as a method of service delivery.		
Groups	Functional groups, activity groups, task groups, social groups, and other groups used on inpatient units, within the community, or in schools that allow clients to explore and develop skills for participation, including basic social interaction skills, tools for self-regulation, goal setting, and positive choice making.	▪ A group for older adults focuses on maintaining participation despite increasing disability, such as exploring alternative transportation if driving is no longer an option and participating in volunteer and social opportunities after retirement. ▪ A community group addresses issues of self-efficacy and self-esteem as the basis for creating resiliency in preadolescent children at risk for being bullied. ▪ A group in a mental health program addresses establishment of social connections in the community.

Source. From *Occupational Therapy Practice Framework: Domain and Process* (3rd ed.), by the American Occupational Therapy Association, *American Journal of Occupational Therapy, 68*(Suppl. 1), pp. 29–31. Copyright © 2014 by the American Occupational Therapy Association. Used with permission.

engagement" (AOTA, 2014, p. S29). The activities used in occupational therapy interventions are often components of occupations that are important to the client. Both occupations and activities are as important in the intervention process as they are in the evaluation process.

Preparatory Methods and Tasks

Preparatory methods used in intervention prepare the client for occupational performance but may not be inherently occupation-based themselves. Preparatory methods include modalities, devices, and techniques that are typically administered by the occupational therapy practitioner without the client's active participation to prepare the client for occupational engagement. Examples of preparatory methods include the use of splints, environmental modifications, positioning, and physical agent modalities (PAMs).

Preparatory tasks used in intervention may be exercises or activities selected to target specific client factors or performance skills. These preparatory tasks involve the client's active participation and may be unrelated to the identified occupational performance outcome. Preparatory tasks are often designed to simulate components of occupations. As noted in the *OTPF–3*, "Preparatory tasks themselves may not hold inherent meaning, relevance, or perceived utility as stand-alone entities" (AOTA, 2014, p. S30). Preparatory tasks and measures typically rely on a reductionistic approach to addressing impairment. This type of approach is sometimes vital to jump-start the rehabilitation or recovery process, but preparatory approaches should actually get the client ready for the occupation-based intervention approaches that follow.

Most people think of direct 1:1 treatment when they consider the occupational therapy profession, but the other categories of intervention—education and training, advocacy, and group intervention—are equally as important in addressing the occupational therapy domain of practice.

Education and Training

Although the *OTPF–3* considers **education** as the "imparting of knowledge" and **training** as "facilitation of acquisition of concrete skills" (AOTA, 2014, p. S30), the terms are considered together here as aspects of client learning. Whether it is learning pain management strategies, new movement patterns, or new ways to perform desired occupations, learning is a client outcome that is consistent across all occupational therapy practice settings. Despite how pervasive the need for learning is in the implementation of occupational therapy, there has been relatively little explicit discussion of education and training in the occupational therapy literature as an occupational therapy intervention.

However, a great deal of research has been done on learning in the field of education. Learning theory has increasingly integrated constructs from cognitive science. Contemporary learning theory argues that "learning entails more than simply filling minds with information; it requires the transformation of naive understanding into more complete and accurate comprehension" (Pellegrino, Chudowsky, & Glaser, 2001, p. 83). Table 9.1 presents 4 perspectives from which to consider learning (Acedo & Hughes, 2014).

Education and training as an occupational therapy intervention should be grounded in strategies to help clients organize new information in a manner that makes retrieval both efficient and reliable. These strategies may include using multiple teaching modalities (e.g., instruction, demonstration, trial and error) and multiple retrieval strategies (e.g., electronic calendars, visual schedules, verbal prompts).

Novice vs. expert learners

Also consider the differences between experts and novices in task-specific learning. Novice learners are likely to take a naive approach that is not critically examined, whereas expert learners draw on a repertoire of learned strategies and experiences that support the approach being

TABLE 9.1.	Perspectives on Learning
PERSPECTIVE	**LEARNING ATTRIBUTES**
Learning as a model of cognition	Short-term memory is limited, but long-term memory can hold an expansive store of knowledge. *Learning* is how well a person can retrieve the knowledge stored in long-term memory and use it to reason efficiently about current information and problems.
Learning as a developmental progression	Learning is supported by the individual's inherent abilities and capacity as these abilities respond to the influence of maturation, experience, and impairment.
Learning as a social activity with societal impact	Therapeutic use of self is an essential aspect of learning. Much learning is inherently social. Aspects of an individual's social context can either support or hinder learning.
Learning as reflection	Clients' ability to see and assess their own performance can support their own learning and provide the occupational therapy practitioner with insight into the client's learning needs.

considered in terms of accuracy, quality, and context. For example, given a new wheelchair, a novice wheelchair user may limit their focus on coordinating arm movements to achieve a smooth forward motion. However an expert user may try out a new wheelchair by executing precise pivots or "wheelies" to explore the potential of the new device to respond to uneven terrain and curbs.

Readiness

People need a basic level of readiness for learning to occur. That readiness may be based on maturation, because some skills, such as riding a bicycle, cannot be taught until the child has gained certain prerequisite physical and cognitive skills. Learning is also developmental in that students learn new content over time that builds on and enriches earlier learning, moving them from the status of novice learner to that of expert. Although practitioners tend to think of the building of educational supports for clients as a measured, step-by-step sequence, the science reflects that the progression of learning is not usually

> a series of smoothly articulated conceptualizations but a series of important moments characterized by understanding and change—"aha moments" . . . they are transformative (occasioning a significant shift in the perception of a subject), irreversible (unlikely to be forgotten, or unlearned only through considerable effort), and integrative (exposing the previously hidden interrelatedness of something). (Land, Cousin, Meyer, & Davies, 2005, p. 53)

Teacher–learner connection

Learning is affected by the student's emotional reaction within social contexts. The therapist as teacher needs to consider how to best engage the student emotionally through the inherent social nature of teaching. The interpersonal context in which teaching occurs can support or hinder the process. Acedo and Hughes (2014) affirmed that "the teacher must share many parts of the learning experience with the students (expectations, criteria for success, feedback on performance) and they need to share their learning with each other in well-designed group work, projects and discussion groups" (p. 510).

The importance of the teacher–learner connection is considered in the occupational therapy process in the focus on the therapeutic use of self. A well-managed teacher–learner connection during intervention results in clients feeling good about the process, understanding the usefulness of what they are learning, and connecting what they are learning to their everyday occupations.

Learner self-reflection

Finally, learning can be viewed as a form of self-reflection. When students think back on what they have learned

and how they learned it, they are able to draw conclusions from the process. These conclusions can lead to the development of important strategies such as selective attention, self-regulation, and strategic planning. In a clinical setting, the occupational therapy practitioner is often focused on the delivery of educational content, and the pragmatics of the setting make client reflection difficult. Reviewing prior learning with clients as a routine part of the intervention process can help encourage this type of supportive reflection.

Practitioners should also build the intervention process in a manner that allows clients to see evidence of progress and achieve some degree of success. Using concepts from the field of psychology such as errorless learning and backward chaining can be very helpful in the delivery of supportive educational interventions.

Error is a natural part of learning just as it is a natural part of clinical reasoning. The occupational therapy practitioner using education and training as intervention tools should provide opportunities for error and for learning through error. This approach supports generalization of learning and helps the client learn problem-solving in the context of task performance.

Advocacy

Advocacy is described in the *OTPF–3* as "efforts directed toward promoting occupational justice and empowering clients to seek and obtain resources to fully participate in daily life occupations" (AOTA, 2014, p. S30). As an intervention tool, advocacy includes those actions performed by occupational therapy practitioners either in collaboration with or on behalf of a client to pursue a change in the environment that will ultimately enhance occupation (Dhillon, Wilkins, Stewart, & Law, 2016). Advocacy offers an approach to intervention that is population focused rather than client centered. Advocacy can occur at the direct service delivery level, but it can also occur at institutional and legislative levels.

Through advocacy, occupational therapy practitioners serve as catalysts for change at both the client and the societal levels. Occupational therapy practitioners must recognize and respond to issues of social injustice they encounter in clinical practice. Some kinds of social injustice encountered in practice are restricted access to occupational therapy services, reimbursement for occupational therapy services that is based on medical diagnosis rather than on functional limitation, and overreliance on rubrics and clinical pathways in determining the focus of interventions.

Practitioners must advocate with and for clients regarding issues that negatively affect their potential for occupational performance and occupational engagement. Stover (2016) stated that

> duties of an effective advocate often expand beyond the traditional elements of most health care professionals'

treatment intervention, but these duties may be required to ensure clients' well-being, safety, and access to necessary care. Advocacy and the ability to interpret and define terms such as medical necessity can be necessary elements of the ethical obligation to exhibit beneficence. (p. 2)

As Stover argued, the simple legalese term *medical necessity* is wielded to limit access to care and to equipment. The definition of this term is vague and varies with each new version of health policy legislation. When the occupational therapy practitioner engages in advocacy activities, the benefit extends beyond individual clients.

In school-based practice, there is a focus on teaching self-advocacy, also called *self-determination,* as part of the process of preparing the student to transition into the community. Interventions to build self-advocacy are prevalent across practice areas but are seldom listed as goals in the formal plan of care. In schools and in many mental health settings, building self-advocacy skills is a valued intervention. However, it is less recognized and therefore less likely to be reimbursed in other practice areas. This may be part of the reason it is so seldom identified as an outcome goal.

Group Intervention

In general, *group intervention* is defined as simultaneous treatment of 2 or more clients who may or may not be doing the same activities. If the occupational therapy practitioner is dividing attention among his or her clients, providing only brief, intermittent personal contact, or giving the same instructions to 2 or more clients at the same time, then group intervention is occurring.

Group interventions are best used when the clients involved benefit from having other clients present and engaged in a shared task. A group intervention is commonly chosen in instances in which the occupational therapy practitioner is able to use peers as models, when the client is working on skills requiring the presence of peers (e.g., social skills, coping or self-monitoring skills), and when the client needs extended access to skill practice. Group interventions, although supported by the evidence, are not consistently reimbursable through third-party payers. For this reason, they may be used less often to address client needs.

Case Example 9.1 describes effective group intervention used in a mental health practice.

CASE EXAMPLE 9.1. GROUP INTERVENTION

In a psychiatric hospital, group intervention was used with **participants with psychiatric diagnoses**. Exhibit 9.3 lists occupational considerations for using the cognitive–behavioral frame of reference as an occupational therapy tool for group intervention. When using group interventions, group members should be working toward similar occupational performance goals.

All group members were able to come up with strengths for both the lion and the ant during the warm-up. This activity helped the group members to relax and begin the process of positive thinking. During the main activity, a few people had some trouble thinking of positive characteristics, although they were able to complete their brochure with prompting

EXHIBIT 9.3.	Group's Occupational Considerations

Referral: Psychiatric hospital weekly occupational therapy group intervention.

Impact on occupation: Group intervention is not only an efficient use of occupational therapy resources but also allows peer feedback in a relatively safe environment. Groups are widely used in psychiatric settings and have been shown to offer members positive experiences interacting with others, as well as greater self-acceptance through group participation.

Medical/functional history: The participants have a range of psychiatric diagnoses; depression and substance abuse are the most prominent ones.

Occupational roles: Varied.

Goals: The goals for this group are written more generally than they would be for individual clients and include
- Group members will recognize and identify positive personal strengths to increase self-esteem.
- Group members will demonstrate positive self-affirmations to increase self-confidence and decrease negative thought patterns.

Frame of reference: Cognitive–behavioral. By changing self-talk, people can change the way they feel about a situation or person, effectively changing their behavior and the accompanying consequences of that behavior.

(Continued)

CASE EXAMPLE 9.1. GROUP INTERVENTION *(Cont.)*

EXHIBIT 9.4.   Group's Occupational Considerations *(Cont.)*

Purpose of group: The purpose of this session is to allow the members to identify and recognize personal strengths that they may typically ignore. By recognizing these strengths and by incorporating peer support, group members can change their thinking to focus on positive aspects of themselves as opposed to weaknesses or negative self-expressions.

Method and procedure: The group begins with an introduction by the group leader, explaining the purpose of the group session, followed by a warm-up activity.

Warm-up: On a white board are pictures of an ant and a lion. Each group member is asked to introduce themselves to the group and to identify 1 strength for both the lion and the ant. The therapist lists these strengths on the white board as each member takes his or her turn. When all members have gone, the therapist reflects on the warm-up, noting that although a lion and an ant are very different from each other, they still have unique characteristics that can be viewed as strengths.

Main activity:

1. Each participant will choose a piece of colored construction paper and fold it twice to make a trifold brochure. They will then decorate the front of the brochure with their name and any other design they would like.
2. Group members will be asked to choose from a few of the following prompts:
   My proudest moment:_____
   My best feature: _____
   My favorite activity: _____
   Something I am good at is: _____
   What makes me happiest: _____
   I feel most valuable when: _____
   My favorite "feel good" song is: _____
3. On the inside of the brochure, participants will write both the prompts and their individual response to each of the prompts. Once they are finished, they will close the brochure and put a paper clip on it to keep it closed.
4. Each participant will then pass his or her brochure to the person on the right. That person will be asked to write down 1 positive thing about the other person. This can be personal or can be as simple as "I like your hair" or "I like your shirt."
5. Each brochure will then continue to be passed to the right until everyone in the group has had a chance to write a positive comment about the person whose name is on the front of it. Participants will then be given an opportunity to review their brochure.

Discussion or closure: The group will be asked to share how it felt to read positive things others had written about them and how difficult it was to come up with responses for the self-prompts.

from the therapist. Most group members were surprised at how easy it was for other group members to write positive statements about them. The brochures served as a medium that had an initial positive effect and could be used in the future to serve as a reminder that how people think about themselves and situations affects how they feel. This activity also allowed for self-expression and self-exploration in a guided, positive manner.

There is often a misconception that group therapy interventions offer less than individual therapist–client interventions. In fact, group-based interventions offer something different altogether. Bullock and Bannigan (2011) noted that in occupational therapy, group work is usually activity based and aims to develop skills or encourage social interaction. Group intervention strategies are complex, and a complete discussion of group interventions is beyond the scope of this text.

Strategic Thinking During Intervention Implementation

Strategic thinking is a reasoning process that involves the generation and application of unique insights and opportunities. Strategic thinking is essential in effective clinical reasoning and considers the significance, logic, and clarity of innovations and ideas. It is strategic thinking when the occupational therapy practitioner considers incorporating a "shiny new thing" into his or her practice. It is also strategic

thinking when the occupational therapy practitioner builds a practice that thoughtfully includes less prevalent interventions such as advocacy activities and group interventions.

Liedtka (1998) observed 5 major attributes of strategic thinking in practice:

1. Having a systems perspective,
2. Being hypothesis driven,
3. Including a focus on intent,
4. Incorporating a historical perspective, and
5. Involving intelligent opportunism.

TABLE 9.2.	Strategic Thinking
STANDARDS	**COMMON PROBLEMS**
Provides clarity of focus on what the innovation actually offers.	May assert claims without considering all relevant information.
Can articulate and evaluate information beyond what the product claims.	Does not subject new products or information to systematic scrutiny.
Draws conclusions to the extent they are supported by the data and sound reasoning.	Makes inferences that go beyond what the data support.
Consistently seeks to discern and understand the assumptions supporting critical reasoning.	Does not question personal assumptions or the claims associated with the innovation or strategy.

Table 9.2 presents the standards and common problems that must be applied to strategic thinking to ensure that it is a useful tool for occupational therapy practice.

Having a *systems perspective* refers to being able to understand the implications that follow from one's reasoning, including the implications of specific actions or problems for the whole situation or system. A strategic thinker using a systems perspective steps beyond intervention algorithms, approaches the client's difficulties from many angles, and incorporates nonlinear thinking.

When Liedtka (1998) stated that strategic thinking must be hypothesis driven, she was noting that a clearly delineated hypothesis focuses the process and incorporates the scientific method into strategic thinking. A focus on intent, as described by Liedtka, means that the thinker is both determined and has an intent to work strategically. This focus on intent allows occupational therapy practitioners to focus attention, to assert a claim only when they have sufficient evidence to back it up, and to be persistent in the reasoning process as they address a specified problem or goal. The intent to support occupation is common to occupational therapy clinical reasoning, and occupational therapy practitioners should evaluate new products or innovations in thinking on the basis of data and sound reasoning relating to their potential impact on occupation.

Although clinical questions occasionally have 1 definitive answer, occupational therapy practitioners commonly must choose between competing approaches, both broadly (in terms of frame of reference) and on a smaller scale (in terms of specific intervention strategies). Clinical questions with arguably more than 1 answer require occupational therapy practitioners to identify the best answer from a range of possibilities.

Intelligent Opportunism

Intelligent opportunism is a less familiar concept than strategic thinking. *Intelligent opportunism* means being responsive to good opportunities (Liedtka, 1998). Strategically thinking, occupational therapy practitioners are able to spot and react to new opportunities and new ideas as they arise. They may change their strategy to assimilate something new in a client's environment, such as a change in living situation or access to a particular community resource. Intelligent opportunism assumes that the reasoning process must have room for flexibility, challenging practitioners to be open to new approaches and innovations that allow them to take advantage of emergent strategies that may be more relevant in a client's social or environmental context. The successful occupational therapy practitioner is action oriented and, as reflected in the quote by Eleanor Roosevelt in Practice Wisdom 9.1, looks toward the horizon and the potential to enhance interventions, programs, and policies.

Bridgette LeCompte is a school-based occupational therapy practitioner who writes the blog "School OT Empowered." She has described intelligent opportunism as "rocking the boat gently." LeCompte (2017) posted,

> I'm here to reassure you that you can and should rock the boat gently, slowly, and steadily. It is our responsibility to carve the path and swim upstream against the designated current. It might be a change for people to get used to, but you will be far more valued and appreciated in the long run for challenging tradition. I'm also here to say that our expertise is NOT in sensory/motor realms (sure, we are excellent in this area), it is in meaningful occupation and participation. We need to remember our roots in occupation as we educate others about our role, model best practices, carry out non-traditional roles, empower others, and continue moving forward.

In her blog, LeCompte (2017) presented a list of steps for school-based occupational therapy practitioners to take to fully transform themselves from "sensorimotor therapists" to occupational therapists. The blog post offered an operationalized plan for intelligent

PRACTICE WISDOM 9.1.	Dreaming

"The future belongs to those who believe in the beauty of their dreams."—*Eleanor Roosevelt (n.d.)*

opportunism. It also offered insight into the everyday clinical challenges that affect clinical reasoning in the intervention stage of the occupational therapy process. One barrier she perceived is that other professionals on her team had a very limited idea of the scope of occupational therapy, and with this viewpoint they boxed in occupational therapy practice. This boxing-in might relegate school-based occupational therapy practitioners to being handwriting teachers and occupational therapy practitioners in rehabilitation to being upper-extremity physical therapists.

Occupational therapy practitioners sometimes box themselves in by repeating what is comfortable and billable. The occupational therapy practitioner working in hand therapy who continues to use PAMs even when the client is no longer reporting pain may be doing so out of habit rather than using clinical reasoning. PAMs play an important role in hand therapy, but they are often also an easy way to have overlapping client times, leading to more billable service hours. If every client has 20 minutes of fluidotherapy before 20 minutes of hands-on therapy, a practitioner can be treating 2 clients at the same time. From a business standpoint, this is beneficial, and this dovetailing of clients is a sound practice if the client is experiencing pain or some other symptom that warrants the use of the modality. However, if it is a routine that is not guided by collaborative client goals, then the occupational therapy practitioner may have fallen into the rut of being a "one-trick pony," as described in Practice Wisdom 9.2.

The school-based occupational therapy practitioner whose whole practice is exclusively focused on handwriting or the occupational therapy practitioner in the skilled nursing unit who only addresses ADLs could also be considered one-trick ponies because they have boxed themselves in, and their practice does not reflect the domain of occupational therapy. Regardless of specialization or advanced training, the occupational therapy practitioner should remain an occupational therapy practitioner in addition to being a certified hand therapist, a driving specialist, or an assistive technology professional.

Algorithms and Clinical Pathways

Interventions are specific actions taken to improve a situation or problem. It is expected that people experiencing the same problems will respond similarly to the same interventions, and this is the idea behind the development of intervention algorithms. An ***intervention algorithm*** is a prescribed sequence of specific actions guided by a set of rules that reflects best practice clinical reasoning. Intervention algorithms are common in practice situations where many clients present with very similar conditions. These algorithms, also called *clinical pathways,* outline a process that can be audited to assure high quality care across practitioners. Case Example 9.2 presents the case of Alice and demonstrates the use of intervention algorithms.

Although Alice was admitted secondary to her hip fracture, a full recovery of hip function is expected with a gradual strengthening and gait-training program. The complicating issue for Alice is her cognitive deficits, and the occupational therapy practitioner is focusing on function related to these deficits while Alice is in rehabilitation. A one-trick pony occupational therapy practitioner would simply address the rehabilitation of the hip fracture using the standard protocol and not consider the other complicating factors, but another occupational therapy practitioner might also integrate consideration of the dementia and its potential impact on the rehabilitation process. A published algorithm for occupational therapy intervention for persons with middle-stage Alzheimer's disease is presented in Table 9.3.

According to the algorithm offered in Table 9.3, the occupational therapy intervention plan should focus on health maintenance and restoration of habits and routines, with compensations and environmental strategies to support occupational performance across all performance areas. This algorithm is sound and offers reasoned approaches to intervention. However, this algorithm is also reductionistic. It offers guidance and supports consideration of issues beyond the hip fracture, but it would still be possible to fully address the identified occupational therapy goals without integrating Alice's interests, values, or priorities. A standard protocol based on this algorithm would likely focus on homemaking tasks that Alice does not value.

Aspects of the occupational therapy domain are interrelated and influence each other in a continuous, dynamic process. If Alice is experiencing pain and disorientation, a focus on ADL tasks that she does not value may lead to a lack of engagement and motivation in the intervention process. Alice's goal is to return to her apartment, and her disengagement may make that outcome impossible to achieve. A practitioner who simply follows protocol is unlikely to give Alice the individualized care she needs.

There is a dynamic interrelationship between evaluation and intervention planning, and this relationship continues throughout the intervention stage of the occupational therapy process. Interventions should be targeted toward goals that were identified in collaboration with the client. If the occupational therapy practitioner working with Alice is a one-trick pony, he or she

PRACTICE WISDOM 9.2.	Etymology: One-Trick Pony

"A performing animal that knows only one trick. (idiomatic, by extension) A person or group noteworthy for only a single achievement, skill, or characteristic."—*"Etymology: One Trick Pony" (2017)*

CASE EXAMPLE 9.2. ALICE: ALGORITHMS AND CLINICAL PATHWAYS

Alice, age 88 years, has Alzheimer's disease. She fell, fractured her hip, had hip replacement surgery, and needed rehabilitation—a common reason for placement in a skilled nursing facility (SNF). Because the condition is common and it is often uncomplicated, hip replacement rehabilitation is an intervention process that lends itself well to the use of intervention algorithms. Exhibit 9.5 provides Alice's occupational profile.

EXHIBIT 9.5.	Alice's Occupational Profile		
Client	**Reason the client is seeking service and concerns related to engagement in occupations**	Referred to occupational therapy in a SNF to evaluate and treat after a fall and a right hip fracture. _Impact on occupation:_ Prior to her injury Alice was functioning in her apartment but was making obvious mistakes around the home, such as putting dirty laundry in the dryer rather than the washing machine and putting coffee grounds into the coffee pot without a coffee filter. Because she had weekly housekeeping services and 1 hot meal provided daily, the family was not overly concerned by these errors. Alice is easily startled, and her fall occurred because she jumped up when the phone rang and lost her balance with the sudden position change.	
	Occupations in which the client is successful	Alice was living on her own in an assisted-care apartment before her fall.	
	Personal interests and values	Alice has never been very interested in homemaking but has been an avid outdoorswoman her whole life. Alice highly values her independence, and even with her current memory difficulties, she always pays careful attention to her personal appearance.	
	Occupational history (i.e., life experiences)	Alice was diagnosed with a Garden Type I incomplete fracture with valgus impaction on the right. Her fracture was surgically stabilized with closed reduction and internal fixation, and she was transferred to skilled nursing for rehabilitation. Alice and her family hope that she will be able to return to her apartment after rehabilitation. Alice has been living with Stage 3–4 Alzheimer's disease.	
	Performance patterns (routines, roles, habits, & rituals)	Alice's valued life roles include her roles as grandmother and mother. She has a large extended family and values her role as an elder in the family. She still enjoys long walks, bird-watching, and talks on natural history. She regularly talks to her 3 children on the telephone, and her daughter lives near her. Alice enjoys interactions with others in her retirement community, but because of her limited memory, she has formed no real friendships in the facility.	
Environment		**Supports to occupational engagement**	**Barriers to occupational engagement**
	Physical (e.g., buildings, furniture, pets)	The SNF is designed to be accessible.	While she is using the walker, Alice is limited by the physical accessibility of the environment.
	Social (e.g., spouse, friends, caregivers)	There are organized social activities available to Alice.	Alice has little access to her friends from the community.

(Continued)

CASE EXAMPLE 9.2. ALICE: ALGORITHMS AND CLINICAL PATHWAYS (Cont.)

EXHIBIT 9.5.	Alice's Occupational Profile (Cont.)	
Context	**Cultural** (e.g., customs, beliefs)	No issues related to culture, customs, or beliefs were identified during assessment.
	Personal (e.g., age, gender, SES, education)	Age 88 years. Female. College educated. Middle income.
	Temporal (e.g., stage of life, time, year)	Late adulthood. Widowed. Retired.
	Virtual (e.g., chat, email, remote monitoring)	This is not one of Alice's interests.
Client goals	**Client's priorities and desired targeted outcomes**	Alice wants to return to her apartment and the routine she is used to keeping.

ANALYSIS OF PARTICIPATION	
Basic ADLs	
Eating/oral–motor	Alice has no difficulty in this area.
Grooming	Alice has no difficulty in this area.
Bathing/transfer	Alice is currently using a walker and has a shower bench and grab bars in the SNF. She is able to bear weight for a moderate assist transfer to the shower bench.
Dressing upper body	Alice has no difficulty in this area.
Dressing lower body	Alice currently needs maximal assistance in this area. She does assist with weight shifts and with extending her legs, but she is unable to use adaptive devices to maintain required hip precautions.
Toileting	Alice is able to bear weight for a moderate assist transfer to the toilet. Before her fall, she had episodes of bladder incontinence, and she is not always aware of the need to toilet. She will use the toilet when prompted.
Problem solving/memory	Alice has difficulty with basic problem solving. She needs help choosing proper clothing for the season or the occasion and does not remember whether she has eaten a meal or taken her medication. When unexpected things happen, she becomes agitated and engages in repetitive hand-wringing.
Comments:	None.
IADLs	
Community mobility	Alice does not drive or own a vehicle. There is a walking trail near her apartment, and she tries to walk at least 1 mile daily.
Health management/ prevention	Alice is largely healthy and takes only a statin medication to lower her cholesterol. Alice's daughter loads a weekly medication dispenser for her, and it is with her breakfast things. Alice still occasionally forgets her medication, but this has not been a concern to date.
Home management	Alice keeps her apartment tidy. Most other home management tasks are completed by others.

(Continued)

CASE EXAMPLE 9.2. ALICE: ALGORITHMS AND CLINICAL PATHWAYS *(Cont.)*

EXHIBIT 9.5.	**Alice's Occupational Profile *(Cont.)***
Financial management	Alice's finances are managed by her daughter. Her daughter recently set up a new checking account for Alice because Alice does not remember what checks she has written. She wrote 4 donation checks to the local library in 1 week, each for $200. Her new account has a $500 limit so she can still donate to charities but on a regulated basis.
Leisure/play	When asked, Alice says that she likes to bird watch, read, and do puzzles. In reality, she does like sitting and reading books, but she does not follow the plot and seems to pick up books and read at whatever point they fall open. She is unable to do even simple jigsaw puzzles on her own.
Safety	Several safety supports are in place in Alice's apartment. She wears an emergency alert bracelet, has grab bars in the bathroom, and has motion detection lights throughout the apartment. All over-the-counter medications have been removed because she once overdosed on ibuprofen.
Comments:	Alice has been very functional in her limited assistive-living environment.
	Motor and Praxis Skills
Sitting—static/dynamic	Alice has some pain with sitting. She has a history of OA and complained of hip pain in sitting before her recent injury. Her sitting balance is good.
Standing—static/dynamic	Alice stands with support. She is able to bear partial weight on her right leg but bears the bulk of her weight on her left leg. Before her injury, her balance was good. At this time, her standing tolerance is poor.
Joint stability and skeletal mobility	Alice has a history of OA, and because of this has pain in her wrists, ankles, and knees. With the exception of her fractured right hip, she has full AROM. She has limited right hip flexion and rotation.
Place can on shelf	Alice currently uses a walker for support, which makes it difficult for her to get close enough to the shelf without challenging her balance.
Retrieve item from floor	Alice currently uses a walker for support, which makes it difficult for her to reach the floor without challenging her balance and breaking her hip precautions.
Screw lid on jar	When seated, Alice has no difficulty in this area.
Comb back of head	When seated, Alice has no difficulty in this area.
Writing	When seated, Alice has no physical difficulty with writing. Her writing is often illegible.
Lift grocery bag	This is not applicable to Alice's current living situation.
Coordination	This is adequate for her age. Alice is able to move limbs independently and engage in both simple and more complex tasks that are familiar.
Manipulation	Alice prefers her right hand for skilled activity and has good grip strength for her age.
Comments:	None.
	Process Skills
Energy for task	Alice is physically able to do most tasks but often seems detached and does not persist in them.
Knowledge/organization of task	Alice is able to function with some error in the familiar environment of her apartment. She does sometimes miss steps of familiar tasks and is unable to organize or initiate novel tasks.
Adaptation/praxis	Alice's praxis is adequate for her age, but she is poor at imitating novel movement patterns (e.g., in dance class).
Comments:	None.

(Continued)

CASE EXAMPLE 9.2. ALICE: ALGORITHMS AND CLINICAL PATHWAYS (Cont.)

EXHIBIT 9.5.	Alice's Occupational Profile (Cont.)
Behavioral and Cognitive Skills	
Communication and following social conventions	Alice's receptive and expressive language is adequate. She follows established social conventions well but does not remember her place in conversations or whom she has already greeted.
Cognitive and emotional regulation skills	Alice is often moody or withdrawn, especially in socially or mentally challenging situations.
Level of arousal/attention	Alice is easily distracted, even in 1:1 settings.
Orientation	Alice knows her name and age but forgets events or aspects of her own personal history. She knows she is in the hospital and what town she is in, but her orientation to time is poor.
Energy and drive	For a person her age, Alice has very high energy. She has remained physically active and without regular activity becomes fidgety and agitated. She feels strongly about being active but has difficulty maintaining her focus.
Memory and understanding	Alice is able to understand simple 1-step instructions but does not anticipate problems and does not problem-solve solutions when familiar strategies do not work.
Higher level cognition	Alice has difficulty with many executive function skills, including keeping track of time, making plans, making sure work is finished on time, and looking for help or more information when it is needed.
Sensory–Perceptual Skills	
Sensory	Alice wears glasses and with them has good functional vision. She has a mild age-related hearing loss.
Self-perception	Alice is aware of her growing limitations and has expressed that she does not want to be a burden.
Pain	Alice has been dealing with mild to moderate intermittent arthritis-related pain for more than 20 years. At this time, she also has acute pain secondary to her hip fracture and surgical repair.
Skin integrity	Alice's skin is intact.
Comments:	None.

Note. Occupational profile template from American Occupational Therapy Association (2017). Analysis of participation format adapted from Skubik-Peplaski, Paris, Boyle, & Culpert (2009). ADLs = activities of daily living; AROM = active range of motion; IADLs = instrumental activities of daily living; OA = osteoarthritis; SES = socioeconomic status; SNF = skilled nursing facility.

TABLE 9.3.	Occupational Therapy Intervention Approaches by Alzheimer's Disease Stage		
APPROACH	**EARLY STAGE**	**MIDDLE STAGE**	**LATE STAGE**
Maintenance	Exercise, nutrition, cognitive stimulation, social relationships, sleep hygiene	Exercise, nutrition, activity engagement, social relationships, sleep hygiene	Exercise, nutrition, sensory stimulation, social relationships, sleep hygiene
Compensation	Memory aids, memory training, environmental modification	Memory aids, environmental modification, habits and routines	Environmental modification, habits and routines
Education	Community mobility, community safety, home safety, caregiver education	Home safety, personal safety, and positive behavioral support, caregiver education	Supervision with positive behavioral support, caregiver education

Source. From Alzheimer's Disease and Related Disorders in Occupational Therapy Practice, by P. Schaber, 2015, Brockton, MA: Western Schools, p. 39. Copyright © 2015 by Western Schools. Used with permission.

will work through an IADLs checklist and not address Alice's love of the outdoors or consider the supports already in place that meet her IADLs. Alice does need support in the form of adaptations or environmental modifications to support her growing difficulty with ADLs and executive functions.

Interventions should be directed toward client goals to meet Alice's desired outcome of returning to her apartment. While she is receiving occupational therapy intervention, Alice's responses and achievements will be monitored and documented. There should be ongoing evaluation of the intervention plan to ensure that it is effectively helping Alice progress toward the targeted outcomes. There is good reason to believe that Alice will be able to return to her apartment, because of her many strengths and family support, but her cognitive difficulties will make her rehabilitation challenging. Alice is likely to be more disoriented than usual because of the sudden changes in her situation, as well as new medication for pain. She is likely to forget instructions and precautions. In addition, she is likely to be in some emotional distress in the socially and mentally challenging environment of the SNF. The algorithm for occupational therapy intervention approaches does not offer guidance for responding to these challenges.

To develop an evidence-informed plan of care that is specific to Alice, the practitioner should pull together information from diverse sources, including the occupational profile, occupation-focused practice models, frames of reference, intervention algorithms, and foundational knowledge through clinical reasoning. This is not only the best practice approach for Alice, it also is the ethical approach. The *Occupational Therapy Code of Ethics (2015)* (AOTA, 2015) indicates that occupational therapy personnel shall "provide appropriate evaluation and a plan of intervention for recipients of occupational therapy services specific to their needs" (p. 3). The use of an intervention algorithm, such as the one presented in Table 9.3, is undeniably useful, but it will not ethically address Alice's specific needs.

Practical Reasoning

Schell and Cervero (1993) introduced the concept of *pragmatic reasoning* as an essential aspect of the clinical reasoning process. The term *pragmatic reasoning* is also used in the field of philosophy, but it has a meaning different than that proposed by Schell and Cervero. To avoid confusion, in this text we use *practical reasoning,* but the aspect of clinical reasoning under consideration is the same as that described by Schell and Cervero as pragmatic reasoning.

Practical reasoning is the use of reason to decide how to act in response to the context and pressures of the clinical environment. Practical reasoning encompasses the thought processes that influence occupational therapy

practitioners, including the impact of reimbursement regulations, productivity standards, and the relative cost to the institution of the type of intervention provided. The decisions occupational therapy practitioners make on the basis of organizational, political, and economic realities are the result of practical reasoning. Upon receiving a referral for occupational therapy services, occupational therapy practitioners are often simultaneously informed of the number of visits for which referred clients are eligible. In many settings, practitioners have little control over the occupational therapy dosage clients receive in terms of time and frequency. Practical reasoning involves making the best use of the time available in a manner that is respectful of clients' own goals.

Practical reasoning is one of the most important skills in ensuring that clients receive the best possible occupational therapy services in the context in which the services are offered. However, although it is vitally important, practical reasoning is one of the most difficult reasoning skills to teach. The difficulty lies in the myriad guidelines and policies that affect service delivery. These are often highly specific to the organization in which the occupational therapy practitioner practices.

Practical reasoning often involves reflection on ethics and ethical practice. In many cases, occupational therapy practitioners can work within institutional guidelines to provide quality ethical care. When occupational therapy practitioners are concerned that the organization's expectations are ethically challenging, they are advised to look for support from other professionals and to use professional organizations such as AOTA as sounding boards and advocates to support ethical occupational therapy practices.

INTERVENTION REVIEW

Intervention review is the iterative aspect of the intervention process. As soon as intervention begins, practitioners must consider and review the strategies used and how they affect the client's progress. The *OTPF-3* (AOTA, 2014) describes intervention review as including the following steps:

1. Reevaluating the plan and how it is implemented relative to achieving outcomes
2. Modifying the plan as needed
3. Determining the need for continuation or discontinuation of occupational therapy services and for referral to other services. (p. S16)

Intervention review is dynamic and may be grounded in activity analysis or on performance data gathered during intervention sessions. Intervention review is a continuous process of reevaluating intervention goals and the strategies used to achieve those goals. Outcome oriented, the process is grounded in data and includes collaboration with the client to achieve outcomes. The intervention review process could be used to determine whether an intervention algorithm is effective with a client or determine the need for outside referrals. In addition, the process of reevaluation and review may lead to change in the intervention plan to help better achieve the desired outcomes.

SUMMARY

Often, novice occupational therapy practitioners consider the foundational knowledge of standard treatments to be the primary resource needed to provide occupational therapy intervention. This chapter focuses instead on the complex clinical reasoning that makes intervention a highly skilled service. A clear presentation of the occupational therapy intervention strategies described in the *OTPF–3* that serve to create or promote, establish or restore, maintain, or modify occupational performance while preventing disability or disease offers the occupational therapy practitioner insight into how to compare, contrast, and integrate frames of reference and occupation-focused models into occupational therapy intervention planning.

The intervention process includes the skilled services provided by occupational therapy practitioners in collaboration with their clients. Intervention requires ongoing and complex clinical reasoning in response to both the client and the practical aspects of providing the needed intervention. The expected outcome of any occupational therapy intervention is to facilitate engagement in occupation related to health, well-being, and participation. This chapter argues that occupational therapy practitioners should not only advocate for clients but also use strategic thinking and intelligent opportunism to support the inclusion of occupational therapy services broadly and in innovative ways to respond to the demands of the practice environment. The intervention process is dynamic and complex and involves ongoing reflection and practical reasoning. Novice practitioners should locate sources of support as they face challenges in the practice setting.

LEARNING ACTIVITIES

1. Choose a case example from this text that you (on the basis of where you are in your occupational therapy education) feel you have enough background for which to build an intervention plan. Outline an occupation-based intervention plan, and clearly label preparatory methods and tasks, occupations and activities, education and training, advocacy, and group interventions. Does your plan have all of these categories? Justify your choices using a client-centered and evidence-driven argument.
2. In a short essay, explain how occupation-based practice incorporating evidence-based frames of reference

supports the position of the occupational therapy practitioner as essential to the health care team.
3. Considering the earlier discussion of expert clinical reasoning, make a table listing what you see as the pros and cons of practicing occupational therapy in a specialty area as opposed to practicing as a generalist.
4. Go to AOTA's evidence-based practice tools and resources web page (https://www.aota.org/Practice /Researchers/EBP-Resources.aspx). Summarize 3 resources that increase awareness of occupational therapy research that are relevant to a practice area of interest to you.
5. Identify a new, innovative, or nontraditional intervention approach of interest to you. Explore the available evidence supporting and refuting the use of this approach. When would you consider using this intervention? Justify your choices using a client-centered and evidence-driven argument.
6. Review the discussion of intelligent opportunism presented in this chapter. Consider current health care service trends, and outline an innovation in occupational therapy service delivery that you feel reflects intelligent opportunism.

REFERENCES

Acedo, C., & Hughes, C. (2014). Principles for learning and competences in the 21-century curriculum. *Prospects, 44,* 503–525. https://doi.org/10.1007/s11125-014-9330-1

American Occupational Therapy Association. (2014). Occupational therapy practice framework: Domain and process (3rd ed.). *American Journal of Occupational Therapy, 68*(Suppl. 1), S1–S48. https://doi.org/10.5014/ajot.2014 .682006

American Occupational Therapy Association. (2015). The occupational therapy code of ethics (2015). *American Journal of Occupational Therapy, 69*(Suppl. 3), 6913410030. https://doi.org/10.5014/ajot.2015.696S03

American Occupational Therapy Association. (2017). AOTA occupational profile template. *American Journal of Occupational Therapy, 71*(Suppl. 2), 7112420030. https://doi.org /10.5014/ajot716S12

Bullock, A., & Bannigan, K. (2011). Effectiveness of activity-based group work in community mental health: A systematic review. *American Journal of Occupational Therapy, 65*(3), 257–266. https://doi.org/10.5014/ajot.2011.001305

Collins, J., & O'Brien, N. P. (2003). *Greenwood dictionary of education*. Westport, CT: Greenwood Press.

Dhillon, S., Wilkins, S., Stewart, D., & Law, M. (2016). Understanding advocacy in action: A qualitative study. *British Journal of Occupational Therapy, 79,* 345–352. https://doi .org/10.1177/0308022615583305

Eleanor Roosevelt. (n.d.). Retrieved from https://www.brainy quote.com/quotes/eleanor_roosevelt_100940

Etymology: One trick pony. (2017). In *English language and usage.* Retrieved from https://english.stackexchange.com/questions/175620/etymology-one-trick-pony

Kielhofner, G., & Forsyth, K. (2009). Activity analysis. In E. Duncan (Ed.), *Skills for practice in occupational therapy* (pp. 91–104). Edinburgh: Churchill Livingstone.

Land, R., Cousin, G., Meyer, J. H. F., & Davies, P. (2005). Threshold concepts and troublesome knowledge: Implications for course design and evaluation. In C. Rust (Ed.), *Improving student learning: Diversity and inclusivity* (pp. 53–64). Oxford, UK: Oxford Centre for Staff and Learning Development.

LeCompte, B. (2017). *Stepping outside of the box into the world of occupation* [blogpost]. Retrieved from https://school otempowered.wordpress.com/

Liedtka, J. (1998). Linking strategic thinking with strategic planning. *Strategy and Leadership, 26*(4), 30–35.

Pellegrino, J. W., Chudowsky, N., & Glaser, R. (2001). *Knowing what students know: The science and design of educational assessment.* Washington, DC: National Academy Press.

Schaber, P. (2015). *Alzheimer's disease and related disorders in occupational therapy practice.* Brockton, MA: Western Schools. Retrieved from https://www.westernschools.com/ce-course/occupational-therapy-ce-course/alzheimers-disease-and-related-disorders-in-occupational-therapy-practice-3615.aspx

Schell, B., & Cervero, R. (1993). Clinical reasoning in occupational therapy: An integrative review. *American Journal of Occupational Therapy, 47,* 605–610. https://doi.org/10.5014/ajot.47.7.605

Skubik-Peplaski, C., Paris, C., Boyle, D., & Culpert, A. (Eds.). (2009). *Applying the* Occupational Therapy Practice Framework: *Using the Cardinal Hill Occupational Participation Process in client-centered care* (2nd ed.). Bethesda, MD: AOTA Press.

Stover, A. D. (2016). Client-centered advocacy: Every occupational therapy practitioner's responsibility to understand medical necessity. *American Journal of Occupational Therapy, 70,* 1–6. https://doi.org/10.5014/ajot.2016.705003

Thomas, H. (2015). *Occupation-based activity analysis* (2nd ed.). Thorofare, NJ: Slack.

Strategic Thinking and Outcomes

Anne Cronin, PhD, OTR/L, ATP, FAOTA, and Garth Graebe, MOT, OTR/L

10

CHAPTER HIGHLIGHTS

- Applies, analyzes, and evaluates models of occupational performance and the identification of occupation-based outcomes throughout the occupational therapy process.
- Introduces the concept of *knowledge translation*, including strategies for the evaluation of information sources.
- Provides an explanation of strategic thinking and reasoning for client-centered programs and program evaluation in occupational therapy.
- Discusses processes for quality improvement (e.g., outcome studies analysis and client engagement surveys) to ensure the quality of occupational therapy services.

KEY TERMS AND CONCEPTS

Criterion reference	Outcome measure	Relative standard
Functional outcomes	Outcomes	Service outcomes
Knowledge translation	Prospective reasoning	Strategic thinking
Normative standard	Quality of life	

Using clinical reasoning strategies introduced in this text, occupational therapy practitioners can combine and synthesize diverse data into clinical hypotheses, understand the use of occupation-focused models of practice and frames of reference, and formulate intervention plans that are client centered and evidence based. Throughout this text, readers have been challenged to adopt a reflective and holistic approach to knowledge and to use science and clinical reasoning to guide practice decisions. This chapter guides practitioners in the application of research evidence to client outcomes by defining and offering examples of knowledge translation in occupational therapy and reflective practice. Issues of accountability and quality assurance and strategic thinking in program development are addressed from a clinical reasoning framework.

OVERVIEW OF OUTCOMES AND OUTCOME MEASUREMENT

The *Occupational Therapy Practice Framework: Domain and Process* (3rd ed.; *OTPF–3;* American Occupational Therapy Association [AOTA], 2014) describes **outcomes** as the end result of the occupational therapy process. Although outcomes are indeed an end result of the occupational therapy process, a focus on desired outcomes is integral to the entire process of occupational therapy from evaluation onward. Outcomes should be a measure of function valued by both the client and the referral source (e.g., ability to dress independently, ability to return to the workplace). The final aspect of the occupational therapy process described in the *OTPF–3* is outcomes.

An **outcome measure** is a measure of the quality of medical care, the standard against which the end result of an intervention is assessed (Cronin & Mandich, 2016). Porter (2010) argued that because "value depends on results, not inputs, value in health care is measured by the outcomes" (p. 2477).

Porter discussed outcomes in health care as the results clients care most about. He noted that outcomes "are inherently condition-specific and multidimensional. For any medical condition, no single outcome captures the results of care" (p. 2477).

Law and MacDermid (2014) identified 3 reasons to measure outcomes in clinical practice:

1. To focus the client–therapist interaction on the achievement of relevant goals,
2. To improve recognition of rehabilitation's role in the health care system, and
3. To support the scientific foundations of the profession.

Including routine outcome measurement into occupational therapy practice supports client-centered care, but it also offers benefits in the areas of quality assurance, reimbursement, and program development. In addition, clearly identifying desired outcomes and the systematically measuring intervention outcomes supports intervention research. Intervention research involves the study of a systematic change in response to treatment. This type of research explores the efficacy and effectiveness of specific treatment strategies and is essential to occupational therapy. To make the outcomes more accessible to professionals outside of occupational therapy, researchers have increasingly been using overarching or global outcomes such as quality-of-life (QoL) measures rather than discipline-specific assessments to allow them to consider participation across different performance contexts.

The outcomes stage of the occupational therapy process relies on reflection. Both consumers and occupational therapy practitioners want evidence of the effectiveness of what they are doing, but many commonly used intervention strategies have limited support. When considering outcomes, practitioners must both look for measurement strategies that are sensitive to the types of performance and participation goals set by the client and reflect on the whole occupational therapy process from a professional perspective in terms of the service delivery process and quality assurance.

Documentation

Outcome measurement can be facilitated by presenting routine client documentation in a manner that allows it to serve as a data set and be used to measure the client's progress over time. Using this approach, the occupational therapy practitioner views each client as though he or she was the subject of a single-subject research design. The initial assessment and clinical hypothesis would inform the intervention decision, and the documentation of the interventions would provide the data set. Through collaborative goal setting, occupational therapy practitioners dynamically and continuously consider the efficacy of selected interventions in helping clients achieve the target goals and carefully document them. The intervention plan and outcome measures can be altered to accommodate the client's changing needs, contexts, and performance abilities. This approach offers clear information about the intervention in process but does not provide a strong form of evidence in the big picture.

Outcome Tiers

Porter (2010) described a 3-tier hierarchy of outcomes in health care:

- *Tier 1:* health status achieved or maintained
- *Tier 2:* process of recovery
- *Tier 3:* sustainability of health.

His model acknowledges the interconnectedness of all the interventions and therapy supports a client receives as a factor in determining outcomes. Although Porter focused on the system as a whole, considering his hierarchy helps occupational therapy practitioners think more broadly about outcome measures. Porter's model, adapted for occupational therapy, is presented in Figure 10.1.

Occupational therapy practitioners working in acute care may be focused on Tier 1 outcomes, which are usually highly medical and focused on impairment-level changes. In Tier 1, improvements in endurance, ADLs and strength are the desired outcomes. These Tier 1 outcomes are supportive of health but may not, by themselves, result in improved performance and participation in the client's natural setting. *Functional outcomes* are

---

FIGURE 10.1.   Occupational therapy adaptation of Porter's (2010) outcome measures hierarchy.

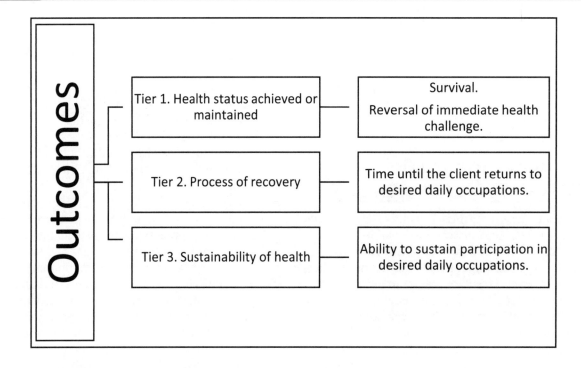

those outcomes that measure the client's ability to return to daily occupations; although Tier 1 outcomes may not be considered functional, outcomes at the remaining levels should be functional.

Tier 2 outcomes focus on recovery and the performance of desired daily occupations, and they include outcomes that are similar across practice areas. Tier 2 includes occupational performance outcomes, which are often focused on working toward the greatest possible level of independence in ADLs and IADLs. Table 10.1 presents this category of outcomes as they are described in the *OTPF–3*.

TABLE 10.1.	Tier 2 Occupational Performance Outcomes	
CATEGORY	**DESCRIPTION**	**EXAMPLES**
Occupational performance	Act of doing and accomplishing a selected action (performance skill), activity, or occupation (Fisher, 2009; Fisher & Griswold, 2014; Kielhofner, 2008) and results from the dynamic transaction among the client, the context, and the activity. Improving or enabling skills and patterns in occupational performance leads to engagement in occupations or activities (adapted in part from Law et al., 1996, p. 16).	See "Improvement" and "Enhancement," below.
Improvement	Outcomes targeted when a performance limitation is present. These outcomes reflect increased occupational performance for the person, group, or population.	▪ A child with autism playing interactively with a peer (person). ▪ An older adult returning to a desired living situation in the home from a SNF (person). ▪ Decreased incidence of back strain in nursing personnel as a result of an in-service education program in body mechanics for carrying out job duties that require bending, lifting, and so forth (group). ▪ Construction of accessible playground facilities for all children in local city parks (population).
Enhancement	Outcomes targeted when a performance limitation is not currently present. These outcomes reflect the development of performance skills and performance patterns that augment existing performance in life occupations.	▪ Increased confidence and competence of teenage mothers in parenting their children as a result of structured social groups and child development classes (person). ▪ Increased membership in the local senior citizen center as a result of expanding social wellness and exercise programs (group). ▪ Increased ability of school staff to address and manage school-age youth violence as a result of conflict resolution training to address bullying (group). ▪ Increased opportunities for older adults to participate in community activities through ride-share programs (population).
Prevention	Education or health promotion efforts designed to identify, reduce, or prevent the onset and reduce the incidence of unhealthy conditions, risk factors, diseases, or injuries (AOTA, 2014). Occupational therapy promotes a healthy lifestyle at the individual, group, community (societal), and governmental or policy level (AOTA, 2001).	▪ Appropriate seating and play area for a child with orthopedic impairments (person). ▪ Implementation of a program of leisure and educational activities for a drop-in center for adults with severe mental illness (group). ▪ Access to occupational therapy services in underserved areas regardless of cultural or ethnic background (population).

Source. From *Occupational Therapy Practice Framework: Domain and Process* (3rd ed.), by the American Occupational Therapy Association, 2014, *American Journal of Occupational Therapy,* Vol. 68, Suppl. 1, p. S34. Copyright © 2014 by the American Occupational Therapy Association. Used with permission.
Note. AOTA = American Occupational Therapy Association; SNF = skilled nursing facility.

TABLE 10.2.   Occupational Performance Outcomes

CATEGORY	DESCRIPTION	EXAMPLES
Quality of life	Dynamic appraisal of the client's life satisfaction (perceptions of progress toward goals), hope (real or perceived belief that one can move toward a goal through selected pathways), self-concept (the composite of beliefs and feelings about oneself), health and functioning (e.g., health status, self-care capabilities), and socioeconomic factors (e.g., vocation, education, income; adapted from Radomski, 1995).	▪ Full and active participation of a deaf child from a hearing family during a recreational activity (person). ▪ Residents being able to prepare for outings and travel independently as a result of independent living skills training for care providers (group). ▪ Formation of a lobby to support opportunities for social networking, advocacy activities, and sharing of scientific information for stroke survivors and their families (population).
Participation	Engagement in desired occupations in ways that are personally satisfying and congruent with expectations within the culture.	▪ A person recovering the ability to perform the essential duties of his or her job after a flexor tendon laceration (person). ▪ A family enjoying a vacation while traveling cross-country in their adapted van (group). ▪ All children within a state having access to school sports programs (population).
Role competence	Ability to effectively meet the demands of roles in which the client engages.	▪ An individual with CP being able to take notes or type papers to meet the demands of the student role (person). ▪ Implementation of job rotation at a factory that allows sharing of higher demand tasks to meet the demands of the worker role (group). ▪ Improved accessibility of polling places to all people with disabilities to meet the demands of the citizen role (population).
Well-being	Contentment with one's health, self-esteem, sense of belonging, security, and opportunities for self-determination, meaning, roles, and helping others (Hammell, 2009). *Well-being* is "a general term encompassing the total universe of human life domains, including physical, mental, and social aspects" (WHO, 2006, p. 211).	▪ A person with ALS being content with his ability to find meaning in fulfilling the role of father through compensatory strategies and environmental modifications (person). ▪ Members of an outpatient depression and anxiety support group feeling secure in their sense of group belonging and ability to help other members (group). ▪ Residents of a town celebrating the groundbreaking of a school during reconstruction after a natural disaster (population).
Occupational justice	Access to and participation in the full range of meaningful and enriching occupations afforded to others, including opportunities for social inclusion and the resources to participate in occupations to satisfy personal, health, and societal needs (adapted from Townsend & Wilcock, 2004).	▪ An individual with an IDD serving on an advisory board to establish programs offered by a community recreation center (person). ▪ Workers having enough break time to have lunch with their young children in their day care center (group). ▪ Increased sense of empowerment and self-advocacy skills for people with persistent mental illness, enabling them to develop an anti-stigma campaign promoting engagement in the civic arena (group) and alternative adapted housing options for older adults to age in place (population).

Source. From "Occupational Therapy Practice Framework: Domain and Process (3rd ed.)," by the American Occupational Therapy Association, 2014, *American Journal of Occupational Therapy,* Vol. 68, Suppl. 1, pp. S34–S35. Copyright © 2017 by the American Occupational Therapy Association. Used with permission.

Note. ALS = amyotrophic lateral sclerosis; CP = cerebral palsy; IDD = intellectual and developmental disabilities; WHO = World Health Organization.

Tier 3 outcomes are also inherently functional. The distinction between the tiers is sometimes blurred; for instance, as you may have noted, ADL performance is included in both Tier 1 and Tier 2 outcomes. The *OTPF–3* defines several additional types of outcomes (see Table 10.2). Note that many of these outcomes, including prevention, health and wellness, participation, and role competence, are commonly a focus of both Tier 2 and Tier 3 outcomes within the occupational therapy process. The remaining outcomes listed in the *OTPF–3* are QoL, well-being, and occupational justice. These outcomes are ideals in all tiers of care and are difficult to capture in Porter's (2010) hierarchy.

Considering Porter's hierarchy and using occupation-based clinical reasoning, the ideal outcome measure is a measure of participation. Although this seems obvious, participation is often difficult to assess, especially for occupational therapy practitioners practicing in Tier 1 medical settings such as hospitals and outpatient clinics. In these settings, the initial evaluation of participation comes from client report, and occupational therapy practitioners in these settings are unable to directly assess participation in natural environments while their clients are involved in the intervention process.

There is a widespread clinical belief that improvement in body structures and functions by itself leads to an improvement in participation, but this has not been convincingly demonstrated in the literature. Sullivan and Cen (2011) reported that the direct effect of impairment on participation was not statistically significant, but its indirect effect through activity was significant. Improved strength or range of motion (ROM) is not a functional outcome.

Similarly, Law and MacDermid (2014) reported that "agreement between clinician-based outcomes (particularly at the impairment level) and self-reported measures of pain and disability has been shown to be only moderate across a wide spectrum of patient problems" (p. 76). This finding suggests that occupational therapy practitioners should take extra care with their planning and choice of outcome measures to be certain that their intervention does have a positive effect on client outcomes.

OUTCOME MEASUREMENT: HYPOTHESES, FRAMES OF REFERENCE, AND THEORY

Selected outcome measures should be directly related to the clinical hypothesis that has been developed and refined throughout the occupational therapy process. The clinical hypothesis is tested and clarified, and measured outcomes reflect this refined hypothesis.

Measurement Standards

Many valid and reliable measurement tools are available to occupational therapy practitioners, but most of these tools measure impairment levels rather than functional outcomes. It is often these measures of impairment that are included in standard documentation. Examples of such measures would be pain scales and measurements of ROM.

Normative standard

One approach to outcome measurement is to assume that if the client's performance on tests of impairment falls within a normative range, called the **normative standard,** then function automatically results. Using the normative standard involves comparing the client's functional performance with that of the population at large. This approach may work in cases of acute injury, but it is less effective in evaluating outcomes for persons with developmental differences or with a chronic condition.

Relative standard

More widely used in rehabilitation and with persons with a disability is the measurement of outcomes on a **relative standard.** In this case, clients serve as their own measure of success, and the data document change from a functional baseline. A widely used measurement associated with the relative standard is the Canadian Occupational Performance Measure (COPM; Law et al., 2014). In this assessment, clients identify personal goals, rate their current performance on those goals, and then set priorities for goal achievement. The COPM allows a basic numerical analysis of progress, but goals are unique to the client and progress is based on self-perception. Clients cannot be compared with each other using this approach because the goals and the values guiding intervention are unique to each client.

Criterion reference

Another measurement option, and one used in all occupational therapy practice settings, is the **criterion reference.** Criterion-referenced measurements are designed to measure performance against a fixed set of predetermined criteria. The easiest example of this is the standard ADL assessment. These assessments often consist of a checklist of skills that the client can or cannot successfully perform. The checklist may include a very general statement, such as "client feeds self independently," or they may include specific details, such as the time needed to complete the task, the ability to manage a variety of food textures, the ability to manage utensils, and the ability to function in different mealtime environments.

Quality of life

A final approach to outcome measurement is the use of QoL outcomes. In general, **QoL** is the self-perceived evaluation of daily life with a focus on the person's expectations and sense of well-being. Typically, QoL scales consider emotional, social, and physical aspects of the client's life rather than specific performance skills or rehabilitation outcomes. In health care, a health-related QoL assessment considers how the client's well-being may be affected over time by a disease, disability, or disorder. This type of measure has been important in research but is less clinically applicable because many factors other than response to intervention may influence the perception of QoL.

Comparison Results

Outcome measurement has become a growing focus of research, program planning, quality assurance, and policy decisions. More so than any other aspect of the occupational therapy process, outcome measures may be assigned at a program or an institutional level. The reason for this is that use of a standardized tool allows the comparison of results across multiple clients and multiple settings. Outcome data can be pooled to create a very large data set that can be used to analyze outcomes with a high degree of statistical confidence. An example of this is the widespread use of the FIM® (Keith, Granger, Hamilton, & Sherwin, 1987; Uniform Data System for Medical Rehabilitation, 1997). The FIM is a brief criterion-referenced test that provides a uniform system of measurement for disability. The FIM specifically measures the level of a person's disability and indicates how much assistance is required for the person to carry out ADLs. The FIM was designed to be used in inpatient rehabilitation settings (Tier 2), and this is the context in which it is most useful.

Using the FIM as an outcome measure in rehabilitation is supported by science, and it is widely promoted at the institutional level because of the rigorous data that can be generated, but it does have many notable limitations. The most widely cited limitation is that it lacks depth and discriminative ability in the areas of communication and cognition (Salter et al., 2017). Human occupation cannot be evaluated without careful consideration of the impact of cognition and communication on performance and participation. This limits the FIM's ability to fully reflect the outcomes of occupational therapy intervention. Because FIM scores are commonly used to evaluate not only clients but also rehabilitation programs, overreliance on this measure may lead to a lack of recognition of occupational therapy's unique contributions. Occupational therapy practitioners should be sensitive to the idea that the FIM may not fully reflect the outcomes of occupational therapy intervention and should consider additional outcome measures to support the client's transition to the community as well as to support the practitioner's own program.

Selecting Outcome Measures

Law and MacDermid (2014) offered guidance for the clinician in selecting outcome measures for clinical practice that are sensitive to practice setting. The process that these authors recommended is summarized in Table 10.3.

The FIM is only one of the widely used functional outcome measures. Like the FIM, the Disabilities of the Arm, Shoulder and Hand (DASH; Hudak et al., 1996) outcome measure is a self-report questionnaire designed to measure physical function and symptoms in patients with any of several musculoskeletal disorders of the upper limb (Institute for Work and Health, 2013). The DASH can be used to measure functional outcomes, but it should be used with specific reflection on the client's identified goals. The use of the DASH as a functional outcome measure is illustrated in the case of Saffiyah (see Case Example 10.1).

TABLE 10.3.   Process of Selecting an Outcome Measure

STRATEGY	JUSTIFICATION
Use a science-driven frame of reference to identify what it is important to measure.	Focuses you on client issues and goals rather than on specific changes in structure or function.
Search for recent scientific articles that address treatment effectiveness in a similar client population, especially those using a congruent frame of reference.	Offers current insights and allows you to learn from the experiences of others.
After completing Step 2, remove any outcome measures reported that are not standardized or clearly not suited to your purpose.	Ensures that the measures you choose will be replicable and that you can compare the results across time and across clients.
Use a standard process to rate the clinical utility of the selected outcome measures.	An example of such a process was published by CanChild (2004), which allows you to determine whether the instrument can evaluate change, discriminate, or predict in the manner required for your population.
Obtain the measures of interest and explore scoring and administration guidelines.	Explores usability and at the same time identifies copyright and cost for clinical use.
Pilot test the selected instruments.	Devises and documents an implementation strategy and ascertains the measure's performance and feasibility in your setting.

Note. Strategies from Law & MacDermid (2014).

CASE EXAMPLE 10.1. SAFFIYAH: RIGHT-WRIST FRACTURE

Saffiyah is age 50 years and is a mother of 3 who has been working as an office manager. Following an injury, her usual occupations were disrupted. Exhibit 10.1 presents Saffiyah's occupational profile.

Saffiyah was seen by an occupational therapy practitioner who is a certified hand therapist. A *certified hand therapist* is a specialized expert clinician who is either an occupational therapy practitioner or a physical therapist with a minimum of 3 years of clinical experience, including 4,000 hours or more in direct practice in hand therapy, and who has passed a comprehensive test of advanced clinical skills and theory in upper-quarter rehabilitation.

Even in highly specialized practices, occupational therapy practitioners consider the domain of occupational therapy and have a focus on occupation in outcome measures. Saffiyah wants to resume full duty at her workplace. The DASH will not measure whether this has occurred. Similarly, she wants to resume cooking, crocheting, and kayaking. An improved score on the DASH may correlate with return to desired activities, but the practitioner should not assume this.

EXHIBIT 10.1.	Saffiyah's Occupational Profile		
Client	**Reason the client is seeking service and concerns related to engagement in occupations**	Referred to occupational therapy hand therapy secondary to right wrist fracture. *Impact on occupation:* Saffiyah reports that she is right hand dominant. She is experiencing limitations in cooking, cleaning, and her job as an office manager.	
	Occupations in which the client is successful	Mother, spouse, friend, and worker.	
	Personal interests and values	Saffiyah enjoys spending time with her family, and she is proud of her work role. Her interests include cooking, crocheting, and kayaking.	
	Occupational history (i.e., life experiences)	Saffiyah reports that the injury occurred when she fell off a motorcycle while riding with her husband. She explained that she immediately went to the emergency department and underwent surgical repair of the distal radius the next day. Saffiyah reports she wore a cast for 6 weeks. The cast was removed 1 week ago, and she is currently wearing a prefabricated wrist immobilization orthosis for support. She noted that her physician instructed her to wear the splint for support when lifting and carrying objects and when out in public. She is permitted to remove the splint for therapy and while at home. While casted, she had to return to the physician's office numerous times because of edema exacerbations, especially in her fingers, which were not casted. She has no other comorbidities.	
	Performance patterns (routines, roles, habits, & rituals)	Saffiyah is a wife and mother; 2 of her 3 children are adults and have moved out of the home. Another child, a teenager, remains at home. Saffiyah's husband and teenage child are available to assist with difficult tasks at this time. She was released to return to work on light duty while the cast was still in place. She remains on light duty at this time.	
Environment		*Supports to occupational engagement*	*Barriers to occupational engagement*
	Physical (e.g., buildings, furniture, pets)	Saffiyah has no mobility limitations.	Managing doors, and carrying things are challenging at this time.
	Social (e.g., spouse, friends, caregivers)	Her family is very supportive. Her husband has taken over most household tasks.	

(Continued)

CASE EXAMPLE 10.1. SAFFIYAH: RIGHT-WRIST FRACTURE *(Cont.)*

EXHIBIT 10.1. Saffiyah's Occupational Profile *(Cont.)*

Context	Cultural (e.g., customs, beliefs)	Naturalized American originally from Pakistan. No issues related to culture, customs, or beliefs were identified during assessment.	
	Personal (e.g., age, gender, SES, education)	50-year-old female with a bachelor's degree.	
	Temporal (e.g., stage of life, time, year)	Middle adulthood. Employed.	
	Virtual (e.g., chat, email, remote monitoring)	Saffiyah uses communication tools such as a smartphone and computer.	She is limited to left-hand use, which is time consuming and frustrating.
Client goals	Client's priorities and desired targeted outcomes	Saffiyah enjoys her job and is currently on light duty. She wants to resume full duty as soon as possible.	

ANALYSIS OF PARTICIPATION

Basic ADLs

Eating/oral–motor	While casted, Saffiyah fed herself with her left hand. She is unable to hold utensils with her right hand at this time.
Grooming	Saffiyah reports that she cannot use a curling iron to style her hair and has been brushing her teeth with her left hand. She noted that she is unable to hold a mascara wand.
Bathing/transfer	Saffiyah reports that she is independent in showering. She cannot take a bath at this time because she is unable to weight bear through her right wrist and therefore cannot stand up from a seated position in the bathtub.
Dressing upper body	Saffiyah reports that she has a difficult time donning and doffing her bra. Her husband has been helping her complete this task, but she is anxious to resume this task herself.
Dressing lower body	Saffiyah is unable to button pants or tie shoelaces.
Toileting	Saffiyah is using her left hand for toilet hygiene.
Problem-solving/memory	Saffiyah has no limitation in this area.
Comments:	Saffiyah's work tasks include computer use, writing checks, and completing paperwork.

IADLs

Community mobility	Saffiyah is able to use her left hand to start the ignition in her car. She feels comfortable driving for short distances.
Health management/prevention	Saffiyah is active and enjoys being outdoors. She strives to achieve 10,000 steps each day.
Home management	Saffiyah requires assistance for home management, including vacuuming and cleaning.
Financial management	Saffiyah's husband is responsible for home finances.
Leisure/play	Saffiyah is currently unable to complete her leisure activities of crocheting and kayaking.
Safety	There are no safety concerns.
Comments:	On initial assessment, Saffiyah scored 82% on the DASH (0%–20% = *normal;* 20%–40% = *mild disability;* 40%–60% = *moderate disability;* and 60%–80% = *severe disability*). Specific hand measures are as follows: Right hand AROM (in degrees): wrist flexion, 10; wrist extension, 5; radial deviation, 0; ulnar deviation, 2; pronation, 75; supination, 10.

(Continued)

CASE EXAMPLE 10.1. SAFFIYAH: RIGHT-WRIST FRACTURE *(Cont.)*

EXHIBIT 10.1. Saffiyah's Occupational Profile *(Cont.)*

	Elbow: WFL in flexion and extension.
	Shoulder: WFL in all planes.
	Digit AROM (recorded in extension/flexion; negative numbers indicate extension lag): Thumb—IP, 0/10; MCP, 0/14; opposition—unable to oppose to any fingertips; Digit 2—MCP, −20/35; PIP, −10/20; DIP, 0/15; Digit 3—MCP, −22/27; PIP, −12/25; DIP, 0/19; Digit 4—MCP, −20/29; PIP, −7/19; DIP, 0/13; Digit 5—MCP, −5/15; PIP, −5/19; DIP, 0/10.
	Circumferential measurements: wrist crease, R = 18.9 cm, L = 16.2 cm; distal palmar crease, R = 24.8 cm, L = 20.9 cm; right middle proximal phalanx Digit 3, R = 7.1 cm, L = 6.0 cm.
Motor and Praxis Skills	
Sitting—static/dynamic	Independent.
Standing—static/dynamic	Independent.
Joint stability and skeletal mobility	No concerns.
Place can on shelf	Saffiyah is able to complete this with her left hand only. She is unable to wrap the fingers of her right hand around the can.
Retrieve item from floor	Saffiyah is able to complete this with her left hand only.
Screw lid on jar	Saffiyah is able to complete this with left hand only. She has very limited AROM in wrist radial and ulnar deviation and limitations with finger AROM secondary to edema.
Comb back of head	Saffiyah is able to complete this with her left hand only because she cannot hold a brush or comb.
Writing	Unable to hold a writing implement.
Lift grocery bag	Unable to carry anything at this time with right hand.
Coordination	Before injury, no coordination limitations. Currently, Saffiyah is unable to complete bilateral hand tasks.
Manipulation	Given significant finger stiffness, Saffiyah is unable to manipulate any objects with her right hand.
Comments:	None.
Process Skills	
Energy for task	No concerns.
Knowledge/organization of task	No concerns.
Adaptation/praxis	No concerns.
Behavioral and Cognitive Skills	
Communication and following social conventions	Saffiyah enjoys texting, emailing, and using social media to keep in contact with her friends and family. She is able to use the touch screen on her iPad.
Cognitive and emotional regulation skills	No concerns.
Level of arousal/attention	No concerns.
Orientation	Alert and oriented to person, place, time, and event.
Memory and understanding	No concerns.
Energy and drive	Saffiyah is very motivated to return to full duty at work. She is also motivated to resume her usual ADLs and IADLs.
Higher level cognition	No concerns.

(Continued)

CASE EXAMPLE 10.1. SAFFIYAH: RIGHT-WRIST FRACTURE (Cont.)

EXHIBIT 10.1. Saffiyah's Occupational Profile (Cont.)

Sensory–Perceptual Skills	
Sensory	Intact basic sensory function.
Self-perception	No concerns.
Pain	Pain 4/10 at rest and 8/10 with use.
Skin integrity	Postsurgical incision well approximated on volar surface of right wrist. No signs or symptoms of infection. Scar is adherent, especially on the distal aspect of the scar. Hypersensitivity along the scar line.
Comments:	None.

Note. Occupational profile template from American Occupational Therapy Association (2017). Analysis of participation format adapted from Skubik-Peplaski, Paris, Boyle, & Culpert (2009). ADLs = activities of daily living; AROM = active range of motion; DASH = Disabilities of the Arm, Shoulder and Hand; DIP = distal interphalangeal; IADLs = instrumental activities of daily living; IP = interphalangeal; L = left; MCP = metacarpophalangeal; PIP = proximal interphalangeal; R = right; WFL = within functional limits.

KNOWLEDGE TRANSLATION

An essential part of the clinical reasoning process is the application of knowledge. Knowledge is acquired throughout life, and the process of occupational therapy education is to build a foundation of knowledge to inform clinical reasoning and critical thinking.

Earlier in this text, we distinguished between novice practitioners, who are new to the field and have only foundational knowledge, and expert practitioners. Experts have accumulated knowledge from a variety of sources and have a richer well of data available to the clinical reasoning process. Experts are more likely to quickly formulate algorithms and heuristics to delve quickly into complex reasoning. Insight is the tool most available to expert practitioners. It is insight that helps bring together seemingly disparate things, such as science and everyday life, as noted in Practice Wisdom 10.1.

Knowledge translation is a "dynamic and iterative process that includes synthesis, dissemination, exchange and ethically-sound application of knowledge to improve the health of [people], provide more effective health services and products and strengthen the health care system" (Canadian Institutes of Health Research, 2010, para. 4). It is a process that converts scientific findings and scholarly knowledge into a form that is meaningful and useful to the occupational therapy practitioner.

Knowledge translation includes any process that contributes to the integration of evidence-based information into the practice of occupational therapy practitioners to improve the health and participation outcomes of their clients. In occupational therapy, knowledge translation maximizes the understanding and appropriate use of occupational therapy in both the health care system and the community.

It is widely accepted that a research–practice gap exists in all aspects of health care, including occupational therapy. Some of the occupational therapy gaps that have been mentioned in this text are the persistence of some older theoretical models (e.g., neurodevelopmental therapy) and hasty generalization that led to the expansion of clinical interventions in the sensory integration frame of reference that are not supported by the evidence. It is likely that these practices persist in part because occupational therapy practitioners view them as the best option in terms of client needs and believe them to be both cost- and clinically effective. However, another reason for their persistence is poor knowledge translation.

Challenges

Although all occupational therapy practitioners are guided in acquiring the skills to locate, analyze, and critique scholarly literature to support evidence-based decision making as a part of their entry-level education, once practitioners are working in a clinical setting, it is often difficult for them to keep up with current literature. Knowledge translation is the process that filters new scientific findings in terms of their utility and applicability in actual clinical settings. Through practical reasoning, occupational therapy practitioners may reasonably reject some science-driven findings because they are based on high-therapy-dose clinical trials that cannot

PRACTICE WISDOM 10.1.   Science and Everyday Life

"Science and everyday life cannot and should not be separated."
—*Rosalind Franklin (as cited in Maddox, 2002)*

be duplicated in the clinic. In other cases, science-driven findings may be rejected because they require additional extra resources, highly specialized training, or specialty certification that is not available to the occupational therapy practitioner. The best approach is to use studies focused on the effectiveness of specific occupational therapy interventions, but these are unfortunately relatively few, and those that exist are seldom done in the usual care environment.

Analyzing Research

A skill basic to knowledge translation is the ability to analyze and assess clinical research. Occupational therapy practitioners seeking to understand and keep up with the growth of science must be able to do more than read research articles. They must analyze them in terms of their utility, assumptions, implications, and ethics. Hawkins, Elder, and Paul (2010) described aspects basic to effective analysis of clinical research (see Table 10.4).

The Internet offers great access to information from diverse sources, but it can be challenging to systematically consider all the information on a specific topic. This is where the support of organizations and practice groups can be of great value. Some clinical settings encourage the development of "journal clubs" so that clinicians can systematically review topics relevant to the interprofessional team in the context of their own practice constraints.

Most professional organizations, including AOTA, are committed to supporting practitioners and provide concise fact sheets and critically appraised topic reviews to help practitioners assimilate research findings. These resources are intended to facilitate knowledge translation and to assist occupational therapy practitioners in identifying clinical outcomes that are valued by the client, the occupational therapy practitioner, and the larger infrastructure supporting service provision. It is important that outcomes be considered in terms of both the individual client and occupational therapy practice in general.

TABLE 10.4. Analyzing Clinical Research		
CRITERIA	**STANDARDS**	**COMMON PROBLEMS**
All clinical research has a purpose.	The purpose should be reflected in the research question or hypothesis and should constrain the scope of the study to an answerable question.	The purpose of the question guiding the study is unclear. The question is insignificant to the clinical problem you are exploring. The scope of the study is insufficient to apply it in a clinical setting.
All clinical research identifies data, information, and evidence relevant to the purpose.	Conclusions should be drawn only to the extent they are supported by data and sound reasoning.	The measurement strategies are unclear or involve tools or approaches that are not widely available or are inconsistent with clinical expectations. Anomalous data are accepted without association to the whole of scientific knowledge.
All reasoning contains inferences from which one draws conclusions that gives meaning to the data.	Reasoning can only be as sound as the inferences it makes, and the conclusions reached should logically follow from the evidence.	Inferences may be based on preexisting assumptions or beliefs rather than the data. Inferences may be superficial rather than inclusive of the scope of current knowledge. Data are excluded because they are not consistent with the beliefs of the thinker.
All reasoning is influenced by the assumptions of the reasoner.	Skilled thinkers constantly seek to discern and understand their own assumptions and how they interface with the point of view of the authors.	Preexisting assumptions are not considered or identified. Thinkers may cherry-pick only those findings that support their established viewpoint. New ideas may be disregarded or dismissed if they are inconsistent with thinkers' assumptions.
All reasoning, when acted on, has consequences.	Skilled thinkers consider both potentially negative and potentially positive consequences of their reasoning.	Thinkers may consider only the consequence or outcome they had in mind at the beginning. There may be unexpected outcomes, such as increased costs to the client.

STRATEGIC THINKING

This text focuses on clinical reasoning, a process by which practitioners collect data, process information, and come to an understanding of a presenting problem or situation. Practitioners then use critical thinking to plan and implement interventions, evaluate outcomes, and reflect on and learn from the process. This reasoning process can be broadened when considering other projects such as program development, quality assurance measures, or prevention programs. The practitioner needs to think strategically. Strategic thinking differs from clinical reasoning in that it focuses on the future rather than the present.

Because outcome measures have so many uses, they are invaluable tools to support **strategic thinking.** Recall the 5 major attributes of strategic thinking Liedtka (1998) proposed: (1) having a systems perspective, (2) being hypothesis driven, (3) including a focus on intent, (4) incorporating a historical perspective, and (5) involving intelligent opportunism.

The first step of problem solving, identifying the problem, aligns with Liedtka's systems perspective. A strategic thinker focuses first on deeply understanding the problem at hand, thinking more broadly than intervention algorithms and approaches, and instead considers ways in which the dysfunction, as experienced by the client, limits engagement in occupational pursuits. Identifying the problem is often the part of strategic thinking that takes the most time, because most clinical problems are multifactorial and involve not just a clinical presentation but also an interprofessional team, institutional policies, and evidence-based practice considerations. Problems to be considered may be client-specific problems, and they may also include problems in service delivery or program implementation. By understanding both desired and actual outcomes, strategic thinkers can aspire to change things for the better.

In clinical practice, occupational therapy practitioners first gain an understanding of clients through the occupational profile. At this point, the practitioner must consider established procedures for responding to specific problems. These procedures may be algorithm-based clinical pathways that reflect scientific reasoning, or they may be less formal guidelines directing the expected intervention process for the client. Effective occupational therapy practitioners must be client centered and as well as able to effectively look beyond the client for conditions that may affect outcomes. Outcomes inform future actions and changes in approaches to improve desired outcomes.

PROSPECTIVE REASONING

Reflective practice melds experiential knowledge with that drawn from science and theory to support professional and personal development. While working in the present, occupational therapy practitioners must be able to evaluate outcomes and project their reasoning into the future to consider and plan specific prospective factors that may affect the client's future. **Prospective reasoning** is small-scale strategic thinking that considers what might be ahead for clients. Using prospective reasoning, occupational therapy practitioners consider a client's condition and how it affects participation in valued occupations. (*Note.* In some occupational therapy literature, this type of reasoning is called *conditional reasoning.* In this text, we have chosen the term *prospective* rather than *conditional* to distinguish it from conditional reasoning as described in the field of logic.)

To bring the unique value of occupational therapy to the client, occupational therapy practitioners focus on what is already known but, more important, seek to know what is not yet known (i.e., what needs to be understood by way of the occupational therapy lens) by using prospective reasoning. The inclusion of prevention and wellness interventions in Porter's (2010) Tier 2 recovery outcomes is an example of this forward-looking prospective reasoning. Prospective reasoning can also support program development, such as the inclusion of occupational therapy services in a cancer survivorship clinic or in advocacy activities to support health care legislation that best meets clients' needs.

Fleming (1994) described *prospective reasoning* (which she labeled *conditional reasoning*) as having 3 aspects:

1. Thought about the whole condition, including the person, the illness, the meaning the illness has for the person, the family, and the social and physical contexts in which the person lives;
2. Informed vision of how the condition could change and become a revised condition; and
3. Client's perspective of personal success, measured on the basis of the mentally constructed image of possible outcomes.

Prospective reasoning is illustrated in Case Example 10.2.

Prospective reasoning requires practitioners to look beyond the immediate and prepare for the "maybe" that the client could face. Clearly, practitioners cannot prepare for all maybes, but when a clear path is expected, such as with a medical diagnosis of a degenerative condition, outcome expectations are affected by the condition's trajectory. Although outcomes reflect the end of the intervention process, outcome measures are selected early in the evaluation stage. These outcome measures should ideally be valid, reliable, and appropriately sensitive to change in clients' occupational performance. Outcome goals should be realistic and congruent with clients' own goals and priorities.

Well-chosen outcome measures can be used to measure progress and adjust both intervention goals and the intervention approach by comparing progress toward goal achievement to desired outcomes. In Chapters 3 and 4 of this text, cases were presented in which the

CASE EXAMPLE 10.2. PATRICIA: AT

Patricia, age 60 years, has ALS. As a person living with a serious and progressive condition, Patricia's goals and values have a different focus than those of someone expecting a return to typical functioning. Exhibit 10.2 details Patricia's occupational profile.

The occupational therapy practitioner must be sensitive to Patricia's psychological needs. Although Patricia and her husband are focused on a short-term solution for Patricia's inability to use their current telephone, the practitioner must take a longer view of her situation because of the progressive nature of her disease. The practitioner's intervention involved 2 basic assumptions: (1) Patricia is motivated to continue to do as much as possible for herself, and (2) Patricia's abilities will deteriorate as her disease progresses. The intervention included a significant amount of education and an emphasis on basic ADLs and IADLs.

The occupational therapy practitioner helped Patricia understand the potential impact of her condition and tools to alter that impact through equipment demonstration. Using this strategy, the practitioner was able to show Patricia that adaptive equipment was simply a tool to help her manage her fatigue. This also helped provide Patricia with an informed vision of how her condition might change, in terms of both disease progression and strategies to maximize occupational participation.

By using work simplification and energy conservation techniques, Patricia was able to engage in more daily activities that were important to her. This helped her to begin to resolve some of the role conflict that she was experiencing. Additionally, by adopting AT early, Patricia had less difficulty learning to use devices and was able to become proficient in less time than if she had waited until they were a necessity. This also gave Patricia some perception of her own potential to affect her own role participation and helped her consider some adapted means of participation as acceptable.

EXHIBIT 10.2.	**Patricia's Occupational Profile**	
Client	**Reason the client is seeking service and concerns related to engagement in occupations**	Referred to occupational therapy for AT evaluation and recommendation. *Impact on occupation:* Patricia has been having difficulty using the telephone and is often home alone, creating a safety concern.
	Occupations in which the client is successful	Spouse, friend, parent.
	Personal interests and values	Patricia has limited her activities but has enjoyed entertaining and hosting parties. She loves reading and enjoys watching sports on TV.
	Occupational history (i.e., life experiences)	Patricia was diagnosed with ALS 12 years ago. The disease has progressed to the point at which she is often unable to use her hands in a coordinated fashion and sometimes requires a manual wheelchair for mobility. At other times, she can ambulate with a front-wheeled walker.
	Performance patterns (routines, roles, habits, & rituals)	*Occupational roles:* Patricia has always been a homemaker. Her 2 children, ages 31 and 28 years, do not live in the same state as Patricia and her husband. Patricia typically did most of the household tasks, but as her disease has progressed, her husband has taken over the cooking, and they have hired a cleaner.
Environment		***Supports to occupational engagement***	***Barriers to occupational engagement***
	Physical (e.g., buildings, furniture, pets)	Patricia manages within her home with a walker. Her home is on 1 floor so that stairs are not a problem.	Patricia tires easily and is dependent in community mobility.
	Social (e.g., spouse, friends, caregivers)	Patricia lives with her husband who has helped adapt the home to meet her needs. Patricia also has a cleaner who comes once a week to help with the tasks that she cannot manage.	Her husband works full-time, which leaves Patricia alone at home during the workday.

(Continued)

CASE EXAMPLE 10.2. PATRICIA: AT *(Cont.)*

EXHIBIT 10.2.	Patricia's Occupational Profile *(Cont.)*		
Context	**Cultural** (e.g., customs, beliefs)	No cultural issues were identified.	Patricia has always been proud of her role as homemaker. She does not like losing this role.
	Personal (e.g., age, gender, SES, education)	60-year-old female. Patricia has a college degree and is in a middle-income bracket.	
	Temporal (e.g., stage of life, time, year)	Middle adulthood.	
	Virtual (e.g., chat, email, remote monitoring)	Patricia uses social media to keep up with friends and family.	
Client goals	**Client's priorities and desired targeted outcomes**	Patricia would like to be as independent as possible for as long as possible.	

ANALYSIS OF PARTICIPATION

Basic ADLs

Eating/oral–motor	Patricia is able to feed herself, but it requires a lot of time, and she has difficulty manipulating utensils.
Grooming	Patricia denies any difficulty in this area, although she clearly struggles with hair care and makeup application.
Bathing/transfer	Patricia sometimes requires her husband's help to transfer in and out of the shower. She has a shower chair and a hand shower and can usually manage her bathing.
Dressing upper body	Patricia cannot manage most clothing fasteners, so she has limited her wardrobe to pullover shirts.
Dressing lower body	Patricia cannot manage most clothing fasteners, so she has limited her wardrobe to pants with an elastic waistband. She wears slip-on shoes and sandals.
Toileting	Patricia has no significant difficulty in this area. She has grab bars and a raised toilet seat that she uses.
Problem-solving/memory	Patricia has no difficulty in this area.
Comments:	Patricia and her husband have been dealing with her disease by addressing each problem as it occurs. She is resistant to using adaptive equipment because it makes her feel as though she is giving up.

IADLs

Community mobility	Patricia no longer drives and relies on her husband for transportation. She does not like to go out except for doctor appointments because she does not want to be seen using her walker or wheelchair in public.
Health management/prevention	Patricia takes a 1-day-at-a-time approach to managing her disease.
Home management	Patricia's husband and hired help do all of the home management tasks.
Financial management	Patricia relies on her husband for financial management.
Leisure/play	Patricia does not engage in any active leisure. She spends most of her day watching television.
Safety	This area is of the most concern for Patricia and her husband because she would have difficulty in an emergency when her husband is at work.

(Continued)

CASE EXAMPLE 10.2. PATRICIA: AT *(Cont.)*

EXHIBIT 10.2.	Patricia's Occupational Profile *(Cont.)*
Comments:	At this time, Patricia and her husband are most concerned about her ability to use the telephone in an emergency. They have a landline phone and do not trust cordless phones or cellphones because the batteries may fail. Patricia has been having greater difficulty pushing the small buttons on their phone to make calls.
Motor and Praxis Skills	
Sitting—static/dynamic	Patricia has good static sitting balance and fair dynamic balance.
Standing—static/dynamic	Standing balance varies from fair to poor depending on Patricia's level of fatigue.
Joint stability and skeletal mobility	Patricia has no difficulty in this area.
Place can on shelf	Patricia has difficulty in this area.
Retrieve item from floor	Patricia has some difficulty in this area.
Screw lid on jar	Patricia has difficulty in this area.
Comb back of head	Patricia has occasional difficulty in this area.
Writing	Patricia has difficulty in this area.
Lift grocery bag	Patricia has difficulty in this area.
Coordination	Patricia has some difficulty in this area.
Manipulation	Patricia has difficulty in this area.
Comments:	Patricia's performance can vary greatly depending on her level of fatigue. She is unable to predict when she will have a good or a bad day.
Process Skills	
Energy for task	Patricia has significant difficulty in this area.
Knowledge/organization of task	Patricia has no difficulty in this area.
Adaptation/praxis	Patricia has some difficulty in this area.
Comments:	None.
Behavioral and Cognitive Skills	
Communication and following social conventions	Patricia has no difficulty in this area.
Cognitive and emotional regulation skills	Patricia has a diagnosis of depression for which she is being treated.
Level of arousal/attention	Patricia has no difficulty in this area.
Orientation	Patricia is alert and oriented to person, place, time, and event.
Energy and drive	Patricia has the drive to be as independent as possible but often lacks the energy because of her significant fatigue.
Memory and understanding	Patricia has no problems in this area.
Higher level cognition	Patricia has no problems in this area.
Sensory–Perceptual Skills	
Sensory	Patricia has no problems in this area.
Pain	Patricia complains of moderate musculskeletal pain, especially after periods of inactivity.

(Continued)

CASE EXAMPLE 10.2. PATRICIA: AT *(Cont.)*

EXHIBIT 10.2. Patricia's Occupational Profile *(Cont.)*	
Skin integrity	Patricia is mobile enough at this time that this is not a problem.
Self-perception	Patricia is often embarrassed by her condition and avoids being around strangers.
Comments:	The occupational therapy practitioner theorizes that Patricia has been experiencing role conflict, and both she and her husband may have been experiencing some denial regarding her prognosis.

Note. Occupational profile template from American Occupational Therapy Association (2017). Analysis of participation format adapted from Skubik-Peplaski, Paris, Boyle, & Culpert (2009). ADLs = activities of daily living; ALS = amyotrophic lateral sclerosis; AT = assistive technology; IADLs = instrumental activities of daily living; SES = socioeconomic status.

data collected in terms of client progress caused reflection on and reconsideration of the guiding frame of reference for intervention. Outcome measurement is a very powerful part of the occupational therapy process.

Chapter 8 discussed the use of promising and emerging practices in occupational therapy intervention. The occupational therapy practitioner using these strategies was challenged to develop skills to support and defend these intervention choices. Clear identification of functional outcome measurement can provide excellent support for the use of innovative, promising, and emerging practices.

SERVICE OUTCOMES

Our focus so far has largely been on client outcomes. *Service outcomes* are those related to management and administration, and they affect how and what occupational therapy services are supported. These broader service outcomes include measures of efficiency, service costs and profits, and patient satisfaction. Health services management must explore service delivery critically in terms of value to clients. In program evaluation, a goal is the identification and elimination of inefficient or ineffective practices. Retrospective reviews of client outcomes in consideration of the specific types and frequencies of services provided are widely used to guide hiring, program development, and strategic planning across the health care delivery system. The FIM is a tool widely used across multiple settings that results in pooled datasets that are used in both planning and health policy decisions.

Howard-Wilsher et al.'s (2016) systematic review examined specific clinical subgroups individually and explored the service delivery value for each of them. An example of the use of service outcomes is illustrated in this excerpt:

- Rehabilitation interventions were associated with both additional costs and improved clinical outcomes (e.g., example, exercise interventions additional to general practitioners' care for back pain).

- Rehabilitation interventions were associated with lower costs and similar clinical outcomes (e.g., early supported discharge of stroke survivors; home-based vs. center-based cardiac rehabilitation).
- Rehabilitation interventions were cost-saving by reducing the costs of other health care services (e.g., home-based programmes for preventing falls in older people), or the costs of social care services (e.g., occupational therapy for older people), or reducing the disability-related productivity loss (e.g., worksite-based disability management). (p. 21)

Howard-Wilsher et al.'s study, although qualified with the statement that the available evidence for their systematic review, was often described as limited, inconsistent, or inconclusive, suggested that some rehabilitation interventions were cost-effective. For example, Howard-Wilsher et al. reported that early supported discharge of stroke patients was cost-effective not in terms of costs but in terms of ADLs and QoL improvements associated with home-based rehabilitation. This finding, based on a systematic analysis of outcome data, could greatly affect occupational therapy service delivery.

OUTCOME MEASUREMENT AND RESEARCH

In service provision to clients, outcome measures should be selected early in the intervention process. The outcome measures selected should be valid, reliable, and appropriately sensitive to changes in clients' occupational performance. Outcome measures can be based on normative standards on criterion-based standards or on a relative standard in which the client serves as his or her own control. Outcome measures, if used uniformly over a period of time, also offer important data for the evaluation and consideration of specific occupational therapy interventions. Of all forms of research, it is outcomes research that is likely to have the most direct impact on clinical practice. Studies of costs versus benefits, such as that of Howard-Wilsher and colleagues (2016), have the potential to influence health policy and funding for services.

Retrospective studies using occupational therapy data can be powerful tools in supporting (or refuting) specific clinical practices. Simon and Collins (2017) effectively used retrospective data to support an occupational therapy intervention for pain management. These authors reported that the Lifestyle Redesign® (Clark et al., 2015) intervention has a significant effect on the QoL, self-efficacy, and functional abilities of people living with chronic pain. They used both the COPM and QoL measures in their analysis. This study not only supported the specific intervention that was targeted but also offered support for occupational therapy's participation in the growing social problem of opioid abuse secondary to chronic pain. Although the study did not address cost-effectiveness, it did provide evidence to support reimbursement for occupational therapy treatment by insurance companies and provided support for the inclusion of occupational therapy in health care policy.

SUMMARY

Many discussions of outcomes in the occupational therapy literature focus on the presentation of specific measurement instruments. The potential impact of using consistent, reliable outcome measures that capture functional and QoL aspects is great and aids in clinical reasoning, strategic thinking, and program planning. Outcomes, although positioned near the end of any discussion, are actually essential in all clinical reasoning and in service delivery, management, research, and policy considerations. As outcome measures guide the provision of occupational therapy services, outcome studies guide the future of the occupational therapy profession.

LEARNING ACTIVITIES

1. Read Simon and Collins (2017). Describe how they used retrospective data to support occupational therapy intervention.
2. Review the prospective reasoning case presented in this chapter. Drawing on your own knowledge, list at least 3 clinical conditions that would require a similar approach to clinical reasoning. Justify your choices.
3. Review recent news about issues in health or in health care that affect your community. In a short essay, explain what functional outcome measures could support policy decision making about this issue. Using evidence and knowledge, include a discussion about why occupational therapy should or should not be part of the discussion about this issue.
4. Go to the American Occupational Therapy Political Action Committee's website (https://www.aota.org /Advocacy-Policy/AOTPAC.aspx), and search on *congressional affairs*. Choose 1 of the issues listed, and

write a short essay advocating support for occupational therapy on this issue.
5. Choose an impairment (or disability) or policy you care about, and identify action steps (including outcome measures) to building the needed resources to ensure that adequate knowledge exists to support ethical and cost-effective clinical reasoning about developing supportive occupational therapy programs.

REFERENCES

American Occupational Therapy Association (2001). *Occupational therapy in the promotion of health and the prevention of disease and disability*. Retrieved from https://www.aota .org//media/corporate/files/practice/health/tools/factsheet _healthpromotion.pdf

American Occupational Therapy Association. (2014). Occupational therapy practice framework: Domain and process (3rd ed.). *American Journal of Occupational Therapy, 68*(Suppl. 1), S1–S48. https://doi.org/10.5014/ajot.2014.682006

American Occupational Therapy Association. (2017). AOTA occupational profile template. *American Journal of Occupational Therapy, 71*(Suppl. 2), 7002420030. https://doi .org/10.5014/ajot.2017.716S12

Canadian Institutes of Health Research. (2010). *Knowledge to action: An end-of-grant knowledge translation casebook*. Ottawa: Author. Retrieved from http://www.cihr-irsc.gc.ca /e/41594.html

CanChild. (2004). *Outcome Measures Rating Form*. Ontario: CanChild Centre for Disability Research, Institute of Applied Health Sciences, McMaster University. Retrieved from https://www.canchild.ca/system/tenon/assets/attachments /000/000/372/original/measrate.pdf

Clark, F.A., Blanchard, J., Sleight, A., Cogan, A., Floríndez, L., Gleason, S., . . . Vigen, C. (2015). *Lifestyle Redesign®: The intervention tested in the USC Well Elderly Studies* (2nd ed.). Bethesda, MD: AOTA Press.

Cronin, A., & Mandich, M. (2016). *Human development and performance throughout the lifespan* (2nd ed.). Boston: Cengage Learning.

Fisher, A. G. (2009). *Occupational Therapy Intervention Process Model: A model for planning and implementing top-down, client-centered, and occupation-based interventions*. Fort Collins, CO: Three Star Press.

Fisher, A. G., & Griswold, L. A. (2014). Performance skills: Implementing performance analyses to evaluate quality of occupational performance. In B. A. Boyt Schell, G. Gillen, & M. Scaffa (Eds.), *Willard and Spackman's occupational therapy* (12th ed., pp. 249–264). Philadelphia: Lippincott Williams & Wilkins.

Fleming, M. (1994). The therapist with the three track mind. In C. Mattingly & M. Fleming (Eds.), *Clinical reasoning: Forms of inquiry in a therapeutic practice* (pp. 119–136). Philadelphia: F. A. Davis.

Hammell, K. W. (2009). Self-care, productivity, and leisure, or dimensions of occupational experience? Rethinking occupational "categories." *Canadian Journal of Occupational Therapy, 76*, 107–114. https://doi.org/10.1177/000841740907600208

Hawkins, D., Elder, L., & Paul, R. (2010). *The thinkers guide to clinical reasoning*. Tomales, CA: Foundation for Critical Thinking.

Howard-Wilsher, S., Irvine, L., Fan, H., Shakespeare, T., Suhrcke, M., Horton, S., . . . Song, F. (2016). Systematic overview of economic evaluations of health-related rehabilitation. *Disability and Health Journal, 9,* 11–25. https://doi.org/10.1016/j.dhjo.2015.08.009

Hudak, P., Amadio, P. C., Bombardier, C., Beaton, D., Cole., D., Davis, A., . . . Wright, J. (1996). Development of an upper-extremity outcome measure: The DASH (Disabilities of the Arm, Shoulder, and Hand). *American Journal of Industrial Medicine, 29,* 602–608. https://doi.org/10.1002/(SICI)1097-0274(199606)29:6<602::AID-AJIM4>3.0.CO;2-L

Institute for Work and Health. (2013). *About the DASH.* Retrieved from http://www.dash.iwh.on.ca/about-dash

Keith, R., Granger, C., Hamilton, B., & Sherwin, F. (1987). The Functional Independence Measure: A new tool for rehabilitation. In M. G. Eisenberg & R. Grzesiak (Eds.), *Advances in clinical rehabilitation* (Vol. 1, pp. 6–18). New York: Springer.

Kielhofner, G. (2008). *Model of Human Occupation: Theory and application* (4th ed.). Baltimore: Lippincott Williams & Wilkins.

Law, M., Baptiste, S., Carswell, A., McColl, M. A., Polatajko, H., & Pollock, N. (2014). *Canadian Occupational Performance Measure* (5th ed.). Ottawa: CAOT Publications.

Law, M., Cooper, B., Strong, S., Stewart, D., Rigby, P., & Letts, L. (1996). The Person–Environment–Occupational Model: A transactive approach to occupational performance. *Canadian Journal of Occupational Therapy, 63*(1), 9–23. https://doi.org/10.1177/000841749606300103

Law, M., & MacDermid, J. (2014). *Evidence-based rehabilitation: A guide to practice* (3rd ed.). Thorofare, NJ: Slack.

Liedtka, J. (1998). Linking strategic thinking with strategic planning. *Strategy and Leadership, 26*(4), 30–35.

Maddox, B. (2002). *Rosalind Franklin: The dark lady of DNA.* New York: Perennial.

Porter, M. (2010). What is value in health care? *New England Journal of Medicine, 363,* 2477–2481. https://doi.org/10.1056/NEJMp1011024

Radomski, M. (1995). There is more to life than putting on your pants. *American Journal of Occupational Therapy, 49,* 487–490. https://doi.org/10.5014/ajot.49.6.487

Salter, K., Teasell, R., Goettl, T., McIntyre, A., Johnson, D., & Jutai, J. (2017). *Assessment of outcomes: Functional Independence Measure.* Retrieved from http://www.abiebr.com/set/17-assessment-outcomes-following-acquiredtraumatic-brain-injury/functional-independence-measure

Simon, A. U., & Collins, C. R. (2017). Lifestyle Redesign® for chronic pain management: A retrospective clinical efficacy study. *American Journal of Occupational Therapy, 71,* 7104190040. https://doi.org/10.5014/ajot.2017.025502

Skubik-Peplaski, C., Paris, C., Boyle, D., & Culpert, A. (Eds.). (2009). *Applying the* Occupational Therapy Practice Framework: *Using the Cardinal Hill Occupational Participation Process in client-centered care* (2nd ed.). Bethesda, MD: AOTA Press.

Sullivan, K. J., & Cen, S. Y. (2011). Model of disablement and recovery: Knowledge translation in rehabilitation research and practice. *Physical Therapy, 91,* 1892–1904. https://doi.org/10.2522/ptj.2011003

Townsend, E., & Wilcock, A. A. (2004). Occupational justice and client-centred practice: A dialogue in progress. *Canadian Journal of Occupational Therapy, 71,* 75–87. https://doi.org/10.1177/000841740407100203

Uniform Data System for Medical Rehabilitation. (1997). *Guide for the Uniform Data Set for Medical Rehabilitation* (including the FIM® instrument, Version 5.1). Buffalo, NY: Author.

World Health Organization. (2006). *Constitution of the World Health Organization* (45th ed.). Retrieved from http://www.afro.who.int/index.php?option=com_docman&task=doc_download&gid=19&Itemid=2111WHO 2006

Complexity and Disruption in Clinical Reasoning

Anne Cronin, PhD, OTR/L, ATP, FAOTA, and Garth Graebe, MOT, OTR/L

CHAPTER HIGHLIGHTS

- Discusses innovation and clinical reasoning.
- Considers data collection needs in both programmatic and client-focused contexts.
- Introduces the concepts of tacit knowledge and clinical expertise.
- Considers underground practice and steps for fostering change.
- Discusses the negative impact of complacency in occupational therapy practice.
- Considers disruptive innovations and the maker movement relative to occupational therapy practice.
- Introduces the use of occupation-based activity analysis as a tool to address clinical complexity.

KEY TERMS AND CONCEPTS

Complacency	Maker movement	Trauma-informed care
Disruptive innovation	Tacit knowledge	Underground practice

This text has challenged readers to reflectively and holistically use clinical reasoning to guide occupation-focused and evidence-informed practice decisions. This chapter returns to some of the concepts presented in the first 3 chapters of this book and builds on them in the context of challenges that extend the clinical reasoning needed to support expert practice and effective interprofessional, collaborative communication.

REVIEW OF THE CLINICAL REASONING PROCESS

Chapter 1, "Overview of the Clinical Reasoning Process," introduced the 5-step clinical reasoning process. To review, this process involves

- *Step 1.* Consider the client and the referral information.
- *Step 2.* Develop clinical hypotheses to guide collection of cues and information.
- *Step 3.* Use targeted data collection and problem-solving strategies to process information and evaluate the hypothesis.
- *Step 4.* Test and refine the clinical hypotheses.
- *Step 5.* Appraise the evidence.

Clinical reasoning is never a linear process; it involves reflection, review, and reconsideration to be effective.

INNOVATION AND THE "SHINY NEW THING"

Occupational therapy practitioners are always looking for new and innovative ways to improve or enhance the occupational therapy process. They gain new information in several ways, including attending conferences, performing online research, and viewing vendor presentations.

Benefits

Occupational therapy practitioners are often introduced to new products and new ideas that might apply to their own practice as a way to provide an existing type of service in a more engaging way (e.g., use of virtual reality to practice specific movements), as an intervention that seems to provide something unique (e.g., therapeutic listening systems), or as something that is more objective and easier to document (e.g., computer-based assessment tools). Innovations are good to explore because they may integrate new science and research and because they may help practitioners be more effective and efficient in service delivery.

Challenges

A clinical reasoning challenge is that many "innovations" are really established treatments that are packaged well (making them easier to use). For example, soft tissue mobilization techniques are widely used to support hand therapy interventions. The general principles and science underlying soft tissue mobilization are common to all techniques, but occupational therapy practitioners can take courses to be "certified" in techniques branded with a particular name. These branded techniques may offer something valuable, or they may just be good marketing. Clinical reasoning is the best tool to help evaluate them.

Similarly, some innovations may lack rigorous research supporting their use. These "new" approaches are prevalent across practice areas, and many do offer something interesting and potentially valuable to the occupational therapy process. However, these new approaches must be categorized as unsupported practices in terms of evidence-based reasoning. The clinical reasoning challenge, therefore, is that occupational therapy practitioners must consider not only any evidence supporting the new intervention but also the intervention's relationship to occupation and participation and the ethics associated with its introduction. Is this intervention logical in light of existing related evidence? New things can and should be tried, but only when the practitioner can create a compelling argument for trying the intervention that is grounded in the principles of evidence-informed reasoning.

In 2017 the American Occupational Therapy Association (AOTA; 2017b) joined the Choosing Wisely® initiative. This national initiative was developed support consumers of health care services in making smart and effective care choices. It helps identify overused and unsupported interventions, especially those that are unnecessary and inconsistent with the ideal of providing cost-effective and evidence-based interventions. This initiative can help practitioners search and ask questions about established and unfamiliar approaches to best meet client needs.

Ethical Considerations

The *Occupational Therapy Code of Ethics* (2015) states that the occupational therapy profession is grounded in 7 long-standing core values: (1) altruism, (2) equality, (3) freedom, (4) justice, (5) dignity, (6) truth, and (7) prudence (AOTA, 2015). These values should be used to help guide clinical reasoning, especially when considering an unsupported practice. Altruism is especially important when considering the use of an unsupported practice because it requires demonstrating concern for the welfare of others. Altruism comes into play when ensuring that interventions promote desired goals in a manner that is respectful of clients in terms of safety, cost, and necessity. In addition, the Code requires that occupational therapy practitioners be prudent and use sound judgment and reflection to make decisions in professional and volunteer roles.

The Choosing Wisely initiative is an example of looking at occupational therapy interventions with the consumers in mind. For example, is the innovation more convenient for the practitioner, but more expensive for the client, with no gain in intervention efficacy? Is the intervention clearly linked to client-established outcomes? Does the use of the innovation replace a more traditional, but also more evidence-based, strategy? Both clients and clinicians are naturally drawn to the shiny new thing, but in many cases that new thing is not a benefit in terms of costs or outcomes. New approaches should be considered critically in terms of their impact on occupational performance; that impact should be measured in practitioners' own practice setting.

Appraisal

Innovations should be scrutinized by reviewing the professional literature. In addition, client-specific data should guide clinical reasoning about what is effective for a particular client, and program (or device) data should guide clinical reasoning in the introduction of clinical innovations. Cost is always a factor when considering an innovation. If the innovation is a change in approach to intervention, it may cost time in staff training and in documentation systems but have little equipment cost. When considering an unsupported practice, planning objective functional outcome measures is essential.

Example of Innovation: Trauma-Informed Care

One innovation that has been widely introduced into mental health practice is ***trauma-informed care,*** which is

> an organizational structure and treatment framework that involves understanding, recognizing, and responding to the effects of all types of trauma. Trauma Informed Care also emphasizes physical, psychological and emotional safety for both consumers and providers, and helps survivors rebuild a sense of control and empowerment. (Trauma Informed Care Project, 2017)

This approach has been highly regarded in the mental health profession, lending support to its consideration, but it is challenging because it requires an organization-wide commitment to enact.

Introducing this innovation would involve continuing education training costs in terms of the occupational therapy practitioner's staff time. It would probably also require the development of an in-service for other organizational leaders who will be "selling" trauma-informed care as a good path for the organization. If the innovation is accepted, an additional time commitment will likely be required to help organize the transition.

This example involves costs in terms of time but few costs in terms of space or materials. Would the innovation of trauma-informed care be worth the cost to you and to your organization? This determination can only made by collecting outcome data to ascertain whether the client outcomes warrant the additional costs.

Along with an evidence-based process to collect client data, actual data are needed to support clinical reasoning as you consider innovations in your practice. It is easier to introduce a sweeping innovation such as trauma-informed care if it is clear that an evidence-based data collection process will be in place

TABLE 11.1. Structure for Program-Level Evidence-Based Data Collection

STRATEGY	ACTION	CLINICAL REASONING
Collect usage data that include not only client numbers but also the response of both clients and staff to the innovation.	Report facts.	Use evidence-based clinical reasoning to make hypotheses about the facts.
Collect data on administration and planning time.	Report time use.	Time has a high cost in most health care settings. The time costs will be essential in determining the innovation's value to the organization.
Measure something that matters.	Report performance, not details of structure or function.	Maintain a client-centered focus. Measurement should relate to client-identified priorities.
Measure outcomes, not interventions.	Measure how the client does rather than what is done to and for the client.	Choose organization-level outcome measures such as days of inpatient care, readmissions, and successful community placement.
Record the process.	Keep a record of what does and does not work.	In program evaluation, these data can be essential in adapting and modifying the new program to meet institutional needs.

to evaluate the new program. The data you will need will be similar to those described in Table 6.2, which has been adapted in Table 11.1 for consideration of program changes.

Apps

The shiny new thing may also be a device or a tool rather than a program. In many school systems, tablet computers that use application programs, or apps, are widely available to both students and occupational therapy practitioners. Apps are often inexpensive and engaging game applications. Many occupational therapy practitioners now use apps in their practice, and some have become app developers. Both positions involve clinical reasoning.

As with any innovation, the decision to alter existing practice should involve balancing the costs of the innovation against the benefits. What benefits should practitioners look for in a therapy tool such as an app? The following list offers some suggestions:

- Are the target skills gained by app use valued by the client and consistent with the occupational therapy intervention plan?

TABLE 11.2. Common Problem-Solving Strategies Applied to Apps

PROBLEM-SOLVING STRATEGIES	APPLICATION TO APPS
Algorithm: a rule that guarantees the right solution by using a formula or step-by-step procedure.	An app that aids activity recording, such as a fitness tracker, could allow measurement of lifestyle changes. An app that presents a letter of the alphabet in a gamelike presentation could support learning.
Heuristics: allows clinicians to simplify complex problems and reduce the total number of possible solutions.	Specialized visual–motor apps can be programmed to offer specific movements or responses in the client's area of need. Video modeling apps can offer structured sequences to guide the client through tasks.
Trial-and-error: often used in cases in which the problem is ill-defined or there are multiple interacting diagnostic conditions or challenging contextual factors.	A fitness tracker or calendar app can be used to keep logs of activity patterns to help understand confounding issues. A familiar game app can be used as an informal assessment tool to compare the client's performance with typical performance.
Insight: grounded in clinician knowledge and experience; more likely to be used by expert clinicians.	Game play or other app use can be analyzed to understand clients' problem-solving challenges. Apps can be used to identify unexplored issues that emerge as difficulty in app use.

- Are the skills gained by app use simply game skills, or do they translate into improved functional performance?
- What adaptability and data-recording features does the app have?
- How easy is the app to use for both the occupational therapy practitioner and client?
- How engaging is the app? Is its use relevant and meaningful to the client?
- Does the app offer something that is in some way better than the original intervention (i.e., does the client stays engaged longer, or can data be collected on performance outside of intervention setting)?
- Is the app at least as effective as the intervention it is replacing?
- Are there ethical concerns about information sharing or public access?

In considering the use of apps, one can also review the common problem-solving strategies presented earlier in the text. As you read Table 11.2, consider that many widely used apps, such as calendars and fitness trackers, can be used to document habits and routines, as assessment tools to consider activity patterns, as interventions to develop time management and self-advocacy, and as problem-solving tools to better understand why the client has not been successful in meeting goals. App use can be entertaining, but the use of client intervention time solely for entertainment would be unethical.

BECOMING AN EXPERT THINKER

Expert occupational therapy practitioners can think outside the box and find ways to take an activity that the client enjoys, such as playing a game app, and use that activity to motivate or support positive therapeutic change. The expert clinician tends to be less bound by algorithms and heuristics and is able to evaluate interventions, programs, and research. Expert thinking allows clinicians to provide interventions and support achievement of functional outcomes in unique and unconventional ways. Expert occupational therapy practitioners reason through a theoretical lens that is supported by experiential learning. Novices can experience insight in clinical reasoning, but it is more likely to be a mainstay in the reasoning of experts. Lurie (2011) wrote,

> Experts solve problems differently than do beginners. They rapidly identify patterns, prioritize available data and seek out the information that will most efficiently allow them to reach a solution. They can identify common scenarios that can be resolved with few additional data, as opposed to those that require deliberate reasoning from first principles. In general, they have efficient problem-solving strategies that allow them to arrive rapidly at the most likely set of diagnoses. (p. 326)

Many studies have characterized the distinctions between novices and experts in clinical reasoning, and many have presented clinical reasoning as a developmental process that expands through practice and actual clinical experience. Fleming (1994) discussed clinical reasoning as a search for tacit knowledge. *Tacit knowledge* is "the knowledge that practitioners have that is known in a direct practical way but is not stated as a formal theory" (p. 23). More simply stated, tacit knowledge includes history and experiences that practitioners cannot easily express because they are often unaware of them as anything other than intuition.

Expert practitioners are efficient. In their store of tacit knowledge, they have knowledge of "underlying principles, assumptions, values, rules of thumb and gut feelings about what we are doing and why we are doing that" (Fleming, 1994, p. 29). It is generally believed that practice in supervised clinical environments is an essential aspect of developing the tacit knowledge that underlies expert clinical reasoning. Assimilation of professional information such as the *Occupational Therapy Practice Framework* (*OTPF–3*; AOTA, 2014) and the frames of reference commonly used in the profession can support and expedite the development of tacit knowledge, but it cannot replace experiential learning.

Fleming (1994) noted that many expert practitioners state that they enjoy having students in their clinical practice because it enhances their own learning. Fleming suggested that clinical teaching was perceived as learning because, in teaching, the expert clinician may be explicitly describing and discussing knowledge that was once implicit, and the process of teaching helps bring it to the forefront to explain clinical reasoning. She noted that "it may be that [in] being forced to explain actions, a practitioner may organize heretofore nonlinguistic experiential knowledge into a verbal description" (p. 26).

UNDERGROUND PRACTICE

Underground practice is a term coined by Fleming and Mattingly (1994) to describe the dilemma of trying to be holistic and occupation based within the very real constraints of the health care system. Underground practice issues also include professional turf boundaries and reimbursement policies that reward the use of discrete procedures rather than interventions that reflect client values and concerns. Some of these issues were touched on in earlier chapters discussing the use of frames of reference that have emerged from outside the field of occupational therapy in a manner consistent with the guidelines of the *OTPF–3*.

The biomechanical frame of reference is one of the more contentious frames of reference when considering underground practice. At some level, and across disciplines, most health practitioners draw from the biomechanical frame of reference to guide practice. It often becomes challenging, especially for outsiders, to understand the roles of different professionals when they all seem to be focused on the biomechanical aspects of care. The biomechanical frame of reference is essential to occupational therapy practice, but to a layperson, it seems logical to see the occupational therapy practitioner as the upper body therapist and the physical therapist as the lower body therapist. When these stereotypes are allowed to persist, practice in both disciplines is diminished.

Fleming and Mattingly (1994) considered the professional image of occupational therapy practitioners in terms of their institutional contexts. These authors stated that

> the institutional context of the hospital is powerfully restrictive of the occupational therapist's practice, funneling therapy into an acceptable biomechanical channel and constraining the sorts of creative alternatives considered. (p. 297)

Institutional values are internalized by occupational therapy practitioners and are often reflected in how the practitioners describe themselves, such as a school-based practitioner who is content to be seen as the handwriting teacher or a nursing home practitioner who is seen as the ADL therapist. These institutional values and traditions are also seen in professional turf boundaries. For example, a manager may determine that occupational therapy practitioners will do all self-care training except eating, and eating will be the exclusive turf of speech therapy practitioners.

In considering underground practice, clinical reasoning is not focused exclusively on the client; external influences have also predetermined which discipline addresses which aspect of the client's needs and what types of interventions are supported by reimbursement standards. When arguing for client-centered evidence-based practice, the occupational therapy practitioner in a restrictive institutional setting may not be able to be holistic without being subject to penalties in terms of reimbursement or scope of practice.

Understanding underground practice is essential to expert clinical reasoning. It is impossible to be an agent for change in an institutional setting if you do not fully understand the world in which health care providers and organizations function and the factors that support the status quo. To take on the role of change agent, the occupational therapy practitioner must first

> assist people (including both health care professionals and consumers), organizations (hospitals, skilled nursing facilities, physician offices, home health agencies) and other stakeholders in understanding why change is needed and, more importantly, understand how it benefits them. (Kennedy, 2014, para. 5)

Although change can be initiated at many levels, this chapter focuses on change that may be initiated at the service delivery level. At this level, relevant changes can most easily occur in clinical practices, health providers' behaviors or practices, management practices, and management systems (Implementing Best Practices Consortium, 2007).

LEADING CHANGE

Kotter and Cohen (2012) identified 8 principles for fostering and leading change that have been widely adopted across disciplines. Table 11.3 presents these principles in an occupational therapy context as action steps.

The biggest barrier to change is *complacency*, which is defined in 2 ways:

1. self-satisfaction, especially when accompanied by unawareness of actual dangers or deficiencies.
2. an instance of usually unaware or uninformed self-satisfaction. ("Complacency," 2017)

It is complacency when an occupational therapy practitioner accepts the narrow role of handwriting teacher or being the person who works with arms while the physical therapist works with legs. The complacent occupational therapy practitioner has a settled routine and a standard set of therapy approaches, and neither questions the status quo nor seeks to learn new approaches. This may seem to be a way to take it easy in one's job, but for most people complacency leads to boredom and burnout (see Practice Wisdom 11.1). *Knobology,* the study of intervention application without theory, is a form of complacency. The 1-trick pony exemplifies another form of complacency.

Llopis (2014) wrote about complacency in the business world. He acknowledged that change is difficult and usually stress producing, so it is easy to grow complacent when the alternative is to tackle change. He offered some early warning signs to avoid the dangers of complacent leadership that are applicable to occupational therapy practitioners and to business leaders. The first warning sign of complacency is feeling fear—fear of what is required to face administrative challenges or fear of being exposed and placed in a vulnerable position.

The next warning sign of complacency is that attention to detail fades. This may mean cutting corners in the clinical setting, a lack of attention to documentation, or a lack of reflection on the potential negative consequences of inaction. Llopis (2014) noted that "when leaders grow fearful of becoming exposed and begin to lose the required attention to detail to effectively perform, they begin to unknowingly create tension with others" (para. 6). So the final warning sign of complacency is tension and unrest in the workplace.

OUT-OF-THE-BOX THINKING AND CLINICAL REASONING

Chapter 10, "Strategic Thinking and Outcomes," introduced strategic thinking as proposed by Liedtka (1998). A strategic thinker focuses first on deeply understanding

---

PRACTICE WISDOM 11.1. Complacency

"If you always do what you've always done, you always get what you've always gotten."—*Attributed to Jessie Potter (as cited in Ahern, 1981)*

TABLE 11.3.   Actions Steps for Fostering Change

ACTION STEPS	GOALS FOR FOSTERING CHANGE
Step 1. Create a sense of urgency (setting the stage).	▪ Get people's attention, and help them to see the need for change and the importance of acting immediately. ▪ Sell the need for change. Describe the consequences of not changing.
Step 2. Build a guiding team.	▪ Change is built on communication and collaboration; it is not easily managed without allies. ▪ Key characteristics that must be represented on the team include leadership, credibility, communication, expertise, authority, and a sense of urgency.
Step 3. Develop the change vision and strategy.	▪ Create a compelling vision—one that answers the questions "What do we want to achieve?" and "Where do we want to be in the future?" ▪ Clarify how the future will be different from the past, drawing support for change from both within and outside the institution. ▪ Outside supports such as professional organizations can also share knowledge about pathways to successful change, and internal supports can offer strategies to support the scale-up to implementation and strategies to enhance the sustainability of the change.
Step 4. Enlist a volunteer army.	▪ Make sure as many others as possible understand and accept the vision and the strategy. ▪ Accept and plan for resistance. Resisters help to clarify the problem. By addressing their concerns, you can actually improve the change.
Step 5. Empower others to act.	▪ Give people freedom and direction so that they can find their own team-driven solutions. ▪ Encourage people to speak up, even to voice differing views. ▪ Affirm and refine the vision, making room for others' ideas. ▪ Provide people with training and support. ▪ Use existing quality improvement methods in your organization to track activities on a daily basis. ▪ Set short-term goals.
Step 6. Produce short-term wins.	▪ Start where you can start now. ▪ Plan and create the wins, and be sure to visibly recognize and reward people who made the wins possible.
Step 7. Don't let up (sustain acceleration).	▪ You may need to reinvigorate the process with new projects, themes, and change agents. ▪ Persevere even if support for institutionalization is not readily forthcoming from all higher level decision makers.
Step 8. Institute change (and make it stick).	▪ Hold on to the new ways of behaving, and make sure they succeed. ▪ Changing culture comes last, not first. ▪ Only after people change their actions can there be a change in culture.

Note. Steps adapted from Kotter and Cohen (2012).

the problem at hand, thinking more broadly than intervention algorithms and approaches and instead focusing on the ways in which the dysfunction, as experienced by the client, limits engagement in occupational pursuits. A strategic thinker is an agent for change.

Developing a strategic plan, whether it is a personal plan or an organizational plan, is a good starting point to combat complacency. In the strategic thinking process, intelligent opportunism is an important tool to help the occupational therapy practitioner step outside the box. Intelligent opportunism can be used in the

clinical encounter when the client's needs are not easily addressed by any of the usual intervention approaches. Consider the case of Anthony in Case Example 11.1.

In Anthony's case, the occupational therapy practitioner invented an unsupported intervention strategy on the basis of information from within the profession that would not typically be considered in the case of a 21-year-old with a history of traumatic brain injury (TBI). The occupational therapy practitioner used ideas from the sensory processing frame of reference because they seemed logical and were acceptable to the client.

CASE EXAMPLE 11.1. ANTHONY: SCHOOL AND WORK PERFORMANCE

Anthony is a 27-year-old veteran who had sustained a TBI during his military service. Since his discharge, he has also been diagnosed with attention deficit hyperactivity disorder (ADHD), predominantly hyperactive type. He has not responded well to medication. Anthony works with a vocational rehabilitation counselor but feels that this is not enough to help him at work. Anthony's occupational profile is presented in Exhibit 11.1.

EXHIBIT 11.1.	Anthony's Occupational Profile		
Client	**Reason the client is seeking service and concerns related to engagement in occupations**	Referred to occupational therapy for interventions to support school and work performance. *Impact on occupation:* Anthony is enrolled in higher education and works with a local company as a software engineer. He has the necessary skills for the job but has difficulty sitting in meetings and contributing meaningfully. He has been reprimanded for fidgeting in meetings and inattention. He has similar problems in his academic work.	
	Occupations in which the client is successful	Anthony is a son, friend, student, and member of a faith community.	
	Personal interests and values	Anthony is interested in succeeding in the workplace.	
	Occupational history (i.e., life experiences)	Anthony is a veteran and sustained a TBI during military service. Since his discharge, he has also been diagnosed with ADHD, predominantly hyperactive type. He worked with computers in the military and is working toward a degree in software engineering.	
	Performance patterns (routines, roles, habits, & rituals)	Academically, Anthony is a good student, but he does best when he can arrange his own work schedule and can avoid long periods in which he has nothing active to do. Anthony enjoys his role as intern but does not feel he is doing well in this capacity. Anthony is also a son and brother and is active with the local veterans support group.	
Environment		***Supports to occupational engagement***	***Barriers to occupational engagement***
	Physical (e.g., buildings, furniture, pets)	Anthony has no accessibility concerns.	Anthony is easily distracted in busy places.
	Social (e.g., spouse, friends, caregivers)	Anthony is single and mostly socializes with other veterans.	Anthony is socially uncomfortable with the younger college students. Anthony lives with his parents.
Context	**Cultural** (e.g., customs, beliefs)	No issues related to culture or beliefs were identified during assessment.	
	Personal (e.g., age, gender, SES, education)	27-year-old male. Anthony has finished 3 years of college.	
	Temporal (e.g., stage of life, time, year)	Early adulthood.	
	Virtual (e.g., chat, email, remote monitoring)	Anthony is very skilled with all types of digital information and communication technologies.	
Client goals	**Client's priorities and desired targeted outcomes**	Anthony wants to be able to sit through and participate productively in meetings at work. He wants to be able to better organize his time to meet expectations in the other areas of his life.	

(Continued)

CASE EXAMPLE 11.1. ANTHONY: SCHOOL AND WORK PERFORMANCE (Cont.)

EXHIBIT 11.1.   Anthony's Occupational Profile *(Cont.)*

ANALYSIS OF PARTICIPATION

Basic ADLs

Eating/oral–motor	Anthony has no problems in this area.
Grooming	Anthony has no problems in this area.
Bathing/transfer	Anthony has no problems in this area.
Dressing upper body	Anthony has no problems in this area.
Dressing lower body	Anthony has no problems in this area.
Toileting	Anthony has no problems in this area.
Problem-solving/memory	Anthony has no problems in this area.
Comments:	None.

IADLs

Community mobility	Anthony is able to drive a car, manage public transportation, and get around in community situations.
Health management/prevention	Anthony enjoys working out and participating in the veterans' support group.
Home management	Anthony lives with his parents and helps around the house as needed. He maintains his own bedroom and laundry and cooks for the family at least once a week.
Financial management	Anthony is able to manage his own finances well.
Leisure/play	Anthony has little leisure time but enjoys hanging out with his friends and the occasional poker game.
Safety	Anthony has no problems in this area.
Comments:	Anthony is on probation at his workplace because of his inconsistent performance and his sometimes disruptive behaviors during meetings.

Motor and Praxis Skills

Sitting—static/dynamic	Anthony has no problems in this area.
Standing—static/dynamic	Anthony has no problems in this area.
Joint stability and skeletal mobility	Anthony has no problems in this area.
Place can on shelf	Anthony has no problems in this area.
Retrieve item from floor	Anthony has no problems in this area.
Screw lid on jar	Anthony has no problems in this area.
Comb back of head	Anthony has no problems in this area.
Writing	Anthony has no problems in this area.
Lift grocery bag	Anthony has no problems in this area.
Coordination	Anthony has no problems in this area.
Manipulation	Anthony has no problems in this area.
Comments:	None.

Process Skills

Energy for task	Anthony has no problems in this area.

(Continued)

CASE EXAMPLE 11.1. ANTHONY: SCHOOL AND WORK PERFORMANCE *(Cont.)*

EXHIBIT 11.1. Anthony's Occupational Profile *(Cont.)*	
Knowledge/organization of task	Anthony has no problems in this area.
Adaptation/praxis	Anthony has no problems in this area.
Comments:	None.
Behavioral and Cognitive Skills	
Communication and following social conventions	Anthony has adequate communication skills but does not always read other people well. He knows basic manners and social expectations but does not always filter what he says.
Cognitive and emotional regulation skills	Anthony has difficulty regulating his attention and is often impulsive. He becomes stressed or anxious easily and has difficulty continuing tasks when he is emotional.
Level of arousal/attention	Anthony is distractible and active. He gets wound up easily and has difficulty calming down so that he can focus.
Orientation	Anthony is alert and oriented to person, place, time, and event.
Energy and drive	Anthony has plenty of energy, but his drive is uneven. He is passionate about some things but unable to sustain any interest in others.
Memory and understanding	Anthony has no problems in this area.
Higher level cognition	Anthony has no problems in this area.
Sensory–Perceptual Skills	
Sensory	Anthony has no problems in this area.
Hearing and vision	Anthony has no problems in this area.
Skin integrity	Anthony has no problems in this area.
Self-perception	Anthony has been criticized at work and at school for his inattention and impulsivity. He sees himself as very creative; he is convinced that his creativity is linked to his impulsivity and is reluctant to change.
Comments:	None.

Note. Occupational profile template from American Occupational Therapy Association (2017a). Analysis of participation format adapted from Skubik-Peplaski, Paris, Boyle, & Culpert (2009). ADHD = attention-deficit hyperactivity disorder; ADLs = activities of daily living; IADLs = instrumental activities of daily living; SES = socioeconomic status; TBI = traumatic brain injury.

During the interview portion of the evaluation, Anthony was asked how he felt about the criticisms of his work behavior. Anthony replied that he really enjoyed software engineering and that the internship was very important to him. He was aware that his behavior needed to change for him to be successful, but he did not know how to make that happen because his intention was always to behave well. He stated that the fidgeting and daydreaming happened to him, and they were not decisions that he made. He said that he usually did fine for the first 30 or 40 minutes, but that the problem occurred in longer meetings.

The occupational therapy practitioner considered the cognitive rehabilitation frame of reference and the social learning frame of reference, but neither seemed to get at the heart of what was going on with Anthony.

To get more insight, the occupational therapy practitioner talked with her coworkers. A pediatric occupational therapy practitioner suggested that it sounded as though Anthony had a sensory processing disorder and became sensory seeking when he was understimulated. This was out-of-the-box thinking, because of Anthony's age (sensory integration theory is classically applied to children); because he had a brain injury, not a developmental problem; and because there is no evidence to support that sensory processing interventions would work under these conditions.

The application of sensory processing interventions should be questioned in this case because there are few empirical data to support them as effective even with traditional populations. In considering this intervention strategy, the occupational therapy practitioner

CASE EXAMPLE 11.1. ANTHONY: SCHOOL AND WORK PERFORMANCE (Cont.)

spent time talking through options with Anthony. Because the sensory strategies the occupational therapy practitioner described to Anthony could do no harm, could be done by him on his own time and thus were not costly, and did not take away from other more empirically supported interventions, they decided to use some sensory strategies to see whether they could help Anthony be more focused and settled during meetings.

Because this was an out-of-the-box trial, the occupational therapy practitioner worked with Anthony to set outcome goals that they could use to objectively measure the effect of the intervention. Goal attainment scaling (GAS) was used to document Anthony's performance after implementing the sensory diet strategies. Intelligent opportunism came into play here, because Anthony wanted to take advantage of resources already available to him in his work environment in hopes that his interventions could be discrete. Meeting this need involved more outside-the-box consideration. In collaboration with the occupational therapy practitioner, Anthony set a goal of sitting in a boring meeting for 1 hour without engaging in fidgeting that distracted others.

The practitioner set a 5-point GAS to measure the degree of attainment captured relative to the intervention:

Anthony is able to attend for 30 minutes without fidgeting = 0 (this was his performance baseline). Additional scoring:

- +1 (somewhat better) = *40 minutes without fidgeting*
- +2 (much better) = *60 minutes without fidgeting*

- –1 (somewhat worse) = *20 minutes without fidgeting*
- –2 (much worse) = *10 minutes without fidgeting.*

Because Anthony was looking for sensory strategies that he could use discretely in the workplace, he wanted to test them privately before trying them there. Anthony decided to measure his own ability to attend to boring work by using some tasks he had long put off. He chose 4 different sensory strategies and, with his father's help, drew 1 randomly to try for a day before the boring task. When he had tried every strategy twice and scored his own on-task performance, he came back to the occupational therapy practitioner to review them and plan for the workplace.

Through GAS, Anthony learned that although he enjoyed sitting on a squishy gel cushion, it distracted rather than improved his performance. He found that drinking ice water through a straw somewhat improved his behavior, as did performing isometric exercise every 5 minutes during the boring task. Anthony had no change in his performance when he ran in place for 30 seconds before the task, but he was consistently able to stay on task for 50–60 minutes if he ran up and then down 2 flights of stairs before the meeting.

Armed with these data, Anthony had 3 strategies to try for his next meeting. As planned, he ran up and down the stairs before the meeting and came to the meeting with a bottle of ice water. Anthony was successful in regulating his behavior in the meeting, and he found that these strategies were consistently helpful for him.

Although there are times when using an out-of-the-box unsupported practice is worth exploring, it is essential that the client know that the intervention is unsupported, and the occupational therapy practitioner must be careful to identify functional outcomes that help the client know what the intervention is intended to achieve and whether progress is occurring. In the case of Anthony, the occupational therapy practitioner also took the additional step of teaching the client how to trial the sensory interventions himself so there was no added cost to the client. This not only helped Anthony address his immediate problem, but it also gave him the basic tools to explore new sensory strategies on his own. In this case, out-of-the-box thinking was used to address a client need.

Out-of-the-box thinking can also be used to solve program-level clinical needs. An example of out-of-the-box thinking at the programmatic level is illustrated in the work of Verdonck and Maye (2016). These scientists considered the challenges of using smart information technologies after a spinal cord injury and addressed something that has become an essential of everyday life but is not recognized on outcome performance measures.

Verdonck and Maye (2016) first collected data on how their clients had used their devices in everyday occupations and found a wide variety of smart device occupations, including making phone calls, text messaging, reading books and newspapers, checking email and the Internet, recreational music and games, sports updates, and social networking. Exploring this further, Verdonck and Maye identified both common difficulties with smart device task performance and performance goals to address these problems.

Expanding their assessment strategies to explore details in smart device use needs and impairments,

Verdonck and Maye (2016) demonstrated out-of-the-box thinking to meet a perceived client and programmatic need. Through a systematic approach to data collection and problem solving, they also helped other occupational therapy practitioners to consider and address the problems they identified.

DISRUPTIVE INNOVATION

Disruptive innovation is a term widely used in business. It refers to an innovation that both creates a new market and, while doing this, disrupts an existing market.

An example of a disruptive innovation is *cloud computing,* which is the use of a network of remote servers linked to the Internet to store, manage, and process data. Cloud computing is intended to replace a local server or a personal computer. Cloud computing is what allows your smartphone to show which of your emails is unread, based on the last time you logged in on any device (not just your phone). Similarly, it is cloud computing that keeps your place in an online game so you can return to play on another device.

Cloud computing is not really replacing personal computers, but it is disrupting all information technology–related products because consumers like having mobile access to their information. Cloud computing has created many new markets, ranging from wearable fitness monitors and remote health-monitoring devices and data sources to everyday applications such as the palm-sized devices that allow vendors to process credit card payments at places such as farmers' markets.

Disruptive innovations are game changers that make the status quo obsolete. Telehealth, using cloud computing, has the potential to be a disruptive innovation. Rural school districts that have difficulty attracting occupational therapy practitioners are now hiring them to provide virtual therapy services through telehealth and e-learning platforms.

Although video game–based interventions have been around for a long time, Reifenberg and colleagues (2017) have taken them a step further and explored the feasibility of implementing game-based neurorehabilitation intervention with children with cerebral palsy using telehealth technologies. Although they found this approach both feasible and promising, many practitioners find the idea of having only virtual contact with a client worrisome. As occupational therapy practitioners explore telehealth and e-learning technologies, they must also disrupt their ideas about the therapeutic use of self and the ethics and security of cloud-based supports for interventions.

Just as cloud computing has allowed extensive development of telehealth tools and offered the potential of occupational therapy intervention via telehealth, other disruptive innovations have the potential to change occupational therapy more broadly. One example is the growing *maker movement,* a grassroots initiative in which individuals or groups of individuals use do-it-yourself and do-it-with-others techniques and processes to develop unique technology products. This movement is best known for its success in creating sophisticated devices and gadgets out of recycled or scrap materials.

The maker movement is active in the field of assistive technology (AT), and many occupational therapy practitioners have been involved in this growing initiative. This movement, along with another disruptive idea, crowd funding, has the potential to change how AT and assistive devices are developed and customized to client needs. It also makes AT device fabrication available to the average occupational therapy practitioner through open-source documentation of how to build and adapt devices.

COMPLEXITY

Activity analysis is a basic tool used by occupational therapy practitioners in all stages of the occupational therapy process. Chapters 1 and 2 used the case of Matthew. This case was complex because of the combination of impairments that he presented with and the interactions between these impairments that caused additional disability. This case demonstrated that although algorithms and heuristics are valuable tools to move the assessment process forward quickly, these tools are at times not effective in addressing the problem. In this case, the occupational therapy practitioner should return to occupation-based activity analysis. This assessment process is also illustrated by Billy in Case Example 11.2.

During the process of activity analysis, the occupational therapy practitioner used occupation awareness, the understanding of the meaning behind an activity that has meaning to the client, to address Billy's needs. Sometimes when a performance pattern fits a heuristic, as when Billy's performance mirrored that expected of a child with a sensory processing disorder, it is tempting to rush past the basics, which in this case was that Billy valued the occupations associated with independent computer play more than those associated with recess.

SUMMARY

This chapter addressed the issues of meeting client and organizational needs through expert thinking and by using the tools introduced in earlier chapters, such as the use of outcome data when considering the use of unsupported practices and strategies for considering new approaches and innovations in the clinical setting. The term *underground practice* was introduced to reflect the influence of factors unrelated to clinical reasoning that affect the occupational therapy practitioner's decision making. The negative impact of complacency on occupational therapy practice and the occupational therapy profession was also considered. Strategies were included to counteract complacency by taking on the role of change agent.

CASE EXAMPLE 11.2. BILLY: BEHAVIOR PROBLEMS

Billy is an 8-year-old boy diagnosed with ADHD and is having sensory and self-regulation issues that may be affecting his behavior at school. Billy's occupational profile is presented in Exhibit 11.2.

The occupational therapy practitioner spent some time observing Billy in the classroom. In her activity analysis, she noted that Billy had no functional limitations in terms of specific body structures, body

EXHIBIT 11.2.	Billy's Occupational Profile		
Client	**Reason the client is seeking service and concerns related to engagement in occupations**	Referred to occupational therapy to assess and treat sensory and self-regulation issues that may be leading to behavioral problems in school. Billy's parents have asked for a sensory processing assessment in the hope that the OT can remediate the effects of his ADHD, because he is reaching the maximum dosage of his medication. *Impact on occupation:* Billy gets into trouble daily at school. He is very bright and usually finishes class assignments and tests before most of his classmates. He becomes disruptive if he is not engaged in a task he enjoys.	
	Occupations in which the client is successful	Billy is a son, Lego builder, and brother.	
	Personal interests and values	Billy loves building with his toy bricks. He is very creative and builds complex constructions that he works on for days at a time.	
	Occupational history (i.e., life experiences)	Billy was diagnosed with ADHD, predominantly hyperactive type, at age 3 years. He has had various trials of ADHD medication and is currently taking methylphenidate 3 times per day. His behavior at home is similar to that at school. He fights with his younger sister and is argumentative with his parents, especially if he is interrupted when playing with his toy building bricks.	
	Performance patterns (routines, roles, habits, & rituals)	Billy's daily routines are largely managed by his parents and teacher. He has the skills to perform the needed tasks but is very disorganized. Billy is a student, son, brother.	
Environment		*Supports to occupational engagement*	*Barriers to occupational engagement*
	Physical (e.g., buildings, furniture, pets)	Billy does not have limitations in physical accessibility.	Billy is easily distracted and becomes anxious easily.
	Social (e.g., spouse, friends, caregivers)	Billy has a supportive family and an older sister who stands up for him at school.	Billy has immature social skills and does not have any friends at school.
Context	**Cultural (e.g., customs, beliefs)**	No issues related to culture or beliefs were identified during assessment.	
	Personal (e.g., age, gender, SES, education)	Billy is an 8-year-old boy.	
	Temporal (e.g., stage of life, time, year)	Childhood.	
	Virtual (e.g., chat, email, remote monitoring)	Billy is able to manage a smartphone, has access to a school computer, and can play computer games.	Billy has had his phone and gaming device taken away because of his poor school performance.

(Continued)

CASE EXAMPLE 11.2. BILLY: BEHAVIOR PROBLEMS *(Cont.)*

EXHIBIT 11.2.	**Billy's Occupational Profile** *(Cont.)*	
Client goals	**Client's priorities and desired targeted outcomes**	Billy's parents want him to be more attentive and less disruptive at school and at home.
		Billy wants his parents "off his case" and wants to have friends at school.

ANALYSIS OF PARTICIPATION	
Basic ADLs	
Eating/oral motor	Billy has no problems in this area.
Grooming	Billy has no problems in this area.
Bathing/transfer	Billy has no problems in this area.
Dressing upper body	Billy has no problems in this area.
Dressing lower body	Billy has no problems in this area.
Toileting	Billy has no problems in this area.
Problem-solving/memory	Billy has no problems in this area.
Comments:	None.
IADLs	
Community mobility	Billy is able to manage the school bus ride to and from school. He is not involved in other community mobility.
Health management/prevention	This is managed by his parents.
Home management	Billy has no regular chores at home.
Financial management	This is managed by his parents and is age appropriate.
Leisure/play	Billy has no problems in this area.
Safety	Billy has decreased safety awareness as a result of his impulsivity.
Comments:	None.
Motor and Praxis Skills	
Sitting—static/dynamic	Billy has no problems in this area.
Standing—static/dynamic	Billy has no problems in this area.
Joint stability and skeletal mobility	Billy has no problems in this area.
Place can on shelf	Billy has no problems in this area.
Retrieve item from floor	Billy has no problems in this area.
Screw lid on jar	Billy has no problems in this area.
Comb back of head	Billy has no problems in this area.
Writing	Billy has no problems in this area.
Lift grocery bag	Billy has no problems in this area.
Coordination	Billy has no problems in this area.
Manipulation	Billy has no problems in this area.
Comments:	None.

(Continued)

CASE EXAMPLE 11.2. BILLY: BEHAVIOR PROBLEMS *(Cont.)*

EXHIBIT 11.2.	Billy's Occupational Profile *(Cont.)*
Process Skills	
Energy for task	Billy has no problems in this area.
Knowledge/organization of task	Billy has no problems in this area.
Adaptation/praxis	Billy has no problems in this area.
Comments:	None.
Behavioral and Cognitive Skills	
Communication and following social conventions	Billy has age-appropriate verbal communication skills. Socially, he is a loner and is sometimes oppositional when given instructions by an adult.
Cognitive and emotional regulation skills	Billy is highly persistent in performing liked tasks. He does not transition away from these tasks easily and has difficulty organizing and planning unfamiliar tasks. Billy becomes frustrated and distressed easily, resulting in loud vocalizations accompanied by physical actions such as throwing things and slamming them on the floor.
Level of arousal/attention	Billy has significant difficulty in this area. Billy is medicated to manage his attention, but once overaroused he has difficulty regrouping and calming down.
Orientation	Billy is alert and oriented to person, place, thing, and event.
Energy and drive	Billy has plenty of energy, but his drive is limited to self-interests.
Memory and understanding	Billy has no problems in this area.
Higher level cognition	Billy has no problems in this area.
Sensory–Perceptual Skills	
Sensory	Billy has no problems in this area. He has good vision and hearing. An assessment of sensory processing identified no patterns of sensory processing differences.
Hearing and vison	Billy has no problems in this area.
Skin integrity	Billy's skin is intact.
Self-perception	Billy does not think he has any problems.
Comments:	The OT theorizes that sensory processing difficulties are not the underlying cause of Billy's behavior.

Note. Occupational profile template from American Occupational Therapy Association (2017a). Analysis of participation format adapted from Skubik-Peplaski, Paris, Boyle, & Culpert (2009). ADHD = attention-deficit hyperactivity disorder; ADLs = activities of daily living; IADLs = instrumental activities of daily living; OT = occupational therapist; SES = socioeconomic status.

functions, performance skills, or performance patterns in most aspects of the school day. Although he was referred to occupational therapy for assessment of sensory processing, assessment did not support sensory processing disorder as a strong clinical hypothesis in his case.

Because the occupational therapy practitioner had provisionally ruled out a sensory processing explanation for Billy's behavior, she needed a new approach to understand his functional impairments. As noted in Chapter 10, "Strategic Thinking and Outcomes," activity analysis is one theory-driven assessment strategy. Using activity analysis to guide her assessment, the

occupational therapy practitioner noted that Billy's behavior was getting him something that he preferred (computer play). Armed with this information, the occupational therapy practitioner selected the behavioral frame of reference to help organize and plan her intervention strategy.

Reflecting on his strengths, the occupational therapy practitioner felt that Billy should be able to understand the cause-and-effect relationship between his behaviors and punishments. Because he continued to act out in the classroom in the specific ways that the teacher had informed him would result in a loss of recess, the occupational therapy practitioner theorized

CASE EXAMPLE 11.2. BILLY: BEHAVIOR PROBLEMS *(Cont.)*

that Billy might not perceive the consequences as particularly bothersome.

The occupational therapy practitioner followed up the classroom observation by interviewing Billy, and she asked him how he felt about missing recess every day at school. Billy replied that he did not like recess and preferred to stay inside where he could play on the classroom computer. He said that he liked school and enjoyed doing well on tests and assignments. He also revealed that whenever he finished tests and assignments early, his teacher let him play on the computer as a way to keep him from being disruptive. He also indicated that he could usually get his way at home by wearing his parents down. Billy said that his favorite activities were his toy building bricks and the computer.

The desired outcome of occupational therapy intervention in the school setting was participation in the school routine, including recess, and decreased disruptive behavior. The desired outcome at home was for Billy to continue to excel in his schoolwork but to also follow instructions and comply when assigned tasks by his parents. Billy identified goals for himself as getting all the time he wanted to play with the things he likes.

The occupational therapy practitioner's intervention plan was designed to advance the goals of all 3 parties. The main strategy involved helping Billy comply with classroom expectations by establishing a behavioral intervention plan that both the school and his parents could implement. His teacher was educated that although the school viewed withholding recess as a punishment, in Billy's case it was a reward that was reinforcing his negative behaviors. Similarly, at home, Billy's toy building bricks were a powerful motivator. His parents began to use them as a reward for good behavior. They were advised to consistently communicate their expectations to Billy. His desired activities, computer games and playing with his building bricks, were only available as rewards. The consequences of oppositional or noncompliant behaviors were non-negotiable lack of access to these desired activities.

Billy's behavior at school improved almost immediately. At home, he continued to have occasional problems, especially with his little sister, but his parents reported decreased outbursts when he was reminded to settle down. To help Billy build his skills, his occupational therapy practitioner introduced the use of cognitive–behavioral strategies to help Billy problem-solve in challenging situations and learn to regulate his emotions. The desired school outcome of decreased disruptive behavior and participation in the school routine was met quickly, but Billy did seem to continue to struggle with impulses and self-regulation.

At home, Billy showed progress in the desired outcome of following instructions and complying when assigned tasks by his parents. This outcome was slower to develop because his parents had made few demands on Billy in the past as a strategy to avoid meltdowns. Billy knew that his meltdowns were powerful and resorted to them as expectations were raised. His parents needed ongoing support in managing Billy's behavior and moving his performance at home toward age-expected performance of chores. Finally, Billy had identified his goal as getting all the time he wanted to play with the things he likes. Billy did not feel that he got all the time he wanted, but he could articulate what he needed to do to get more time and was pleased that he was in trouble less often.

LEARNING ACTIVITIES

1. Identify a new, innovative, or nontraditional intervention approach of interest to you. Explore the available evidence supporting and refuting the use of this approach. When would you consider using this intervention? Justify your choices using a client-centered and evidence-driven argument.
2. Think of a time in your own life when you achieved an outcome to a problem that was different than the one you expected. Write a brief essay describing the situation, and analyze the logic you used in trying to solve this problem and why it did or did not work as you expected.
3. Cellular telephones are an example of a disruptive technology on many levels. Research how cellular phones have transformed how the telephone is used as a means of communication over the past 50 years.
4. Make a list of favorite apps that you routinely use and compare this list with those of either your classmates or friends. Analyze why you prefer these particular apps, and compare your analysis with that of your peers.
5. From your own experiences in the rehabilitation community, can you think of any instances in which underground practice might have been happening? Write a brief essay about your experience and why you think this may have been the case.

REFERENCES

Ahern, T. (1981, October 24). Search for quality called key to life. *The Milwaukee Sentinel*.

American Occupational Therapy Association. (2014). Occupational therapy practice framework: Domain and process (3rd ed.). *American Journal of Occupational Therapy, 68*(Suppl. 1), S1–S48. https://doi.org/10.5014/ajot.2014.682006

American Occupational Therapy Association. (2015). Occupational therapy code of ethics (2015). *American Journal of Occupational Therapy, 69,* 6913410030p8. https://doi.org/10.5014/ajot.2015.696S03

American Occupational Therapy Association. (2017a). AOTA occupational profile template. *American Journal of Occupational Therapy, 71*(Suppl. 2), 7112420030. https://doi.org/10.5014/ajot.2017.716S12

American Occupational Therapy Association. (2017b). *AOTA's involvement with Choosing Wisely.*® Retrieved from https://www.aota.org/Practice/Researchers/choosing-wisely.aspx

Complacency. (2017). In *Merriam-Webster*. Retrieved from https://www.merriam-webster.com/dictionary/complacency

Fleming, M. (1994). The search for tacit knowledge. In C. Mattingly & M. Fleming (Eds.), *Clinical reasoning: Forms of inquiry in a therapeutic practice* (pp. 22–34). Philadelphia: F. A. Davis.

Fleming, M., & Mattingly, C. (1994). The underground practice. In C. Mattingly & M. Fleming (Eds.), *Clinical reasoning: Forms of inquiry in a therapeutic practice* (pp. 295–315). Philadelphia: F. A. Davis.

Implementing Best Practices Consortium. (2007). *Implementing best practices in reproductive health: A guide for fostering change to scale up effective health services*. Geneva: U.S. Agency for International Development and World Health Organization. Retrieved from http://www.who.int/management/AGuideFosteringChangeScalingUpHealthServices.pdf

Kennedy, K. (2014). *Being a change agent in a dynamic health care environment*. Salt Lake City, UT: Healthinsight.org. Retrieved from https://healthinsight.org/about-us/healthinsight-blog/entry/1-healthinsight-blog/39-being-a-change-agent-in-a-dynamic-health-care-environment.

Kotter, J., & Cohen, D. (2012). *Accelerate: Building strategic agility for a faster-moving world*. Boston: Harvard Business School Press.

Liedtka, J. (1998). Linking strategic thinking with strategic planning. *Strategy and Leadership, 26,* 30–35.

Llopis, G. (2014, August 5). The dangers of complacent leadership. *Forbes*. Retrieved from https://www.forbes.com/sites/glennllopis/2014/08/05/the-dangers-of-complacent-leadership/#319522373de5

Lurie, S. (2011). Towards greater clarity in the role of ambiguity in clinical reasoning. *Medical Education, 45,* 326–328. https://doi.org/10.1111/j.1365-2923.2011.03938.x

Reifenberg, G., Gabrosek, G., Tanner, K., Harpster, K., Proffitt, R., & Persch, A. (2017). Feasibility of pediatric game-based neurorehabilitation using telehealth technologies: A case report. *American Journal of Occupational Therapy, 71,* 7103190040. https://doi.org/10.5014/ajot.2017.024976

Skubik-Peplaski, C., Paris, C., Boyle, D., & Culpert, A. (Eds.). (2009). *Applying the* Occupational Therapy Practice Framework: *Using the Cardinal Hill Occupational Participation Process in client-centered care* (2nd ed.). Bethesda, MD: AOTA Press.

Trauma Informed Care Project. (2017). *What is trauma-informed care?* Retrieved from http://www.traumainformedcareproject.org/

Verdonck, M., & Maye, F. (2016). Enhancing occupational performance in the virtual context using smart technology. *British Journal of Occupational Therapy, 79,* 385–390. https://doi.org/10.1177/0308022615591172

Appendix A. AOTA Occupational Profile Template

According to the *Occupational Therapy Practice Framework: Domain and Process* (3rd ed.; *OTPF–3;* American Occupational Therapy Association [AOTA], 2014), an *occupational profile* is "a summary of a client's occupational history and experiences, patterns of daily living, interests, values, and needs" (p. S13). The information is obtained from the client's perspective through both formal interview techniques and casual conversation and leads to an individualized, client-centered approach to intervention.

Each item in the template provided here should be addressed to complete the occupational profile. Page numbers on the form correspond to the description in the *OTPF–3*. A fillable version of the form is available to AOTA members at http://bit.ly/2F555Vd. Note that the template is a suggested approach; any template that incorporates the elements indicated in the AOTA template is appropriate.

An occupational profile is a requirement of the *CPT®* occupational therapy evaluation codes as of January 1, 2017 (American Medical Association, 2016). See https://www.aota.org/profile for more information on using the Occupational Profile Template in documentation. For more information on coding, visit http://www.aota.org/coding.

REFERENCES

American Occupational Therapy Association. (2014). Occupational therapy practice framework: Domain and process (3rd ed.). *American Journal of Occupational Therapy, 68*(Suppl. 1), S1–S48. https://doi.org/10.5014/ajot.2014.682006

American Medical Association. (2016). *Current procedural terminology: CPT® 2017 professional edition.* Chicago: Author.

AOTA OCCUPATIONAL PROFILE TEMPLATE

"The occupational profile is a summary of a client's occupational history and experiences, patterns of daily living, interests, values, and needs" (AOTA, 2014, p. S13). The information is obtained from the client's perspective through both formal interview techniques and casual conversation and leads to an individualized, client-centered approach to intervention.

Each item below should be addressed to complete the occupational profile. Page numbers are provided to reference a description in the *Occupational Therapy Practice Framework: Domain and Process, 3rd Edition* (AOTA, 2014).

Client Report	**Reason the client is seeking service and concerns related to engagement in occupations**	Why is the client seeking service, and what are the client's current concerns relative to engaging in occupations and in daily life activities? (This may include the client's general health status.)	
	Occupations in which the client is successful (p. S5)	In what occupations does the client feel successful, and what barriers are affecting his or her success?	
	Personal interests and values (p. S7)	What are the client's values and interests?	
	Occupational history (i.e., life experiences)	What is the client's occupational history (i.e., life experiences)?	
	Performance patterns (routines, roles, habits, & rituals) (p. S8)	What are the client's patterns of engagement in occupations, and how have they changed over time? What are the client's daily life roles? (Patterns can support or hinder occupational performance.)	

	What aspects of the client's environments or contexts does he or she see as:		
		Supports to Occupational Engagement	**Barriers to Occupational Engagement**
Environment	**Physical (p. S28) (e.g., buildings, furniture, pets)**		
	Social (p. S28) (e.g., spouse, friends, caregivers)		
Context	**Cultural (p. S28) (e.g., customs, beliefs)**		
	Personal (p. S28) (e.g., age, gender, SES, education)		
	Temporal (p. S28) (e.g., stage of life, time, year)		
	Virtual (p. S28) (e.g., chat, email, remote monitoring)		
Client Goals	**Client's priorities and desired targeted outcomes: (p. S34)**	Consider: occupational performance—improvement and enhancement, prevention, participation, role competence, health and wellness, quality of life, well-being, and/or occupational justice.	

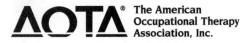

Appendix B. Frames of Reference Summary

FRAME OF REFERENCE	FOCUS	BASIC ASSUMPTIONS	FUNCTION–DISABILITY CONTINUUM	POSTULATES OF CHANGE
Behavioral science	Building of desired behaviors to support occupational participation, which may include the establishment of new behaviors, the modification of existing behaviors, and the extinction of maladaptive behaviors.	Human behavior is deterministic, occurring as a result of intrinsic or extrinsic influences. Because behavior is deterministic, predicting behavior is possible, and behavior can be changed by changing the influences on it.	Function is reflected in socially and developmentally supportive learning that results in effective behavior to support occupation. Dysfunction includes both failure to learn needed behaviors and faulty learning that leads to the development of ineffective or maladaptive behavior.	Behavioral change occurs through learning that is supported by the reinforcement of desired behaviors and the reduction in unwanted behavior by reducing the reinforcement derived from it. It is in defining the behavior of focus and the strategy for delivering supportive reinforcement that the factions within the behavioral frame of reference differ.
Biomechanical	Widely applied in treating musculoskeletal impairments.	Based on scientific knowledge about body function and structure and on the assumption that the voluntary movement that supports human function is built on the interactions of joint ROM, muscle strength, anatomical integrity, and the physiological functions that support endurance.	The typical or average state of bodily function supports engagement in desired movements. Any limitation of movement, strength, endurance, or physiologic stability that limits the use of a limb or produces incapacity to perform desired movements is an impairment.	Exercise or other specific interventions to support improved performance of the musculoskeletal system will result in improved ROM, strength, or endurance. Although specific functional skills and daily occupations are not a part of this frame of reference, it is believed that with improved musculoskeletal function, a person with musculoskeletal impairments will return to desired occupations.

(Continued)

FRAME OF REFERENCE	FOCUS	BASIC ASSUMPTIONS	FUNCTION–DISABILITY CONTINUUM	POSTULATES OF CHANGE
Cognitive rehabilitation	Emphasizes the neuroscientific understanding that every intentional act results from a dynamic balance among all brain structures and the functional nervous system as a whole can be disturbed by a lesion in one area.	Addresses cognition (i.e., acquisition, organization, and use of knowledge), perception, visual–motor organization, thinking operations (i.e., EF), memory, attention, and concentration.	Function is reflected in effective cognitive function for the tasks of everyday life. Dysfunction occurs following injury or disease and results in poor performance because of poor cognitive function.	Improvements in function can be achieved through a combination of cognitive retraining and use of compensation for cognitive deficits.
Developmental	Knowledge of human maturation and development, including the contributions of genes, environment, and factors within individuals that affect participation in daily occupations.	Individual development occurs over changing times and places within an individual's lifespan that can be assessed in terms of health trajectories—predicted pattern of health or disablement that is likely given the internal and external influences on the individual as they develop and mature. Development occurs within a specific point in history that affects the developmental process. Health trajectories may start or change over the life course on the basis of individual, social, and economic influences. Early experiences can "program" an individual's future health and development in a positive or negative manner. Although adverse events can negatively affect any point in a person's life course, the impact will be greatest if the adverse event occurs during a sensitive period of development. Choice and personal motivations are essential influencers on development throughout the lifespan.	This frame of reference considers function to be successful physical maturation and acquisition of skills to allow performance of skills and community participation at the level expected on the basis of the individual's chronological age. Dysfunction is reflected in patterns of developmental delay or atypical developmental trajectories that do not support age-appropriate performance and participation.	Change can occur by offering contextual supports to maturation and development, including actions that improve or restore health and function, improve or restore supportive aspects of the individual's environment (including family support), and increase opportunities for learning needed skills.

(Continued)

FRAME OF REFERENCE	FOCUS	BASIC ASSUMPTIONS	FUNCTION–DISABILITY CONTINUUM	POSTULATES OF CHANGE
Motor learning	Actual movement itself and the functional end goal of the movement—in other words, not just moving to move but moving with a purpose, because that is what will allow the person to learn.	Motor learning results from practice and is supported by active movement, error detection, and error correction. Motor learning may be enhanced through visual imagery in addition to active practice. In addition to motor capability, motor learning requires attention, memory, and motivation to support learning.	Optimal functional movements are efficient and support the performance of daily occupations. Inefficient or impaired movement can be improved through the use of feedback and practice.	Through repetitive movements, the body builds a memory of that movement and can then refine movement patterns to greater efficiency. Movement can be learned and practiced by using different degrees of freedom to create a more efficient movement pattern. Uncoordinated or inefficient movements can be relearned and changed to develop into coordinated functional movements. Practice can be performed in various ways: massed, distributed, whole or part practice, mental, variable, or scheduled. Feedback, either intrinsic or extrinsic, is another important component of success.
Psychodynamic	In occupational therapy, focuses on emotional expression and motivation for engagement in occupation. Of the Freudian concepts, it is the ego with which occupational therapy practitioners have been most concerned.	Individuals' occupational behavior reflects their interaction with the external world and internal forces. By focusing on activities to support aspects of ego functioning, improved performance can be elicited in the areas of social participation, relationship development and maintenance, self-awareness, and clarification of occupational goals and priorities.	Function is portrayed by a strong sense of self that is free from conflicts and fixations, functioning well in the environmental contexts. *Dysfunction* is defined in terms of conflicts among the id, ego, and superego. These conflicts can manifest as neurosis, psychosis, or character disorders that interfere with the ability to complete ADLs and to function as a participating member of society.	Through engagement in structured activities, occupational therapy practitioners strive to alter the function of the client through developing ego skills that enable clients to function optimally. Occupational therapy interventions guided by this frame of reference are based on activities that foster self-expression and motivation for engagement in occupations. They also focus on stress and coping skills to enable clients to express feelings in a safe environment and develop a positive self-efficacy.

(Continued)

FRAME OF REFERENCE	FOCUS	BASIC ASSUMPTIONS	FUNCTION–DISABILITY CONTINUUM	POSTULATES OF CHANGE
Sensory integration	A child's ability to discriminate, modulate, and integrate the sensory information needed for developmentally appropriate tasks (i.e., fully participate in daily life).	SI is an active developmental process that mirrors human development. The brain serves as an information processor that transforms sensory data into meaningful information that supports function and participation. Errors in sensory information processing can occur as errors of input, errors of encoding for memory, and errors of output. • Problems processing and modulating sensory input contribute to deficits in the ability to organize the behavior needed for developmentally appropriate tasks. • Problems storing the information for later use in the form of mental schema make it hard to retrieve the information and to support function. • Problems in how the brain decides what to do with the information and how it will react to the stimulus can lead to inappropriate or dysfunctional behavior. Children have an inborn drive toward higher development and are motivated to explore sensory challenges to advance their own development. Active engagement of the child is essential for developmental change. Using neurobiological and developmental science foundations to plan and engage the child in behaviors that provide organized sensory information tailored to the child's needs can lead to improved sensory processing and adaptive behaviors.	Function occurs through adaptive responses that result from effective sensory modulation, discrimination, and integration. Dysfunction, in the form of sensory defensiveness, avoidance, underregistration of sensation, or poor modulation, manifests as maladaptive behaviors such as poor postural control, praxis or bilateral integration, and participation. Function–dysfunction continua are relevant within each sensory system.	Active engagement in a sensory-rich environment entices the child to play and motivates adaptive responses. Child-directed activity taps into the child's inner drive for developmental advancement. If occupational therapy practitioners increase the complexity of challenge so that the child needs to exert some degree of effort, then the child will be more likely to master challenge and move to a higher level adaptive response. If practitioners present or facilitate challenges in which the child is successful in areas of sensory modulation; discrimination; postural, ocular, or oral control; and praxis, then the child will be more likely to develop skills in the challenged area.

Note. ADLs = activities of daily living; EF = executive function; ROM = range of motion; SI = sensory integration.

Citation Index

Note. Page numbers in *italic* refer to exhibits, figures, and tables.

Citation Index

Note. Page numbers in *italic* refer to exhibits, figures, and tables.

Subject Index

Note. Page numbers in *italic* refer to exhibits, figures, and tables.